Principles of
PHARMACOLOGY
for Athletic Trainers

Principles of
PHARMACOLOGY
for Athletic Trainers

Gary L. Harrelson, EdD, ATC
Director, Organizational Development and Education
DCH Health System
Tuscaloosa, Alabama

Deidre Leaver-Dunn, PhD, ATC
Director, Undergraduate Athletic Training Education Program
University of Alabama
Tuscaloosa, Alabama

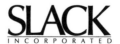

An innovative information, education, and management company
6900 Grove Road • Thorofare, NJ 08086

The work SLACK Incorporated publishes is peer reviewed. Prior to publication, recognized leaders in the field, educators, and clinicians provide important feedback on the concepts and content that we publish. We welcome feedback on this work.

Published by: SLACK Incorporated
                  6900 Grove Road
                  Thorofare, NJ 08086 USA
                  Telephone: 856-848-1000
                  Fax: 856-853-5991
                  www.slackbooks.com

Houglum, Joel.
   Principles of pharmacology for athletic trainers / Joel Houglum,
Gary Harrelson, Deidre Leaver-Dunn.
      p. ; cm.
   Includes bibliographical references and index.
   ISBN-13: 978-1-55642-594-3 (pbk.)
   ISBN-10: 1-55642-594-5 (pbk.)
   1. Pharmacology. 2. Athletic trainers.   I. Harrelson, Gary L.
II. Leaver-Dunn, Deidre. III. Title.
   [DNLM: 1. Sports Medicine--methods. 2. Drug Therapy--methods.
3. Pharmaceutical Preparations. 4. Pharmacology--methods.
QT 261 H8385p 2005]
RM300.H68 2005
615'.1--dc22
   2004024578

Printed in the United States of America.

Contact SLACK Incorporated for more information about other books in this field or about the availability of our books from distributors outside the United States.

For permission to reprint material in another publication, contact SLACK Incorporated. Authorization to photocopy items for internal, personal, or academic use is granted by SLACK Incorporated provided that the appropriate fee is paid directly to Copyright Clearance Center. Prior to photocopying items, please contact the Copyright Clearance Center at 222 Rosewood Drive, Danvers, MA 01923 USA; phone: 978-750-8400; website: www.copyright.com; email: info@copyright.com.

Last digit is print number: 10   9   8   7   6   5   4   3   2   1

DEDICATION

To my wife, Rita, who I can't imagine being without.

To our children and their families, Dan and Becki; Andy, Michelle, and Samuel; and Cate, all of whom have given us more pride and joy than they can imagine.

To my parents, sisters, and brother who gave me a home of security and tons of fond memories.

To the God of my salvation, for His mercy, love, and the blessings above.

JEH

To my mother and late father, who gave to each of us boys in a loving and unselfish way. I never knew nor appreciated the sacrifices I know you made for each of us until I became a father and husband myself—thank you for your unconditional love, it did and does today make a difference in me. And to my heavenly Father who has blessed me with talents that I could never have imagined. May I glorify your kingdom with what you have so richly blessed me with.

GLH

CONTENTS

ABOUT THE AUTHORS

Joel E. Houglum, PhD received a Bachelor of Science in Pharmacy from the University of Minnesota and a PhD in Pharmaceutical Biochemistry from the University of Wisconsin. He is Assistant Dean and Professor of Pharmaceutical Sciences in the College of Pharmacy at South Dakota State University where he has taught courses in pharmacology and pharmaceutical biochemistry for over 25 years. His other publications have been in the areas of leukotrienes, analytical chemistry, curriculum planning and evaluation, and pharmacology for athletic trainers.

Gary L. Harrelson, EdD, ATC, received his BS in athletic training, MS in Exercise Physiology, and EdD in Administration and Teaching all from the University of Southern Mississippi. He is the Director of Organization Development and Education for the DCH Health System in Tuscaloosa, Alabama. Gary has taught in athletic training curriculums at the University of Alabama and University of Southern Mississippi. He has been an Associate Editor for the *Journal of Athletic Training* and is currently an Associate Editor for *Athletic Therapy Today.* Additionally, he has been the coauthor of several books and multimedia projects. His current publications center around the cognitive science of learning.

Deidre Leaver-Dunn, PhD, ATC received her BS from East Carolina University, MEd from the University of Virginia, and PhD from the University of Alabama/the University of Alabama at Birmingham. Currently, Dr. Leaver-Dunn is the Director of the Undergraduate Athletic Training Education Program at the University of Alabama. Previously, Dr. Leaver-Dunn worked as a Research Assistant and ATC at DCH SportsMedicine in Tuscaloosa and as Sports Medicine Coordinator at Upstate Therapy Services, Inc. in Greenville, South Carolina. She has published articles in the the *Journal of Athletic Training* and was a contributor to the latest edition of *Physical Rehabilitation of The Injured Athlete* and *Athletic Training and Sports Medicine.* In addition, Dr. Leaver-Dunn serves as a manuscript reviewer for *Athletic Therapy Today* and the *Journal of Athletic Training,* and a grant reviewer for the National Athletic Trainers' Association Foundation Research Committee.

CONTRIBUTING AUTHORS

Cindy Thomas, ATC has over 23 years of experience in collegiate athletic training, academics, and athletics administration. An active member in the National Athletic Trainers' Association for over 25 years, Cindy completed her undergraduate degree from Longwood College and her Master's Degree in Physical Education with a specialization in Athletic Training from Indiana State University. She served as NCAA Assistant Director of Sports Sciences administering the organization's drug testing programs before joining The National Center for Drug Free Sport.

Robert P. Nickell, RPh, FACA, FAPO grew up working in his father's corner drugstore in Norwalk, California. Since that time, he has become the leading expert in the practice of Sports Pharmacy. In his practice, he represents greater than 60% of every professional sports team in the nation, as well as many colleges and universities. Robert is the first pharmacist to receive Honorary Membership in the National Athletic Trainers' Association, and the first pharmacist to officially serve on the USA Olympic Sports Medicine Team in Athens, Greece. He is the founder and lead course instructor for the USC School of Pharmacy Pharmaceutical Compounding Lab, teaching beginning and advanced compounding. He is the father of four children and lives happily in Hermosa Beach, California.

Michael E. Powers, PhD, ATC, CSCS is an Assistant Professor and the Academic Coordinator of Clinical Education in the Division of Athletic Training at Shenandoah University. Dr. Powers received his Bachelor's and Master's degrees in Athletic Training from Northeastern University and the University of Florida respectively and went on to receive his Doctoral degree in Sports Medicine from the University of Virginia. He is a certified athletic trainer through the National Athletic Trainers' Association and a certified strength and conditioning specialist through the National Strength and Conditioning Association. In addition to his academic duties, Dr. Powers serves as the Head Athletic Trainer with the Department of Athletics and is responsible for overseeing all aspects of health care provided to the university athletes.

Preface

A more drug-using and drug-aware society requires that athletic trainers have an appropriate understanding of pharmacology, especially related to drugs being used by the athlete. This textbook provides the basic principles of pharmacology specifically aimed at the needs of the athletic trainer. Consequently, the drug categories that are included are primarily those that may be pertinent to the treatment of athletic injuries or that may impact athletic performance. A discussion of pharmacological principles of other drug categories, as well as detailed and methodical listings of all available drugs, can be obtained from other references, examples of which are discussed at the end of the first chapter.

The athletic trainer cares for the physically active, but the employment opportunities for the athletic trainer are broader in scope than they once were; athletic trainers are now treating patients across a wide age range. No longer are athletic trainers only providing care for a young physically healthy population, but also for the aging, yet physically active, who have diseases that are being treated with physical activity as well as drug therapy. For example, an athletic trainer may be treating an older patient for a musculoskeletal injury, but must be aware that the patient is also taking a β-blocker medication that reduces cardiac output; thus the athletic trainer may need to adjust the exercise prescription accordingly. This text addresses the diseases and drug treatment options for the physically active population treated by athletic trainers.

The challenge of writing a textbook such as this is identifying the "need to know" information for the targeted audience. Pharmacology is based in biochemistry and knowing that athletic trainers' background in biochemistry is limited we have attempted to present the information as best we can for the athletic trainer. We have used several strategies to help in this quest, which include...

- Summaries that are not at the end of the chapter, but after each major topic within the chapter. This is an attempt to help manage cognitive overload and aid the reader in understanding what was just read.
- Advanced organizers are used at the beginning of each chapter in order for the reader to see what the chapter contains and get a sense of how the chapter is structured, which ultimately also helps manage cognitive overload.
- Key words are in italics and are defined in the glossary.
- Concept maps graphically present important, yet complex, processes in a concise way.
- Textboxes (shaded) throughout the text either add additional information to the topic or help the reader to recall a key concept or process that was addressed in an earlier chapter.
- Very specific learning objectives are stated at the beginning of each chapter.

Finally, even though this textbook provides drug information that will be useful for the athletic trainer in professional practice, caution is also warranted: *the athletic trainer will not be transformed into a drug expert through a study of this textbook.* The athletic trainer should have sufficient knowledge about drugs to provide basic information, to improve compliance with therapy, and to identify drug-related problems in the athlete. Just as important, however, is the ability to realize one's own limitations and to appropriately identify the need to refer the athlete. The expertise of the physician and pharmacist regarding drug information should be among the resources utilized by the athletic trainer. Frequent contact with the athlete provides the opportunity for the athletic trainer to assist the athlete with drug-related issues; this textbook will help provide the knowledge to do it.

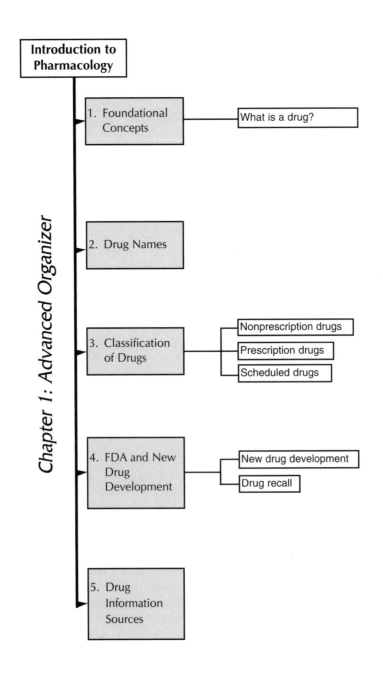

INTRODUCTION TO PHARMACOLOGY

CHAPTER OBJECTIVES

At the end of this chapter, the reader will be able to:

- Define what a drug is.
- Differentiate between a drug's chemical, generic, and trade names.
- Explain the difference between a generic name and a generic drug.
- List the differences between a generic name and trade name drug.
- List and explain the four ways drugs are classified.
- Explain the United States Food and Drug Administration's (FDA) role in new drug development and the recall of drugs.
- Locate drug information sources for prescription and nonprescription medication.
- Employ the use of drug information sources to locate specific drugs.

The availability and use of drugs for therapeutic purposes continues to rise. The number of prescriptions dispensed has increased at an average annual rate of about 6% since 1992. In 2000, there were nearly 3 billion prescriptions dispensed. New drugs have been developed in the past several years to treat diabetes, gastrointestinal ulcers, infection, inflammation, mental disorders, hyperlipidemia, and asthma to name a few. In recent years, the number of drugs and therapeutic categories available without a prescription has also increased and thus the retail sales of over-the-counter (OTC) drug products continue to rise. Society, including athletes, have many more options for self-therapy, which complicates the task for athletic trainers to monitor the drugs being used by the athlete.

FOUNDATIONAL CONCEPTS

A good starting point for foundational concepts is to define pharmacology. Simply put, human *pharmacology* is the effect of drugs on the body and the effect of the body on drugs. Drugs interact with the cells and extracellular components on a molecular level to produce beneficial and detrimental responses. At the same time, other molecular interactions between the drug and body components will determine how, when, and where the action of the drug will be terminated. Consequently, pharmacology encompasses the therapeutic responses and adverse effects of drugs as well as the absorption, metabolism, and excretion of drugs.

Subdivisions of pharmacology include pharmacokinetics and pharmacodynamics. A study of the factors that affect the time course of drug events is called *pharmacokinetics*. The rate at which drugs begin to take effect, the duration of the effect, and factors that impact the rate of change in concentration of drugs at the site of action are included in pharmacokinetics. These parameters impact the optimal dosage schedule and route of administration for the drug and will be discussed in Chapter 2. *Pharmacodynamics* is the study of the mechanism of action of drugs. Some drugs, for example, combine with an enzyme to inhibit the enzymatic process whereas others combine with receptors to either initiate or inhibit a particular effect. A more detailed discussion of pharmacodynamics is the focus of Chapter 3.

What Is a Drug?

Asking the question, "What is a drug?" can spark a philosophical discussion. All drugs are chemicals. Arsenic trioxide is a chemical but is very toxic with no therapeutic application—is it a drug? In the realm of therapeutics, drugs are chemicals that are used to treat or prevent disease. Table sugar (sucrose) is typically not considered a drug, but what if a diabetic is experiencing the sweating, tachycardia, and jittery feeling associated with hypoglycemia and uses table sugar as treatment; is the sucrose a drug? What about vitamin supplements being used by a person in whom there is no evidence of dietary deficiency? Herbal products are chemicals, many of which have unproven claims of effectiveness in preventing or treating disease; is a chemical a drug if it has no therapeutic benefit but is used for a perceived benefit? Legal, ethical, and therapeutic issues all enter the discussion to obtain an all-encompassing definition. For the purpose of this text, a suitable definition of a *drug* is a chemical that has demonstrated to be effective for preventing or treating a disease.

DRUG NAMES

Because drugs are chemicals, they each have a chemical name that specifies the chemical structure. The chemical name often is much too cumbersome for common usage and thus a shorter generic name is also assigned to each drug entity (ie, each chemical compound). For example, 4-(dimethyl-amino)-1,4,4a,5,5a,6,11,12a-octahydro-3,5,10,12,12a-pentahydroxy-6-methyl-1,11-dioxo-2-naphthacenecarboxamide is the chemical name for the generic name doxycycline. The generic name is also known as the nonproprietary name as the name is not the property of any company. The proprietary name, more commonly known as trade name or brand name, is selected by the company that markets the drug. There is only one generic name for each drug but there may be more than one trade name if the drug is marketed by more than one company (Table 1-1). Doxycycline has more than 10 trade names and is also marketed under the generic name by a few other companies.

There is a difference between the generic "name" and a generic "drug." Although every drug has a generic name, not all drugs are marketed as generics. When the patent for the drug expires, companies other than the owner of the patent can market the drug, but these other companies cannot use the trade name owned by the original manufacturer. Consequently, most of these drugs are marketed by one or more companies using the generic name. These generic drugs are typically less expensive than the corresponding trade name drug because they bring price competition to the marketplace and because the companies marketing them have not invested the initial research and development costs necessary to originally obtain FDA approval to market the drug (see below). The average retail price of a prescription for a trade name drug in 2001 was 4.3 times the average retail price of a generic drug. Similarly, drugs with expired patents can be marketed by other companies under new trade names owned by these companies. For example, since the patent is expired for ibuprofen (generic name), this drug is now marketed by several compa-

Table 1-1. Different Names for Chemical Structure

Type of Name	Example(s)
Chemical name	4-(dimethyl-amino)-1,4,4a,5,5a,6,11,12a-octahydro-3,5,10,12,12a-pentahydroxy-6-methyl-1,11-dioxo-2-naphthacenecarboxamide
Generic name	Doxycycline
Trade names	Vibramycin
	Periostat
	Monodox
	Doryx
	Vibra-Tabs

nies under this generic name and by other companies under various trade names (Advil, Medipren, Motrin, Nuprin, Rufen).

Besides cost, there are other notable differences between using a generic name versus a trade name product. Typically, trade names are shorter and easier to pronounce than the generic name.

Patents last for 20 years but it takes approximately 8.5 years for an experimental drug to move through the FDA approval process, leaving about 11.5 years for the marketing of the drug to be protected by the patent.

However, because there can be multiple trade names it is more difficult to remember all of them. Also, unlike the generic name, which refers to one chemical entity, the trade name refers to the entire product contents, which may include more than one active ingredient. For example, Vanquish is the trade name for a product that contains the drugs acetaminophen, aspirin, and caffeine. As evident in Table 1-2, there is no way of knowing from the trade name the number of drugs contained in the product.

When generic or trade name products contain the same quantities of the same drug(s), they usually do not differ significantly in the observed therapeutic response. Companies that market generic drugs must obtain FDA approval through an abbreviated new drug application process. The abbreviated process does not require the company to repeat all of the clinical trials that were conducted by the company that first obtained FDA approval to market the drug. Rather, the approval process focuses on demonstrating that the generic product is bioequivalent to the trade name product.

This approval can be obtained while the trade name drug is still under patent, thus allowing the generic product to be marketed immediately after the patent expires. As more trade name drugs go off patent, the number of generic drugs increases. Although the cost of generic drugs is significantly less than trade name drugs, companies that market generic drugs have the potential to gain significant profits because they do not have to recoup costs associated with research, development, and a lengthy approval process. Consequently, profit margin and availability of off-patent drugs are among the driving forces that will continue to increase

Bioequivalence is discussed in the next chapter. Two drug formulations are bioequivalent if the amount and rate of the drug entering the blood stream is approximately the same.

Table 1-2. Contents of Selected Product Combinations

Trade Name	Contents	Classification
Darvocet-N	100 mg propoxyphene napsylate 650 mg acetaminophen	Controlled Substance C-IV
Excedrin Migraine	65 mg caffeine 250 mg acetaminophen 250 mg aspirin	OTC
Excedrin P.M.	38 mg diphenhydramine citrate 500 mg acetaminophen	OTC
Exedrine P.M.	25 mg diphenhydramine 500 mg acetaminophen	OTC
Hista-Vent DA	20 mg phenylephrine HCl 8 mg chlorpheniramine maleate 2.5 mg methscopolamine nitrate	Prescription
Nucofed Capsules	20 mg codeine phosphate 60 mg pseudoephedrine HCL	Controlled Substance C-III
Rynatuss Tablets	5 mg chlorpheniramine tannate 10 mg phenylephrine tannate 10 mg ephedrine tannate 60 mg carbetapentane tannate	Prescription
Vicodin Tablets	5 mg hydrocodone bitartrate 500 mg acetaminophen	Controlled Substance C-III

See also Tables 7-2, 7-3, and 10-2 for additional examples of products that contain multiple components.

C=category, referring to category of the controlled substance, OTC=over the counter, HCl=hydrochloride.

the number of generic drugs. Table 1-3 provides a summary of the difference between trade name and generic name drugs.

CLASSIFICATION OF DRUGS

Drugs may be classified in a variety of ways. Because all drugs are chemicals, they can be grouped based on their chemistry (Figure 1-1). For example, the tetracyclines are a group of antibiotics that chemically each contain four rings linked together. Although each of the individual tetracycline compounds such as doxycycline (Vibramycin), minocycline (Minocin), and oxytetracycline (Terramycin) have some unique chemical characteristics, they all have a four-ring core structure and share the same mechanism of action. Other examples of drug categories based on chemical structure are the penicillins, cephalosporins, benzodiazepines, and corticosteroids.

Table 1-3. Difference Between Trade Name and Generic Name Drugs

Trade Name Drug

- Can be multiple trade names.
- Names are shorter and easier to pronounce.
- Trade name refers to the entire product, which may include more than one active ingredient.

Generic Name Drug

- Only one generic name.
- Refers to one chemical entity.
- Less expensive.
- Not all drugs are marketed as a generic drug.
- Generic drugs can be marketed by one or more companies.
- Must obtain FDA approval, but through an abbreviated process.
- Must be bioequivalent to the trade name.

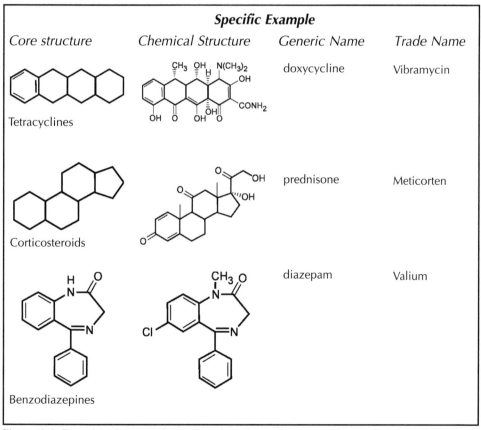

	Specific Example		
Core structure	*Chemical Structure*	*Generic Name*	*Trade Name*
Tetracyclines		doxycycline	Vibramycin
Corticosteroids		prednisone	Meticorten
Benzodiazepines		diazepam	Valium

Figure 1-1. Examples of groups of drugs based on chemical structure. The drugs in these three chemical categories (tetracyclines, corticosteroids, benzodiazepines) have the core chemical structure shown, but each specific drug also has additional smaller chemical groups attached at various places on the core structure.

Table 1-4. Examples of Therapeutic Categories and Subcategories

Therapeutic Category	Examples of Subcategories	Chapter Reference
Analgesics	NSAIDs	7
	Opioids	
Antibiotics	Tetracyclines	5
	Penicillins	
	Cephalosporins	
Antihypertensives	β_2-blockers	12
	Diuretics	
	ACE inhibitors	
Anti-inflammatory drugs	NSAIDs	6
	Corticosteroids	
Asthma drugs	β_2-agonists	9
	Corticosteroids	
	Leukotriene modifiers	

Abbreviations: NSAIDs=nonsteroidal anti-inflammatory drugs, ACE= angiotensin-converting enzyme

Sometimes drug categories are based on the mechanism of action such as the protein synthesis inhibitors, beta (β)-blockers, proton pump inhibitors, H_2-blockers, and β-adrenergic agonists. A broader means of categorizing drugs is by therapeutic effect. As shown in Table 1-4, there are generally several subcategories within the therapeutic category.

Another means of categorizing drugs is by their legal classification. Several federal laws have created three classifications: OTC drugs, prescription drugs, and controlled substances (Table 1-5). The federal laws that led to these classifications are summarized in Table 1-6 (see also Box 4-2 for other federal acts related to the control and distribution of drugs).

Protein synthesis inhibitors is a term used to describe the mechanism of action of several antibiotics, including the tetracyclines and macrolides, as discussed in Chapter 5. β-blockers are a group of drugs used to treat hypertension and certain heart diseases, as discussed in Chapter 12. Proton pump inhibitors and H_2-blockers are groups of drugs used to treat gastrointestinal disorders as discussed in Chapter 11. β-adrenergic agonists are drugs used to treat asthma and are discussed in Chapter 9.

Nonprescription Drugs

Drugs that do not require a prescription are also referred to as OTC drugs. There are an estimated 1000 active ingredients used in over 100,000 OTC products on the market. Some of these products contain a single drug as the active ingredient, whereas many others contain combinations of active ingredients. Table 1-2 lists a few OTC products and their active ingredients.

Several OTC drugs were originally available only by prescription, but were later approved for use in nonprescription products, usually at a lower amount of drug per dosage unit. Motrin (400, 600, or 800 mg per tablet) and naproxen (250 or 500 mg per tablet) are prescription nonsteroidal anti-inflammatory drugs (NSAIDs) that are also available as OTC medications at a maximum of 200 mg per tablet. It is the responsibility of the FDA to approve a drug in the OTC classification. Many factors are considered including: evidence that there is a relatively low fre-

Table 1-5. Classification of Drugs

Classification	Characteristics
OTC drugs	Drugs that do not require a prescription.
	Usually contain a lower amount of drug per dosage unit compared with the corresponding prescription drug.
	Often contain multiple active ingredients in the same dosage form.
Prescription drugs	Prescription drugs generally have a greater potential for adverse effects than OTC drugs, require monitoring for interactions with other medications, should only be used for a restricted time period, or have other problems that necessitate the enhanced restrictions associated with prescription drugs.
	Medical supervision is mandated through the physician writing the prescription and the pharmacist filling it.
Controlled substances	Also referred to as scheduled drugs. They have an abuse potential and thus have more restrictive requirements regarding distribution, storage, and record keeping compared with prescription drugs.
	Schedule I controlled substances (or C-I drugs) have the greatest potential for abuse whereas Schedule V (C-V) drugs have the lowest abuse potential.

quency of toxic and other adverse effects; no need for periodic medical examination or laboratory work to monitor the effectiveness or toxicity; and demonstration of effectiveness in a significant proportion of patients at the dosage recommended on the OTC product label.

Prescription Drugs

Compared to OTC drugs, prescription drugs generally have a greater potential for adverse effects, require monitoring for interactions with other medications, should only be used for a restricted time period, and have other problems that necessitate the enhanced restrictions associated with prescription drugs. Medical supervision is mandated through the physician writing the prescription and the pharmacist filling it. Refilling the prescription is allowed only if it is specifically authorized by the prescriber.

These drugs are also referred to as legend drugs because the Durham-Humphrey Amendment required the label of the prescription drug container prior to dispensing (typically from the manufacturer) to contain the legend, "Caution: Federal law prohibits dispensing without a prescription." The FDA Modernization Act of 1997 changed this labeling requirement so that the drug container now must bear, at a minimum, "Rx only" (Figure 1-2).

Table 1-6. Federal Laws Leading to the Three Classifications of Drugs

Act	Purpose	Comment
Federal Pure Food Act of 1906	Prohibited adulteration and misbranding of medications.	The label had to accurately reflect the strength, quality, and purity of the contents. However, the Act did not require the drug to be safe or effective. *The United States Pharmacopeia/ The National Formulary* were also established by this act as the official standards for drug quality. Drugs that meet the standard can have "USP" placed on the label after the name of the drug.
Food, Drug, and Cosmetic Act of 1938	Required that the safety of new drugs be reviewed and approved by the FDA before the drug could be marketed for interstate commerce.	This Act was the beginning of the New Drug Application (NDA) process. However, efficacy was not addressed.
1952 Durham-Humphrey Amendment of the 1932 Act	Differentiated between prescription and nonprescription drugs.	Drugs that were determined to be unsafe without medical supervision required a prescription. The amendment also prohibited certain drugs, such as opioids and hypnotics, to be refilled without a new prescription.
1962 Kefauver-Harris Amendment of the 1938 Act	Required that the effectiveness of new drugs, whether prescription or nonprescription, be reviewed and approved by the FDA prior to the drug being marketed.	Drugs marketed between 1938 and 1962 were also included in this amendment. Consequently drugs now had to be approved as safe and effective before available to the public.
Comprehensive Drug Abuse Prevention and Control Act of 1970	Established categories designated C-I to C-V (see Table 1-7), for drugs with an abuse potential.	Drugs in schedule C-I have the highest abuse potential and greatest restriction for use. This portion of the Act is referred to as the Controlled Substances Act and thus these drugs are also referred to as controlled substances. The Act regulates the manufacture, distribution, and dispensing of controlled substances. The Drug Enforcement Agency (DEA), a part of the Department of Justice, was designated the responsibility of enforcing the Act.

Abbreviation: USP=United States Pharmacopeia

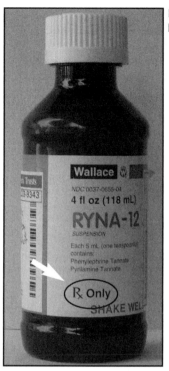

Figure 1-2. Example of "Rx Only" labeling that must appear on the label of the prescription drug container prior to dispensing.

Scheduled Drugs

Scheduled drugs have an abuse potential and, thus, have more restrictive requirements regarding distribution, storage, and record keeping compared with prescription drugs. Table 1-7 provides some examples in each schedule and differentiates the characteristics of the five schedules based on their potential for abuse. Schedule I controlled substances (or C-I drugs) have the greatest potential for abuse whereas Schedule V (C-V) drugs have the lowest abuse potential. Anabolic steroids are C-III drugs. Individual states can move drugs to a more restrictive schedule. The law in some states permits a limited amount of certain Schedule V controlled substances to be distributed without a prescription, usually only by a pharmacist, as long as certain record keeping requirements are followed; codeine-containing cough medication is an example.

FOOD AND DRUG ADMINISTRATION AND NEW DRUG DEVELOPMENT

In 1930, the Food Drug and Insecticide Administration was changed to the Food and Drug Administration (FDA) and is now a component of the Department of Health and Human Services. The FDA is responsible for the review and approval of all new drugs before they are available to the public. New drugs proceed through a rigorous process of testing before they can be marketed. Figure 1-3 is a flow chart of this process; an interactive flow chart is also available at www.fda.gov/cder/handbook/develop.htm. Safety and effectiveness must be demonstrated in clinical trials before approval is granted. Prior to the clinical trials, it often takes testing of hundreds of compounds before one emerges with the potential of therapeutic effectiveness. After sufficient data are obtained in animal studies regarding the use, dosage, and toxic effects, and ade-

Table 1-7. Classification of Controlled Substances

Schedule	Characteristics	Examples (Trade Name)
I	High abuse potential. No accepted medical use in the United States. May be used for research purposes.	Heroin Lysergic acid diethylamide (LSD) Marijuana Mescaline Peyote Tetrahydrocannabiol (THC)
II	High abuse potential. Accepted medical use in the United States. Broad range of drugs.	Amobarbital (Tuinal) Amphetamine (Dexedrine) Cocaine Codeine Hydromorphone (Dilaudid) Meperidine (Demerol) Methadone Methamphetamine (Desoxyn) Methylphenidate (Ritalin) Morphine Opium tincture Oxycodone + acetaminophen (Percocet) Phenmetrazine (Preludin)
III	Lower abuse potential than C-II. Accepted medical use in the United States.	Anabolic steroids Butalbital (Fiorinal) Codeine with acetaminophen or aspirin Dronabinol (Marinol) Hydrocodone with acetaminophen Propoxyphene (Darvon) Propoxyphene + aspirin or acetaminophen Thiopental (Pentothal)
IV	Lower abuse potential than C-III. Accepted medical use.	Alprazolam (Xanax) Chlordiazepoxide (Librium) Diazepam (Valium) Fenfluramine (Pondimin) Flurazepam (Dalmane) Lorazepam (Ativan) Phenobarbital (Luminal)
V	Lowest abuse potential of controlled substances. Preparations contain smaller quantity of controlled substance. Some products are nonprescription in some states.	Cough mixtures containing codeine (Robitussin A-C) Antidiarrheal mixtures with opium (Kapectolin PG)

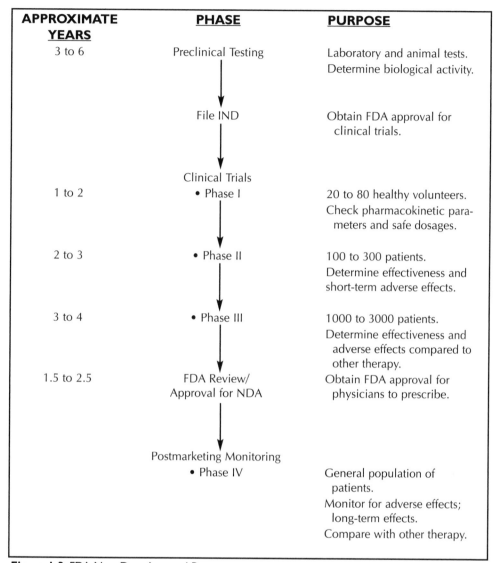

APPROXIMATE YEARS	PHASE	PURPOSE
3 to 6	Preclinical Testing	Laboratory and animal tests. Determine biological activity.
	File IND	Obtain FDA approval for clinical trials.
	Clinical Trials	
1 to 2	• Phase I	20 to 80 healthy volunteers. Check pharmacokinetic parameters and safe dosages.
2 to 3	• Phase II	100 to 300 patients. Determine effectiveness and short-term adverse effects.
3 to 4	• Phase III	1000 to 3000 patients. Determine effectiveness and adverse effects compared to other therapy.
1.5 to 2.5	FDA Review/ Approval for NDA	Obtain FDA approval for physicians to prescribe.
	Postmarketing Monitoring	
	• Phase IV	General population of patients. Monitor for adverse effects; long-term effects. Compare with other therapy.

Figure 1-3. FDA New Drug Approval Process.

quate safety and effectiveness have been demonstrated, the FDA grants Investigational New Drug (IND) status. Clinical trials (ie, human studies) can only begin after IND status is granted. Alternatively, clinical trials may also begin if the FDA does not reject the IND application within 30 days of it being submitted.

Clinical trials include three phases before a New Drug Application (NDA) is submitted (see Figure 1-3). Phase I includes tests on a small number (20 to 80) of healthy volunteers who are not taking other medications. The intent is to assess drug toxicity, absorption, metabolism, excretion, and dosage. Phase II uses a larger number of volunteers (100 to 300) who have the disease. The intent of Phase II is to study the drug's effectiveness and short-term safety, usually by comparing the patients with a control group. Phase III involves 1000 to 3000 patients at various clinics and hospitals. These patients are monitored closely for effectiveness and adverse effects of the drug compared with existing treatments for the same disease. Some patients in this phase may be receiving additional treatment for other diseases. The NDA is granted if the studies demonstrate adequate safety and effectiveness. The drug is then available for physicians to prescribe. Phase IV includes the collection of postmarketing data regarding the effects of the drug on the general population, as reported by physicians who prescribe the drug. Some studies may include a comparison with other drugs in the same therapeutic category.

The FDA also reviews drugs that were on the market prior to 1962, including OTC drugs and drug combinations, in an attempt to determine effectiveness of drugs that were already on the market prior to the 1962 Kefauver-Harris Amendment.

Another important responsibility of the FDA is to recall drugs and drug products from the marketplace that are unsafe. Drug recalls are divided into three classes:

1. Class I recalls are those in which there is a reasonable possibility that there is a serious threat to the health of the consumer. For example, the need to add additional cautionary labeling on the manufacturer's packaging because of a life-threatening adverse effect that has been discovered in selected patients, or the color-coded oral contraceptive tablets are in the wrong sequence in the packaging.

2. Class II recalls are those in which the use of or exposure to the product in violation may cause a temporary health problem that is reversible or the probability of serious health effects is remote. For example, microbial contamination is discovered in certain lots of an oral dosage form, or an oral suspension antibiotic is found to contain less than the labeled amount of antibiotic.

3. Class III recalls are those in which the use of or exposure to a product that is in violation is not likely to cause a health hazard. For example, certain batches of an oral product are found to contain traces of iron, the manufacture packaging does not contain the "Rx only" labeling, or the manufacture mislabels the package indicating the drug to be C-IV instead of a C-III scheduled drug.

Occasionally there is a need to withdraw from the market all dosage forms that contain a certain drug because postmarketing data or additional research information indicates a serious threat to the consumer. Most recalls, however, are to remove certain products (ie, specific formulations produced by a specific manufacturer) or batches of the product. A list of recalls for the previous 60 days is available at www.fda.gov by selecting *Recalls and Safety Alerts. The FDA Enforcement Report Index* is also available through this Web site, which provides a weekly listing of recalls. Information regarding recalls is also distributed to physicians, pharmacists, and patients by the manufacturer through letters, fax, e-mails, listings in professional publications, and announcements through the general news media.

DRUG INFORMATION SOURCES

The public is better informed about names and actions of drugs than ever before. Advertisements of prescription and nonprescription drugs are commonplace in newspapers and magazines, and on television and radio. The widespread use of the Internet has provided pharmaceutical companies with another avenue to provide information about their products to the public. Physicians and pharmacists also provide verbal information regarding the appropriate use and storage of drugs, and pharmacies provide product information sheets when new prescriptions are filled. Clearly, the philosophy of the medical community is that the public should be educated regarding the drugs they are taking.

There are many sources of drug information available to the health care professional, examples of which are discussed below and summarized in Table 1-8. These include books that pro-

Table 1-8. Selected References and Description of Contents

Reference	Type of Information
AHFS Drug Handbook. American Society of Health-System Pharmacists: Bethesda, Md and Lippincott Williams & Wilkins: Springhouse, Pa.	Alphabetical listing of drugs by generic name. Provides quick view of trade names, pharmacologic classification, therapeutic classification, pregnancy category, OTC/prescription classification, and dosage units supplied for each drug. Also includes summary of pharmacokinetics, mechanism of action, uses, dosages, adverse effects, and patient counseling.
DiPiro JT, Talbert RL, Yee GC, Matzke GR, Wells BG, Posey LM, eds. *Pharmacotherapy: A Pathophysiologic Approach.* Stamford, Conn: Appleton Lange.	Extensive and detailed discussion of drug therapy by disease state with discussion of pharmacologic drug categories. Includes extensive discussion of pathophysiology and clinical presentation for each disease. Extensive references for each chapter.
Drug Facts and Comparisons. St. Louis, Mo: Facts and Comparison.	Comprehensive source of drug information. Generic name of drugs listed alphabetically by therapeutic category. Includes uses, pharmacology, adverse effects, pregnancy risk category, and dosages. Each trade name and corresponding dosage form is listed. Some comparison of uses and effects of drugs within the category are provided at beginning of sections. Available as loose-leaf and bound.
Fetrow CW, Avila JR. *Professional's Handbook of Complementary & Alternative Medicines.* Springhouse, Pa: Lippincott Williams & Wilkins.	Alphabetical listing of herbal compounds. Provides results of scientific studies, common names, chemical components, actions, uses, and dosages.
Handbook of Nonprescription Drugs. Washington, DC: American Pharmaceutical Association.	Textbook-like reference with chapters by disease state that includes discussion of pathophysiology, epidemiology, symptoms, and pharmacology of OTC. Provides examples of drugs but not comprehensive lists.
Hardman JG, Limbird LE, eds. *The Pharmacological Basis of Therapeutics.* New York, NY: McGraw-Hill.	Comprehensive and detailed explanation of the pharmacological effects by drug category followed by discussion of individual drugs for each category. Extensive bibliography for each chapter. Includes history and chemistry for many drugs. Includes chapters on general principles.

continued

Table 1-8. Selected References and Description of Contents (continued)

Reference	Type of Information
Herfindal ET, Gourley DR, eds. *Textbook of Therapeutics: Drug and Disease Management.* Baltimore, Md: Lippincott Williams & Wilkins.	Extensive and detailed discussion of drug therapy by disease state with discussion of pharmacologic drug categories. Includes extensive discussion of pathophysiology and clinical presentation for each disease. Extensive references by chapter.
Lacy CF, Armstrong LL, Goldman, MP, Lance, LL, eds. *Drug Information Handbook.* Hudson, Ohio: Lexi-Comp Inc.	Alphabetical listing of drugs by generic and trade name. Includes summary of uses, pronunciation, pregnancy risk factor, effects, dosages, adverse effects, and patient information in 1-2 pages for each drug. Includes an index by therapeutic category and key word.
Lance LL, Lacy CF, Armstrong, LL, Goldman MP, eds. *Drug Information Handbook for the Allied Health Professional.* Hudson, Ohio: Lexi-Comp Inc.	Alphabetical listing of drugs by generic and trade name. For medical, technical, and other health professionals. Includes summary of uses, pronunciation, pregnancy risk factor, effects, dosages, and adverse effects in 1 to 2 pages for each drug. Includes an index by indication/therapeutic category.
PDR for Nonprescription Drugs and Dietary Supplements. Montvale, NJ: Medical Economics Co, Inc.	Contains FDA approved description of OTC products. Includes ingredients, uses, drug interactions, and color photographs of many OTC products. Also information on vitamins, nutritional supplements, and herbal products.
Physician's Drug Handbook. Baltimore, Md: Lippincott Williams & Wilkins.	Alphabetical listing by generic name. Includes trade names, pharmacologic classification, therapeutic classification, pregnancy category, OTC/prescription classification, dosage units supplied, pharmacokinetics, pharmacodynamics, uses, dosages, adverse effects, and information for the patient.
Physicians' Desk Reference. Montvale, NJ: Medical Economics Company, Inc.	The PDR. Trade names of drugs listed alphabetically by manufacturer. Contains FDA approved labeling (package insert) information including pharmacology, uses, warnings, adverse effects, pregnancy risk category, dosage, dosage forms, and some chemical structures. Drugs indexed by manufacturer, trade name, generic name, and product category. Includes many colored product identification photos. Information regarding some OTC drugs and contents of some combination products.
Skidmore-Roth L, ed. *Nursing Drug Reference.* St Louis, Mo: Mosby, Inc.	Contains section of general pharmacological information regarding major drug categories. Drugs listed alphabetically by generic name. Includes pronunciation of generic names, trade names, actions, dosages, adverse effects, pharmacokinetics, uses, and nursing considerations.

vide a listing of drugs along with their respective uses, adverse effects, and other pharmacological information. As an example, the *Physician's Desk Reference* (PDR) contains information about drugs listed alphabetically by trade name according to manufacturer. The information includes chemical properties of the drug; a physical description of the trade name product; pharmacology and clinical data; and information about precautions, adverse effects, indications, dosage, and routes of administration. Diagrams are sometimes included to serve as special instructions for administration. An example of this would be a diagram describing the use of an inhaler or the application of transdermal medication. The information in the PDR is provided by the manufacturer and contains information from the official FDA approved package insert. The PDR also includes indices by manufacturer, trade name/generic name, and product category, which are helpful as a means to locate a drug. For example, if the generic name is known, the trade name/generic name index can be used. Doxycycline, for example, can be found under "doxycycline," under "Monodox" (or any of other trade names), or under "Oclassen Dermatologics" in the manufacturers' index. Alternatively, the page for the doxycycline information can also be found by using the product category index, under the "Tetracyclines" group of the "Antibiotics" section. The PDR also includes color pictures of many products listed in a separate section by manufacturer. A picture of Monodox capsules is among those included and therefore, regardless of which index is used to locate Monodox, the page for the color picture is included with the page for the product information. The PDR is over 3500 pages long and is approximately 9 x 11 inches—too large to conveniently carry as a reference. The information is in much greater detail than needed for a quick reference. PDR Supplements are published twice annually.

There is an array of pharmacology textbooks specifically tailored for pharmacy, nursing, and medical students. These texts typically address general pharmacology principles along with a systematic discussion of every therapeutic drug category with relevance to the respective professional practice. The long-standing authority in the arena of pharmacology textbooks is Goodman and Gilman's *The Pharmacological Basis of Therapeutics*. This reference provides an in-depth presentation of the principles of pharmacology and discussion of drugs by pharmacological category. It also includes a broad base of pharmacological information in each category followed by a discussion of individual drugs in the respective pharmacological category. History, chemistry, and toxicology are provided for many drugs and each chapter ends with an extensive bibliography of original research and review articles. Textbooks of therapeutics usually discuss drugs by disease category along with a discussion of the pathophysiology, clinical presentation of the patient, and means of diagnosis. The focus is the drug therapy for treating the disease rather than a study of each drug by pharmacological category. A highly regarded comprehensive therapeutics textbook is *Pharmacotherapy: A Pathophysiologic Approach* (see Table 1-8).

Drug Facts and Comparisons is a reference that lists drugs alphabetically by therapeutic category. Each section discusses and compares therapeutic uses, pharmacology, contraindications, adverse effects, and patient information regarding the drugs in that category. All available trade names and dosage forms are listed, along with the name of the manufacturer. Many nonprescription products are also included as well as a section of color photographs of tablets and capsules. *Drug Facts and Comparisons* is available in a bound format, or in loose-leaf form so that monthly supplements can be included throughout the year.

The official pharmacopeia in the United States is the *United States Pharmacopeia/National Formulary* (USP/NF). This reference provides the official standards for the purity, strength, quality, and analysis of drugs. The only drugs included in this reference are those for which standards have been developed and approved by the USP Convention. It is not a reference routinely useful for the athletic trainer, but it is noteworthy that products that have met these standards, including OTC products, have "USP" on the label (Figure 1-4) after the name of the drug (eg,

Figure 1-4. Example of "USP" denoted on label. This means that the medicine has met the official standards for purity, strength, and quality set forth by the United States Pharmacopeia/National Formulary.

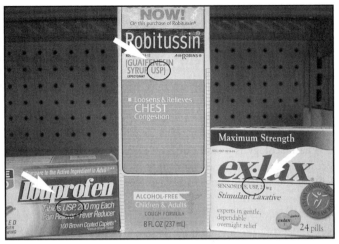

aspirin, USP).

There are sources of information that focus exclusively on OTC products and their uses. Some OTC medications are also available as prescription drugs and are typically discussed in pharmacology texts, but many OTC medications and combination products are exclusively OTC. *The Handbook of Nonprescription Drugs* contains a comprehensive discussion of OTC products by disease state, pathophysiology, symptom, and pharmacological effects of drugs. All of the references mentioned above extensively discuss drugs from one aspect or another but none are convenient reference guides that are easily carried around. However, there are many drug handbooks available (see Table 1-8). These handbooks typically contain a comprehensive alphabetical listing of drugs along with a summary of pharmacological information, uses, adverse effects, description of the dosage forms, trade names, and instructions to the patient. These handbooks provide a quick reference for succinct information but do not typically include explanation of drug action principles, pathophysiology, or basis for specific therapeutic uses. In general, drug handbooks are designed with the assumption that the reader has foundational knowledge regarding pharmacology. Similar handbooks are also available regarding herbal products.

An even more compact source of drug information involves the use of a personal digital assistant (PDA). Some drug references are now available for use with a PDA, including drug handbooks and a version of the PDR. Although more expensive than the texts themselves, the use of PDAs is becoming very popular as they provide a convenient means of carrying and accessing drug information. The Internet is another electronic source of a seemingly unlimited amount of drug information. For example, the National Institutes of Health (NIH) Web site (www.nih.gov) provides health topics by disease and organ systems, which include vast information regarding pathophysiology, symptoms, and drug therapy. Also, the FDA Center for Drug Evaluation and Research (CDER) provides information on regulatory issues, newly approved prescription drugs, lists of approved drugs, and OTC drug information, and can be accessed at www.fda.gov/cder/drug/default.htm. Both the NIH and FDA sites have "search" capability.

Besides information regarding the pharmacology of drugs, it is also important for the athletic trainer to have access to laws that regulate the handling of drugs by the athletic trainer and the policies regulating drug use and drug testing as established by the International Olympic Committee (IOC), National Collegiate Athletic Association (NCAA), and other groups regulating competitive athletics. Chapters 4 and 14 discuss these issues and provide practical information for the athletic trainer. The current policies of the IOC and NCAA regarding banned substances and antidoping are available through the following Web sites: www.usantidoping.org/prohibited_sub/index.htm and www.ncaa.org, respectively. Athletic trainers should check with their respective state high school athletic association and their local school board regarding drug use and drug testing in their respective state regarding the policies regulating drug use in high school students.

SUMMARY

Pharmacology is a study of how drugs affect the body and how the body affects the drug. Because the therapeutic use of drugs (or lack of use) can affect athletic performance, it is important for the athletic trainer to have knowledge of pharmacology that will be useful in the professional practice setting; an understanding of the terminology and classifications of drug names is a starting point for this knowledge. The trade name (or brand name) is a name that is owned by a pharmaceutical company, whereas a generic name is not owned by anyone and refers to one specific chemical compound. Drugs can be categorized by the mechanism of action (eg, all β-agonists combine with the β-receptor), by their chemical structure (eg, all corticosteroids have a similar chemistry), or therapeutic category (eg, all asthma drugs are used to treat asthma, but they are not all β-agonists or corticosteroids). Drugs can also be grouped as to their legal classification of OTC, prescription, or scheduled drugs. The laws regarding the purchase, storage, and distribution differ for these three categories of drugs.

Regardless of the classification of a drug, all drugs must obtain approval of the FDA to be marketed. New compounds must go through a rigorous process of animal testing, followed by three phases of clinical (human) tests before they can be approved for general use. A drug that goes off patent protection can be marketed by other companies after demonstrating that their product is bioequivalent to the original product. This abbreviated approval process helps expedite the marketing of drugs (generic drugs) by companies other than the initial patent holder.

This textbook includes basic pharmacology of drug categories pertinent to the certified and/or licensed athletic trainer and the athletic training student, but does not supply a comprehensive list of drugs. There are, however, numerous drug handbooks available that are convenient to use as a quick reference regarding specific drugs. Comprehensive textbooks and references are also readily available if a more intensive study of the effects and uses of drugs are desired. Programs are available for use with PDAs and an immense amount of information is also available via the Internet. All of these sources of information, along with the availability of pharmacists and physicians for individualized assistance, provide excellent resources for the athletic trainer who has a foundational understanding of basic pharmacology.

BIBLIOGRAPHY

Fetrow CW, Avila JR. *Professional's Handbook of Complementary & Alternative Medicines*. 2nd ed. Springhouse, Pa: Springhouse Corp; 2001.

Fink JL III, Vivian JC, Reid KK, eds. *Pharmacy Law Digest*. 36th ed. St Louis, Mo: Facts and Comparisons Publishing Group; 2001.

Generic drugs. *The Medical Letter*. 1999;41:47-48.

US Food and Drug Administration, Center for Drug Evaluation and Research. The new drug development process: steps from test tube to new drug application review. Available at: www.fda.gov/cder/handbook/develop.htm. Accessed May 22, 2003.

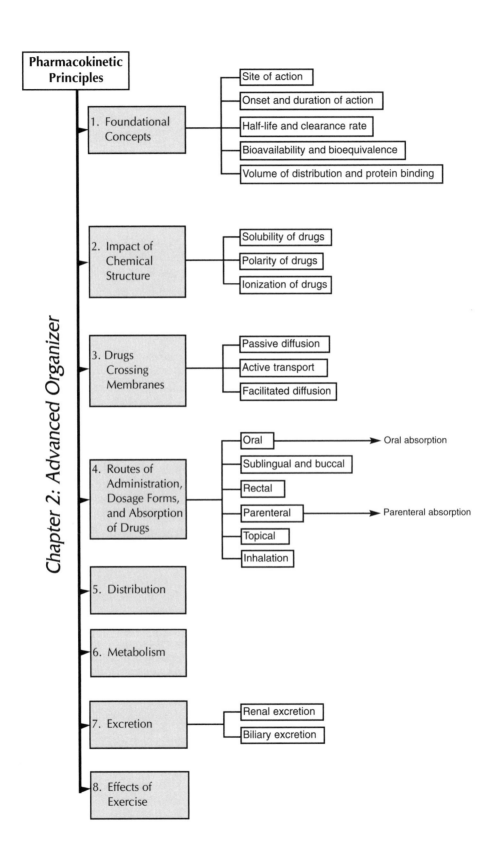

PHARMACOKINETIC PRINCIPLES
Processes That Affect Drugs From Entry to Exit

CHAPTER OBJECTIVES

At the end of this chapter the reader will be able to:

- Apply the concepts of site of action, onset and duration of action, half-life, clearance rate, bioavailability, bioequivalence, volume of distribution, and protein binding to the pharmacokinetic action of drugs.
- Apply the concepts of bioavailability and bioequivalence to the biological effect of drugs.
- List and explain the variables that impact the volume of distribution of a drug.
- Explain how a drug's chemical structure determines its biological effects.
- Explain how the polarity and ionization of a drug affects the ability of the drug to cross cell and tissue membranes.
- Describe three primary mechanisms by which drugs cross membranes to reach their site of action.
- List and describe the major routes in which drugs can be administered.
- Explain what factors affect the distribution of drugs throughout the body.
- Describe the primary ways drugs are metabolized through oxidation, conjugation, hydrolysis, and reduction.
- List the ways drugs are excreted from the body.
- Describe how drugs are excreted from the body by the kidneys.
- Explain the potential impact of exercise on the pharmacokinetics of drugs.

Pharmacokinetics is the study of the impact of the body on a drug. The primary focus of pharmacokinetics is on the rate and extent to which the drug is absorbed into the blood stream, distributed throughout the body, metabolized, and finally excreted. These processes will affect the magnitude and duration of the biological responses, the therapeutic (desirable) effects as well as adverse (undesirable) effects. As will be discussed, the chemical structure of the drug will determine how the body will interact with the drug to dictate the rates of absorption, distribution, metabolism, and excretion.

FOUNDATIONAL CONCEPTS

It is necessary to understand some foundational concepts and terminology to fully grasp the discussion of pharmacokinetics. These concepts and terminology include site of action, onset and duration of action, half-life, clearance rate, bioavailability, bioequivalence, volume of distri-

Figure 2-1. Concentration-time curve following a single oral dose of a drug. The onset of action occurs when the concentration is above the level needed to produce an effect (minimal effective concentration). Duration of action (4 hours in this example) is the time between onset and termination of action. The half-life ($t\frac{1}{2}$) is the time it takes for the concentration of the drug to be reduced by one-half after it has reached peak concentration. In this example, $t\frac{1}{2}$ = 1 ½ hours; the time it takes for the concentration of drug to decrease from 15 to 7.5.

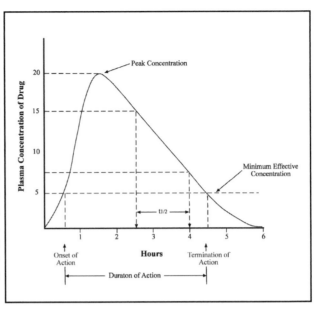

bution, and protein binding. Some of these concepts and terms will not necessarily be used frequently by the athletic trainer, but they are used throughout this textbook and are useful for understanding other drug-related literature.

Site of Action

For any drug to have an effect it must reach its *site of action*. This is the molecular site where the drug has a significant chemical interaction to produce a biological effect. The site of action for most drugs is either a receptor (usually a protein) on the cell surface or inside a specific cell type, or an enzyme within a cell. For example, the site of action may be receptors on the surface of smooth muscle, enzymes within nerve fibers, or receptors on the surface of platelets. The receptor theory of drug action will be discussed in the next chapter.

Onset and Duration of Action

The *onset of action* (Figure 2-1) is the time it takes for the concentration of drug molecules at the site of action to become large enough to cause a noticeable biological response. This response will continue as long as the minimum effective concentration of drug is maintained at the site of action. The minimum effective concentration varies from one drug to the next. As the drug is metabolized and excreted, the drug molecules dissipate from the site of action. This process continues until an insufficient number of drug molecules are present to cause an observable response and action is therefore terminated. The *duration of action* is the time between onset and termination of action and represents the length of time the drug produces its effect.

Half-Life and Clearance Rate

The *half-life* ($t\frac{1}{2}$) of a drug is the time required for the amount of drug in the blood to be reduced by one-half. The two mechanisms that "clear" the drug from the body are *metabolism* and *excretion*. The *clearance rate* is a measure of the efficiency of these two mechanisms. When drugs are metabolized they are considered to be cleared from the body in the sense that they are chemically modified to form a different compound.

An accurate assumption for most drugs is that the drug in the blood is in equilibrium with the drug at the site of action. Therefore, the concentration of drug in the blood is a direct reflection of the concentration at the site of action. The t½ can be determined by measuring the blood (or plasma) concentration of the drug at time intervals after it has reached the peak level and no additional doses of drug are given (see Figure 2-1). For example, if the t½ of a drug is 2 hours and the concentration in the blood is 100 µg/mL it will decrease by 50 µg/mL in 2 hours; if the same drug exists at 10 µg/mL, it will decrease by only 5 µg/mL (ie, 50%) in 2 hours. The rate of decrease is a percentage, not an amount, because the mechanisms by which drugs are removed from the blood are usually not working at their maximum. Thus, the rates at which these mechanisms function are a linear relationship to blood concentration in that they function twice as fast if the concentration is twice as much. Using the example above and assuming no additional drug is given, the 100 µg/mL concentration will be at 25 µg/mL after 4 hours, 12.5 µg/mL after 6 hours, and 6.25 µg/mL after 8 hours.

Drugs with a longer t½ have a longer duration of action. A significantly longer duration of action provides an advantage to the patient in that the drug does not have to be administered as often each day, thus making it easier for patients to remember to take the medications at the appropriate time. For example, naproxen, a NSAID, has a t½ of about 14 hours and is recommended as twice per day dosing. Ibuprofen, by comparison, is another NSAID but has a t½ of 2 hours and, therefore, a more frequent dosing interval of 3 to 4 times per day.

Bioavailability and Bioequivalence

The amount of drug administered has no therapeutic relevance if the drug does not reach the general circulation and have the opportunity to reach the site of action. To be bioavailable, the drug must reach the systemic circulation. There are two components to bioavailability: the amount of drug absorbed and the rate of absorption. *Bioavailability* will be reduced if a tablet or capsule incompletely dissolves in the gastrointestinal tract, or if the drug is inactivated by intestinal enzymes (Figure 2-2). Bioavailability is also diminished if the drug is absorbed from the intestine and directly enters the portal (liver) circulation where it first passes through the liver. As will be discussed later, the liver is the major organ for drug metabolism and may inactivate a portion of the drug before it enters the systemic circulation. This is referred to as the *first pass effect* and has a significant impact on the bioavailability of some, but not all, drugs. Enzymes in the intestinal cells may also participate in drug metabolism, which contributes to the first pass effect and thus, diminished bioavailability. For drugs that have a first pass effect, the manufacturers recommended dose compensates for this characteristic. Calcium channel blockers used to treat angina and hypertension (see Chapter 12) are examples. Also nitroglycerin sublingual tablets (discussed later in this chapter) undergo significant first pass effect and thus are not effective if swallowed. As a result of the first pass effect, less than half of orally administered morphine is bioavailable. To compensate for the first pass effect, the oral dosage range of morphine is increased from the normal adult dose of 2 to 10 mg intravenously to 5 to 30 mg orally.

The other component of bioavailability is the rate at which the drug enters the general circulation (see Figure 2-2). As shown in Figure 2-3, if 100% of orally administered drug A and drug B enter the general circulation but drug A is absorbed quickly and drug B is absorbed gradually over a longer time, the peak blood concentration will be greater for drug A. This also means that the biological effect is greater for drug A. The peak blood concentration for drug B will be lower because, as it enters the blood slower, it does not have as much of a chance to accumulate before

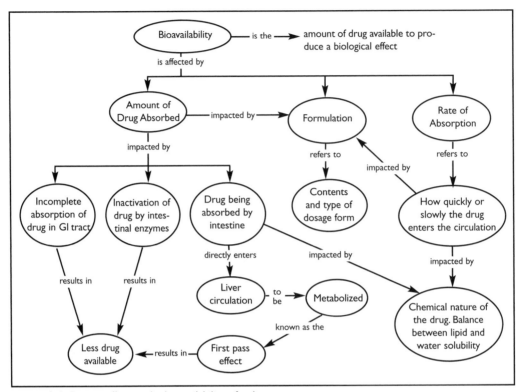

Figure 2-2. Factors affecting the bioavailability of a drug.

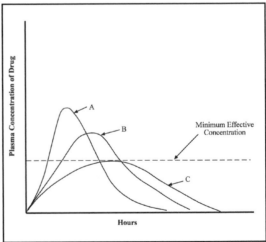

Figure 2-3. Bioavailability and bioequivalence. Concentration-time curve for two drugs, A and B, illustrates a difference in bioavailability. Bioavailability of drugs can differ because of differences in the rates at which they dissolve in the gastrointestinal tract, extent of the first pass effect, extent to which they are affected by the presence of food, and other factors. Lack of bioequivalence is illustrated in the comparison of two formulations, A and C, of the same drug. In this case, formulation C is absorbed more slowly than formulation A, and thus C never reaches minimum effective concentration although approximately the same amount of drug is absorbed.

the clearance rate exceeds the absorption rate. Therefore, the bioavailability of these two drugs is not equivalent. The *formulation* can have a significant impact on bioavailability (see Figure 2-2). The formulation is also called the product and refers to the total contents of the dosage form (active and inert ingredients) and the type of dosage form (eg, tablet, capsule, suspension). Other factors that affect the absorption of drugs are discussed in this chapter.

Bioequivalence is similar to bioavailability, but refers to a comparison of the amount and rate of drug entering the general circulation for two or more similar formulations of the same drug. This concept is used when a company wants to demonstrate that its generic product is equivalent to a trade name product. In other words, two products (ie, different formulations of the same drug) are bioequivalent if the bioavailability of the two products are equivalent. Figure 2-3 illustrates the bioavailability of two formulations (A and C) of the same drug. The total amount of drug absorbed is approximately the same, but the absorption of the drug from formulation C is so slow that the minimum effective blood concentration is not attained; the bioavailability of drugs A and C are significantly different and thus they are not bioequivalent. Therapeutic equivalence refers to the same clinical response when two products are compared. It is similar to bioequivalence except a specific clinical response (eg, pain relief) is measured rather than blood concentration. Because therapeutic response is determined by bioavailability, two drug products that are therapeutically equivalent will be bioequivalent.

Volume of Distribution and Protein Binding

After a drug is absorbed into the blood, it distributes throughout the body. The extent of distribution in various fluids and tissues depends largely upon the drug's lipid solubility and protein binding characteristics. The *volume of distribution* is the apparent space in the body that is available to the drug; the more extensive distribution, the larger the volume of distribution. Drugs that distribute into adipose tissue, bind to muscle tissue, or bind to plasma protein will have a larger volume of distribution. As drugs distribute into these tissue sites, there is less drug available in the blood circulation and thus there is less drug available to reach the site of action. The extent to which a drug binds to tissue and plasma protein is documented prior to its entry into the market and the normal dosage range is established based on this information. *As the volume of distribution increases, the dose needed to get a sufficient concentration of drug to the site of action also increases.*

Another factor affecting the volume of distribution is the physical size of the patient. Body weight is the most common indicator, although body surface area is also used. Obviously, a larger patient has more body tissue into which the drug can distribute. Obese patients have a larger percentage of total body weight in adipose tissue and thus have more tissue into which lipid soluble drugs can distribute. If the drug resides in body fat, the concentration of drug available to reach the site of action is diminished. *Volume of distribution increases with body weight* and is the basis for adjustment of drug dosage according to weight. See Chapter 3 for additional discussion regarding dose calculations.

Binding of the drug to plasma protein also increases the volume of distribution. Albumin is the plasma protein with the largest concentration in the blood (39 to 50 gm/L). The percentage of drug that binds to albumin is a constant for any given drug. Some drugs do not bind significantly to albumin but for many drugs the percentage of the protein-bound drug is quite significant; >99% in some cases. Examples of drugs that are ≥90% bound to protein are shown in Table 2-1. Because albumin is a protein, it is much larger than drug molecules and it does not penetrate through the capillaries. Therefore, drugs bound to albumin also do not leave the capillary and thus are not available to bind at the site of action in the tissue (Figure 2-4). Unlike binding to a receptor site, binding to albumin is nonselective in that many drugs with similar chemical characteristics will bind at the same site on the albumin; this can cause a potential for drug interaction, which will be discussed in the next chapter. The extent and strength of the binding to albumin depends on the chemical structure of the drug. Usually, the binding forces usually weak bonds and consequently protein binding is almost always reversible (ie, the drug

Table 2-1. Examples of Drugs That Exhibit ≥ 90% Protein Binding

Generic Name	Trade Name	Drug Classification
atorvastatin	Lipitor	antilipidemic
celecoxib	Celebrex	NSAID
cerivastatin	Baycol	antilipidemic
diazepam	Valium	muscle relaxant
diclofenac	Voltaren	NSAID
flurbiprofen	Ansaid	NSAID
fluvastatin	Lescol	antilipidemic
glipizide	Glucotrol	antidiabetic
glyburide	DiaBeta	antidiabetic
ibuprofen	Motrin	NSAID
indomethacin	Indocin	NSAID
lovastatin	Mevacor	antilipidemic
montelukast	Singulair	asthma therapy
naproxen	Naprosyn	NSAID
phenytoin	Dilantin	anticonvulsant
pioglitazone	Actos	antidiabetic
rosiglitazone	Avandia	antidiabetic
simvastatin	Zocor	antilipidemic
tolbutamide	Orinase	antidiabetic
valproic acid	Depakene	anticonvulsant
warfarin	Coumadin	oral anticoagulant
zafirlukast	Accolate	asthma therapy
zileuton	Zyflo	asthma therapy

Figure 2-4. Drug binding to plasma protein. Albumin is the most abundant protein in the plasma and many drugs bind to this protein. Drug molecules that are bound to albumin cannot penetrate through the capillary because the albumin is too large. Only unbound (free) drug can leave the capillary circulation, enter the tissue, and reach the site of action.

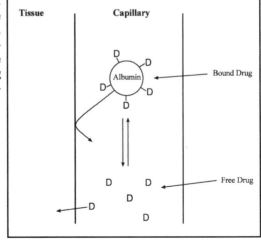

binds and then releases from the albumin back and forth). When the drug is not bound to albumin, it is called unbound drug or *free drug*; only free drug can bind to the receptor and cause a biological effect. The ratio of free drug to bound drug is a constant for that drug and is determined by the drug's chemical characteristics.

Although bound drug cannot reach the site of action, the extent of protein binding is of little consequence with respect to attaining the therapeutic effect because the protein binding is taken into account when the recommended dosage regimen is established before the drug is marketed. Protein binding does have significant therapeutic implications, however, related to the potential for drug interactions (see Chapter 3).

Summary

The study of the effects of the body on drugs is pharmacokinetics. The purpose of giving a drug is for the drug to reach the site of action where it can produce the desired response. As the drug enters the blood, the concentration of drug at the site of action becomes high enough to cause a noticeable biological response; the time it takes for this to occur is the onset of action. The action of the drug is diminished as the drug is cleared (removed) by metabolism and excretion processes. The clearance rate will determine how quickly the drug is removed from the blood. As long as the rate of absorption of the drug is faster than the rate of clearance, the blood level will continue to increase. The time it takes for half the drug to be cleared is the half-life of the drug. As the drug is cleared, eventually the concentration at the site of action is not sufficient to cause a noticeable biological effect and the action of the drug is terminated.

The entire dose of a drug will not necessarily reach the general circulation. If the drug is administered orally, the liver may metabolize some of the drug as it first passes to the liver from the gastrointestinal tract (first pass effect), and thus a portion of the drug dose never reaches the site of action. The more body fluids and tissues that the drug distributes into (volume of distribution), the lower the concentration of drug that will exist at the site of action. If a portion of the drug molecules bind to plasma protein, those molecules are not free to reach the site of action.

IMPACT OF CHEMICAL STRUCTURE

To understand the principles of drug action, it is important to realize that the chemical structure of the drug determines its characteristics. Although acetaminophen and aspirin are both over-the-counter (OTC) analgesics, they are not the same drug because they have unique chemical structures (Figure 2-5). The chemical structure of the drug is the factor that determines the chemical binding forces between the drug and all of the extracellular and intracellular structures with which it interacts. Consequently, the chemical structure determines the biological effects of a drug, whether good or bad, the rate of absorption, excretion, and metabolism (ie, pharmacokinetics). The chemical structure can even influence the types of *dosage forms* available to administer the drug. For example, it is of no value to make a *transdermal* dosage form for a drug that requires a dose of 250 mg twice a day because that amount of drug cannot penetrate through the skin.

Small changes in chemical structure can produce significant changes in the biological effects. This is the principle reason there is such an array of drugs in some drug categories. Many drugs have been developed through slight modifications of the prototype drug known to produce significant therapeutic effects. The prototype drug often is a naturally occurring compound produced by plants or microorganisms or is *endogenous* in humans. For example, numerous modifi-

Figure 2-5. Chemical structure of aspirin and acetaminophen. Two different analgesic drugs with some similar characteristics. The chemical structure determines all aspects of the drug activity.

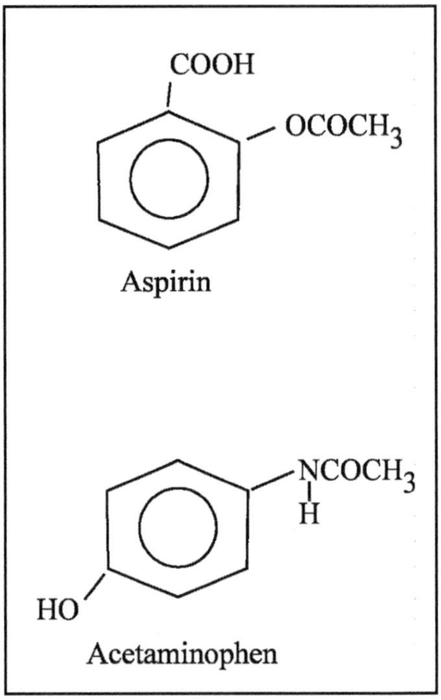

cations have been made to the endogenous neurotransmitter *epinephrine* in an effort to produce drugs that mimic one or more actions of epinephrine. Relatively slight changes in chemical structure can impact not only pharmacokinetic parameters but also therapeutic uses. Modifications of the epinephrine structure have resulted in drugs that are useful as bronchial dilators, nasal decongestants, and central nervous system stimulants. In a similar manner, a microorganism produces penicillin G (Pentids), which was the first penicillin for clinical use. It was the prototype for penicillins and now there are a dozen drugs available that are modifications of penicillin G. The chemical modifications to penicillin G were made in anticipation of improving its characteristics (eg, to prevent stomach acid from destroying the molecule, to improve effectiveness against various microorganisms, or to increase the duration of action). Other examples of naturally occurring prototypes are morphine as an opiate analgesic, testosterone as an anabolic steroid, and cortisone as a steroidal anti-inflammatory drug.

The chemical structure obviously determines the size and chemical shape of each drug molecule. With the exception of drugs that are *polypeptides* and proteins (eg, insulin and glucagon), most drugs have a *molecular weight* of <1000 and are regarded as small compounds. For these small molecular weight compounds, size itself does not have a direct bearing on the site of action or ability to penetrate membranes, but for most drugs the solubility of the drug plays the most important role.

Solubility of Drugs

The solubility of drugs is important because it affects how quickly a drug is dissolved in the gastrointestinal tract, how quickly it is absorbed into the bloodstream, the rate and location of distribution throughout the body, the rate of excretion, and the type of liquid dosage form in which it is available.

The two categories of solubility are water solubility and lipid solubility. Drugs that are water soluble are referred to as *hydrophilic* ("love water"). Drugs that are lipid soluble are referred to as *hydrophobic* ("fear water") or *lipophilic* ("love lipid"). In reality, most drugs have some water solubility characteristics and some lipid solubility characteristics. The more water soluble the drug, the more readily it will dissolve in the gastrointestinal tract (a necessity for absorption into the blood). However, lipid solubility is also important for absorption because the more lipid soluble the drug, the more readily the drug will cross membranes to move from the gastrointestinal tract into the blood. Drugs that are more lipid soluble will penetrate the central nervous system (CNS) more readily; drugs that are more water soluble will be excreted by the kidney faster. It is evident that a combination of these characteristics, water solubility and lipid solubility, play a significant role in the pharmacokinetic and pharmacodynamic parameters of drugs.

Two chemical characteristics that affect solubility are polarity and ionization. The greater the extent of polarity and ionization of a molecule, the greater the water solubility (less lipid solubility), whereas a molecule with less polarity or ionization will have less water solubility (greater lipid solubility). All drugs have one or more portions of their chemical structure that are polar and/or nonpolar, and some also have a portion that can ionize. As the number of polar components increase compared to nonpolar, the molecule becomes more water soluble. If a drug also has a portion of the molecule that is ionized, its water solubility increases greatly.

Polarity of Drugs

Molecular polarity exists when a portion of the molecule has an uneven distribution of electrons; the more areas of uneven electron distribution, the more polar the molecule. Water molecules (H-O-H) also have uneven electron distribution because the oxygen tends to pull electrons toward it. Therefore, polar molecules are attracted to the water molecules and are more soluble in water or in any other aqueous environment such as blood or urine. Thus, the greater the polarity, the more water soluble the drug. In contrast, drugs that are very polar will not dissolve readily in lipid (fat-like) environments (eg, membranes).

If a drug has no areas of uneven electron distribution, it is referred to as nonpolar and will not be very water soluble. Nonpolar drugs will be lipid soluble because lipids are also nonpolar. Remember that most drugs have some water solubility and some lipid solubility characteristics; in other words, most drugs have some areas of the chemical structure that are polar and some areas that are nonpolar. Therefore, the terms polar and nonpolar are usually used in a relative sense when comparing drugs; one drug being more or less polar than another, and thus more or less water soluble than another.

Ionization of Drugs

Another chemical characteristic that can make a drug more water soluble is the degree of ionization. Ionization means that the drug has a portion of the structure that can form either a negative charge or positive charge (Figure 2-6). Drugs that can ionize are acids and bases. Ionization occurs when an extreme uneven distribution of electrons exists, which causes the molecule to either attach a positive charge or release a positive charge (thereby becoming negatively charged). Like polar molecules, molecules with an ionic charge are also attracted to water molecules. Therefore, if a drug is ionized, the drug will be significantly more water soluble because the ions form bonds with water molecules. For example, it takes 120 mL of water to dissolve 1 g of un-ionized codeine whereas it only takes 2.5 mL of water to dissolve 1 g of ionized codeine. In fact, the impact of ionization is greater than the impact of polarity on water solubility.

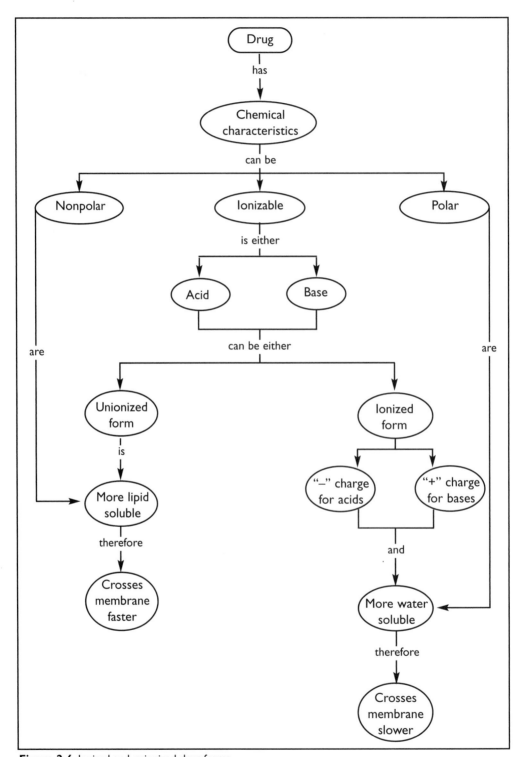

Figure 2-6. Ionized and unionized drug forms.

Box 2-1. pH Scale

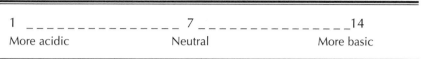

1	7	14
More acidic	Neutral	More basic

When acids or bases are in solution, a portion of the molecules will be in the ionized state whereas the remainder will not be ionized. Each molecule of drug alternates from the ionized to the unionized form (ionized ◄─► unionized). At any given time, the percentage of drug molecules in the ionized form will depend on two things: the chemical structure of the drug and the pH (Box 2-1) of the aqueous environment the drug is in.

If DH represents an acid drug such as aspirin, then the following equation shows the ionization of the aspirin in which a hydrogen ion (also called a proton, H^+) separates from the rest of the aspirin leaving the negatively charged aspirin (D^-). The ratio of $DH:D^-$ depends on the pH of the environment that it is in (eg, urine, blood, stomach). Acids will be more ionized the more basic the environment.

Ionization of an acid drug: $$DH \longleftrightarrow D^- + H^+$$

If DN represents a base such as codeine, then the following equation shows the ionization of the codeine (DNH^+) in which a hydrogen ion attaches to the codeine molecule making it positively charged. The ratio of $DN:DNH^+$ depends on the pH of the environment that it is in. Bases will be more ionized the more acidic the environment.

Ionization of a base: $$DN + H^+ \longleftrightarrow DNH^+$$

The extent to which ionization and polarity dominate the chemical nature of the drug will significantly impact the pharmacokinetic parameters discussed later in this chapter.

Summary

Every characteristic of a drug molecule is determined by its chemical structure. The chemical structure will determine the biological activity at the site of action as well as rates of absorption, excretion, distribution, and metabolism. An important aspect of the chemical characteristics is the relative degree of water solubility and lipid solubility. Polar chemical characteristics and ionic chemical characteristics that comprise the molecular structure of the drug will make the molecule more water soluble (hydrophilic). Ionizable structures can exist in either the ionized or unionized forms. Drugs that can ionize are acids and bases. Molecules that have fewer polar structures or have an ionizable portion in the unionized form are more lipid soluble (lipophilic). The pH of the solution in which acids and bases exist will determine the proportion of the drug molecules that exist in the ionized versus unionized form. Drugs that are bases are more ionized the more acidic the pH of the solution, and drugs that are acids are more ionized the more basic the solution.

DRUGS CROSSING MEMBRANES

Regardless of the chemical structure, every drug must reach the site of action to produce the therapeutic effect. This *site of action* may be on skin cells or within the cells of a specific organ. To reach the site of action, drugs must pass through one or more membranes: gastrointestinal, vascular, cellular, or intracellular. Factors that affect the transport of drugs across membranes will

Box 2-2. Factors That Impact Passive Diffusion of a Drug

Factor	Comment
Concentration gradient of the drug	Drug moves from a level of higher concentration to a level of lower concentration.
Lipid solubility of the drug	Because lipids are the major constituents of cell membranes, the greater the lipid solubility of the drug, the greater the diffusion rate.
pH levels on both sides of the membrane	Acids and bases move across a membrane faster in one direction than the other if the pH differs on the two sides of the membrane.

also influence the absorption, distribution, metabolism, and excretion rates of the drugs. Therefore, the ability of a drug to cross membranes has a very important impact on the pharmacokinetics and pharmacodynamics (see Chapter 3) of the drug.

Lipids, primarily *phospholipids*, and *cholesterol* are the major constituents of cell membranes. The amount of specific phospholipids and cholesterol varies among the various vascular, cellular, and *organelle* membranes. Lipids provide the structural integrity of the membrane and impact the ease with which drugs pass through it. Proteins, which are imbedded in the sea of lipid, comprise the second most abundant membrane component. These proteins serve numerous functions such as receptors, transport mechanisms, enzymes, and cell surface recognition sites. Some proteins transverse the entire membrane, whereas others protrude only on one side or the other. Typically, there are multiple copies of each protein within the membrane. Another characteristic of the membrane is that it is a dynamic structure; the proteins are in constant motion within the sea of lipid due to its fluidity. This movement increases the likelihood for drugs and endogenous compounds to come in contact with the proper protein (eg, receptor) so that the appropriate biological action can be initiated.

There are three main mechanisms for transport of drugs across membranes: passive diffusion, active transport, and facilitative diffusion. In addition, pores in the membranes allow small polar molecules to penetrate. Ion channels are also present in membranes and these transport inorganic ions such as calcium. Although their ability to transport ions may be affected by some drugs (eg, calcium channel blockers), ion channels likely have little impact on the transfer of drugs across membranes.

Passive Diffusion

Passive diffusion refers to the drug penetrating through the membrane due to the solubility of the drug in the membrane (Box 2-2). This transport mechanism has the greatest impact on the pharmacokinetics and pharmacodynamics for most drugs. As membranes are primarily lipids, drugs that are more lipid soluble will diffuse across the membrane quicker than less lipid soluble drugs. The other driving force for the net transfer of drugs from one side of the membrane to the other is the concentration gradient (ie, the difference in concentration of the drug on the two sides of the membrane) (Figure 2-7). Molecules in solution are in random motion. Thus, the likelihood of a drug encountering the membrane is directly proportional to the concentration of the drug on that side of the membrane. Drugs that diffuse in one direction can also diffuse in the other direction at a rate dependent upon the concentration of the drug on that side

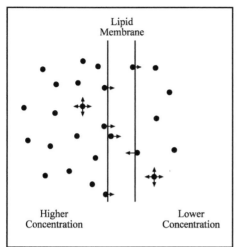

Lipid
Membrane

Higher
Concentration

Lower
Concentration

Figure 2-7. Passive diffusion. Drug molecules are in random motion and thus the probability of drug encountering the cellular membrane is based on the concentration of the drug and solubility in the membrane. Net movement of drug will be down the concentration gradient from the side of higher concentration to the side of lower concentration.

of the membrane. Therefore, the net movement of drug will be in the direction of higher concentration to lower concentration (see Figure 2-7). When the concentration of drug is equal on both sides, a concentration gradient no longer exists and the rate of diffusion of drug in one direction is equivalent to the rate in the opposite direction.

Acids and bases will move across a membrane faster in one direction than the other if the pH differs on the two sides of the membrane. As shown in Figure 2-8, this difference in diffusion rate occurs because the percentage of the unionized drug molecules will be greater on the pH 5-side of the membrane than on the pH 8-side. Because unionized molecules are more lipid soluble than the ionized, the unionized molecules will cross the membrane faster. As the drug moves to the opposite side of the membrane, a greater proportion of ionized drug molecules exists on that side. As a result, movement back across the membrane will be slower because there is more ionized drug trapped on that side. This impacts the rate at which drugs move from the small intestine to the blood or the extent to which acids and bases are reabsorbed from the renal tubule back to the blood (Figure 2-9). The urinary excretion rate of aspirin, for example, is significantly decreased if the urine is pH 6 because the higher percentage of unionized (more lipid soluble) aspirin will exist on the urine side and thus cross to the blood side of the membrane faster compared to urine pH of 8. This enhanced reabsorption could cause increased adverse effects or toxicity in patients on chronic aspirin therapy. Urine pH normally fluctuates throughout the day but may be lower and more persistently acidic due to metabolic or respiratory acidosis, some urinary tract infections, use of vitamin C supplements, and drinking cranberry juice. On the other hand, raising the urinary pH with intravenous sodium bicarbonate can be used as treatment for aspirin toxicity by increasing the rate of excretion. This in turn increases the ionized form of the drug on the urine side and prevents it from being reabsorbed back into the blood.

> *Recall that when an acid drug (DH) is in a more acidic pH (5 versus 8) that a larger percentage of the drug molecules will exist as unionized (free acid), which is more lipid soluble than the ionized form of the drug.*

Figure 2-8. Drugs that are acids and bases will exist in the unionized and ionized forms. If a hydrogen ion (H+) separates from the unionized acid drug (DH), the remaining drug molecule becomes ionized because it has a negative charge (D⁻). The ratio of unionized:ionized will depend on the pH of the solution. For an acid drug, there is more unionized drug (DH) if the pH is acidic. Unionized drug (DH) crosses the membrane by passive diffusion faster than the ionized drug (D⁻) because the unionized form is more lipid soluble (nonpolar) than the ionized drug. Therefore, a net movement will occur of acid drugs from the acidic pH side to the basic pH side of the membrane.

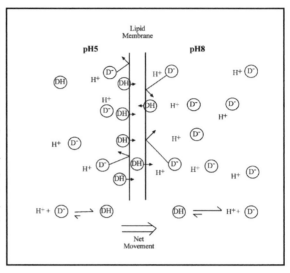

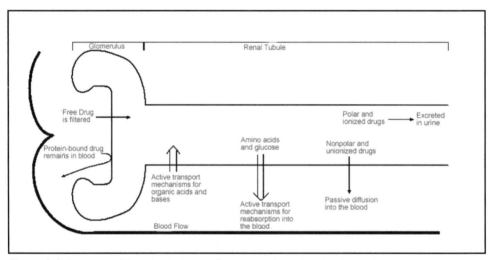

Figure 2-9. Excretion of drugs by the kidney. Free drug is filtered at the glomerulus and enters the renal tubule. Active transport systems for acids and bases also facilitate drugs entering the tubule. Reabsorption from the renal tubule into the blood occurs primarily by passive diffusion. Consequently, drugs that are more nonpolar or in the unionized form will be reabsorbed to a greater extent than drugs that are more polar or in the ionized form.

Active Transport

Active transport mechanisms have a protein with a binding site to which the compound being transported attaches. The transport mechanism facilitates the movement of the compound across the membrane. Active transport mechanisms have the characteristics listed in Box 2-3.

The advantages of the active transport system are the selectivity, which will allow only some compounds across the membrane, and the ability to move the compound against a concentration gradient (from a position of lower concentration on one side of the membrane to a higher concentration on the other side of the membrane). Active transport plays an important role for the transport of some drugs into the urine or secretion into the bile.

Box 2-3. Characteristics of Active Transport Mechanism

- Requires energy
- Requires a carrier protein to transport the drug across the membrane
- Is relatively specific for selected compounds
- Transports the compound in only one direction across the membrane
- Can be saturated to the point where an increased concentration of drug does not increase the rate of transport
- Can be competitively blocked by compounds with similar binding characteristics

Facilitated Diffusion

Facilitated diffusion combines the characteristics of passive diffusion and active transport. It requires a carrier protein and thus selectivity and system saturation are possible, but it does not use energy. Therefore, drugs or other compounds cannot be moved against a concentration gradient by facilitated diffusion and a high to low concentration gradient must be present for net diffusion to occur.

Summary

Drugs must cross membranes to reach the site of action. The main mechanisms that allow molecules to cross membranes are passive diffusion, active transport, and facilitated diffusion. Passive diffusion occurs when the drug becomes dissolved in the membrane and passes through to other side of the membrane. Because membranes are comprised primarily of lipid, the concentration of drug and its lipid solubility combine to dictate the rate of passive diffusion. Active transport and facilitated diffusion require a protein carrier on the membrane that has specific binding characteristics for the drug and will then facilitate the movement of the drug across the membrane. In contrast to passive and facilitated diffusion, active transport uses energy for the transport and can move drugs from a side of low concentration to a side of higher concentration. The predominant transport mechanism for drugs is passive diffusion and, therefore, drugs with a higher degree of lipid solubility will cross membranes faster and drugs with a higher degree of water solubility will cross membranes slower by passive diffusion.

ROUTES OF ADMINISTRATION, DOSAGE FORMS, AND ABSORPTION OF DRUGS

Routes of administration describe the means by which drugs are put in contact with the body for the purpose of reaching the site of action (Box 2-4). There are advantages and disadvantages to each route. The *dosage form* refers to the physical form in which the drug exists for administration. Oral is a route; tablet is a dosage form. Not all drugs administered by the oral route are tablets, and not all tablets are administered by the oral route. In some cases, the physical or chemical characteristics of the drug dictate the route of administration and may also limit the type of dosage form options available. For example, insulin is a protein that is destroyed by digestive enzymes. Because insulin is therefore not effective orally, injectable dosage forms are used. On the other hand, many drugs are available in several dosage forms and selection is based on many

Box 2-4. Routes of Drug Administration

- Oral
- Sublingual and buccal
- Rectal
- Parenteral
- Topical
- Inhalation

factors, including the personal preference of the patient, age (oral liquids swallowed more readily than solids by infants), cost, and desired speed of administration.

Absorption refers to getting the drug into the bloodstream. There is no absorption phase for the intravenous route as the drug is injected directly into the blood. *Some factors that affect the rate of absorption by all other routes of administration are lipid solubility of the drug, blood flow to the site of drug administration, and surface area from which the drug can be absorbed.* Regardless of the route of administration, drugs must cross membranes for absorption, and drugs that are more lipid soluble will diffuse through membranes faster. When the tissue has a rich capillary blood supply, the distance will be shorter for the drug to travel in the extravascular space before contact with a capillary, and thus absorption rate will be increased. Faster blood flow also carries the drug from the absorption site quicker for distribution to the site of action. Exercise increases blood flow to muscle and skin and increases the absorption of drugs administered by intramuscular and topical routes. Obviously, the greater the tissue surface area with which the drug is in contact, the greater the chance for it to come in contact with the membrane and ultimately reach the site of action.

Oral

The oral route is the most common means of drug administration. The drug is swallowed to obtain a systemic effect, or in some cases, to stay in the gastrointestinal tract for a local effect. Aspirin can be used orally to obtain the systemic effect of pain relief; laxatives (see Chapter 11) are used orally for a local effect in the gastrointestinal tract.

There are several reasons why the oral route is the most common route of administration. It is certainly the cheapest and most convenient, as technical assistance or instruction is typically not needed by the patient for self-administration. It is also the safest route as no special equipment or devices are needed, and for at least a short time after administration, the drug can be retrieved by inducing emesis (vomiting).

There are several limitations to the oral route. First of all, not all drugs are effective when given orally. The stomach acid inactivates some drugs and some drug molecules are physically too large to be absorbed. Proteins such as insulin, erythropoetin, and glucagon are inactivated by intestinal enzymes and are too large to be absorbed from the gastrointestinal tract. Other drugs, such as aminoglycoside antibiotics, do not penetrate the intestinal cell membranes efficiently and are thus incompletely or erratically absorbed. Patients who are nauseous or unconscious cannot be given oral dosage forms. NSAIDs are examples of drugs noted for their gastrointestinal irritation and potential for causing gastrointestinal ulcers. Compared to parenteral routes (intravenous, subcutaneous, intramuscular), it takes longer for drug absorption by the oral route.

Table 2-2. Summary of Dosage Forms for Oral Administration

Dosage Form	*Description*
Tablets	Solid dosage forms, most of which are prepared by compressing the powders into the desired shape and usually combined with "inactive" ingredients.
Capsules	Two-piece gelatin containers that are oblong or bullet-shaped. The drug and inactive ingredients are placed in one piece of the container and the second piece acts as the cap.
Syrups	Sweetened and flavored aqueous solutions containing one or more drugs and little or no alcohol.
Elixirs	Sweetened and flavored solutions of ethanol and water containing one or more drugs.
Suspensions	Liquids consisting of a two-phase system in which a solid is dispersed throughout a liquid.
Emulsions	Liquids usually consisting of small droplets of oil dispersed in water.

There are several dosage forms available for use by the oral route (Table 2-2) and drugs often are available in more than one oral dosage form. For example, ibuprofen is available in tablets, capsules, chewable tablets, as an oral suspension, and as oral drops.

Tablets are solid dosage forms, most of which are prepared by compressing the powders into the desired shape (Figure 2-10A-C). The drug usually is combined with "inactive" ingredients that do not have therapeutic activity, but they may impact the effectiveness of the drug by altering the amount of drug absorbed or altering the duration of action. Additives such as lactose or starch may also pose a concern for patients with special dietary restrictions. To some extent, therefore, it is a misnomer to refer to these additives as "inactive" or "inert" ingredients. Nonetheless, these additives are relatively inert compared to the drug and are essential in the formulation for one or more of the purposes listed in Box 2-5.

Capsules are two-piece gelatin containers that are oblong or bullet-shaped (Figure 2-10D). The drug and inactive ingredients are placed in one piece of the container and the second piece acts as the cap. Gelatin is made from chemically processed animal bone and skin to obtain an aqueous soluble, but suitably durable, product. Capsule sizes for human dosage forms range from 000 (the largest), which can hold approximately 600 mg, to 5 (the smallest), which can hold approximately 30 mg. Some patients believe it is easier to swallow capsules rather than tablets and thus prefer capsules. As with tablets, capsules can be manufactured in such a way to give a controlled-release of the drug.

Syrups are sweetened and flavored aqueous solutions containing one or more drugs. They contain little or no alcohol and thus are particularly suitable for children, as well as for adults who have difficulty swallowing tablets or capsules. Syrups are effective in masking the taste of water soluble drugs. Because of the high sugar content, syrups may not be useful for patients who require a calorie restricted diet, especially if the drug is required for daily, long-term use. Syrups may contain preservatives to prevent growth of microorganisms.

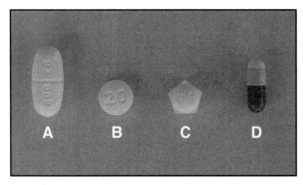

Figure 2-10. Tablets can come in various shapes (A to C); capsules (D) are oblong. Tablets and capsules are the most common solid oral dosage forms.

Box 2-5. Purposes of Inactive Ingredients Contained Within Tablets

- Holding the powders together (binders)
- Increasing the bulk of the tablet to make it a convenient size (diluents)
- Releasing the drug slowly over several hours (controlled-release polymers)
- Breaking the tablet apart in the gastrointestinal tract to increase dissolution rate (disintegrants)
- Enhancing the physical appeal of the product (coloring and flavoring agents)

Elixirs are sweetened and flavored solutions of ethanol and water containing one or more drugs. The alcohol is added to dissolve the drug and may contain anywhere from a few percent to >70% ethanol. Elixirs are less viscous than syrups and are clear in appearance.

Suspensions are liquids consisting of a two-phase system in which a solid is dispersed throughout a liquid. When the solid drug cannot be dissolved in water, use of a suspension is an option. Some drugs that are unstable in water are more suitable when formulated for use as a suspension. Additionally, the unpleasant taste of some drugs is diminished when in suspension form. As with other oral liquid dosage forms, suspensions typically have sweetening and flavoring agents added. Viscosity enhancing agents are added to diminish the rate at which the particles settle to the bottom, but suspensions should be shaken before use to ensure a more homogenous mixture. Table 2-3 lists some examples of drugs that are available as solutions, suspensions, syrups, and elixirs. Most of these drugs are also available as tablets or capsules.

Emulsions are liquids usually consisting of small droplets of oil dispersed in water. The oil may be the drug or may be used to dissolve a lipid soluble drug. Dispersing the oil in water masks the unpleasant taste of the oil, and sweetening or flavoring agents may also be added to the aqueous phase. Emulsifying agents have a degree of attraction for the oil as well as for the water and thus are used to keep the droplets of oil evenly dispersed throughout the aqueous phase. Viscosity enhancing agents may also be added to prevent oil droplets from coalescing. To ensure a homogenous distribution of drug, all emulsions should be shaken before use. Oral emulsions are not used much any more because suspensions are more efficiently produced and are generally more palatable.

Oral Absorption

The rate and extent to which drugs are absorbed from the gastrointestinal tract depends on many factors, including *rate of solubility*, rate that it passes from the stomach into the gastrointestinal tract, lipid *solubility*, and stability with other gastrointestinal contents.

Table 2-3. Examples of Drugs Available as Oral Liquid Dosage Forms

Generic Name	Trade Name	Therapeutic Category	Dosage Form
cefaclor	Ceclor	antibiotic	suspension
clindamycin	Cleocin	antibiotic	solution
cloxacillin	generic	antibiotic	solution
codeine phosphate	generic	analgesic, antitussive	solution
dexamethasone	generic	anti-inflammatory	elixir, solution
dexchlorpheniramine	Polaramine	antihistamine	syrup
dextromethorphan	generic	antitussive	syrup
doxycycline	Vibramycin	antibiotic	syrup, suspension
dyphylline	Lufyllin	bronchodilator	elixir
erythromycin	Ilosone	antibiotic	suspension
ibuprofen	Children's Advil	NSAID	suspension
naproxen	Naprosyn	NSAID	suspension
oxycodone	Roxicodone	analgesic	solution

For a drug to be absorbed by the oral route, it must be in solution. The quicker the drug dissolves, the quicker it can be absorbed. Consequently, a drug administered in solution is absorbed faster than if in a solid dosage form. The bioavailability can also be significantly altered by the formulation. Tablets and capsules must break apart for the drug to readily dissolve. The formulation of the product plays an important role in determining how quickly the tablet falls apart and dissolves; two products from different manufacturers, but containing the same amount of drug, can differ in bioavailability (see Figure 2-3).

Once the drug is dissolved in the aqueous environment of the intestinal tract, it must pass through the intestinal cell membrane to be absorbed into the blood. The small surface area of the stomach and structure of the stomach membrane prevents effective absorption of drugs. However, the villi and microvilli of the small intestine results in a tremendous surface area compared with the stomach and thus almost all drug absorption occurs from the small intestine. Consequently, drug absorption can be expedited by fast movement of the drug from the stomach to the small intestine. Most drugs are absorbed from the intestinal tract by passive diffusion. Therefore, lipid solubility is a major factor affecting rate and extent of drug absorption. Ionizable drugs are absorbed better if they exist in the unionized form.

Considering that drugs must be dissolved to be absorbed and that most drug absorption occurs from the small intestine, it is easy to understand why the use of a glass of liquid with oral drug administration generally is recommended. The liquid moves the drug more quickly from the stomach to the small intestine and expedites the rate at which the drug dissolves. On the other hand, because solid food takes longer to move into the small intestine, the administration of a drug with food will generally delay its absorption. Slower absorption can significantly reduce the peak blood concentration because as the rate of absorption becomes similar to the rate of clearance, less drug accumulates in the blood. Gastric emptying time can range from 10 minutes on an empty stomach to hours following a heavy meal. Depending on the amount of food in the stomach, the change in absorption rate can be similar to the change shown for A to that shown for B in Figure 2-3. It is noteworthy that in some instances the presence of food in the gastroin-

Figure 2-11. Example of packaging indicating enteric coating.

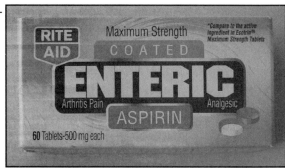

testinal tract is an advantage as a protectant from drugs, such as the NSAIDs, that have a local irritation effect on the gastric mucosa. Exercise can also impact gastric emptying time; strenuous physical activity can increase gastric emptying time whereas light exercise, compared to no exercise, can decrease gastric emptying time.

Other contents of the stomach and gastrointestinal tract can also influence absorption. Some drugs, although administered by the oral route, are not very stable to stomach acid and/or intestinal enzymes. Gastric acidity destroys penicillin G so that only about one-third of an oral dose of penicillin G is absorbed. To compensate for the poor gastrointestinal stability, the usual oral dosage regimen of penicillin G is higher than the intramuscular dose. Some foods may also interact with a drug to prevent absorption. For example, calcium ions can bind to the tetracycline antibiotics and prevent the absorption of the tetracycline. Thus, the use of dairy products should be avoided for 1 to 2 hours before and after the oral administration of these antibiotics.

Sometimes the rate of *dissolution* and absorption is intentionally delayed to give a slower but longer *duration of effect*. These are often referred to as sustained-release, prolonged-release, or controlled-release tablets or capsules. These dosage forms contain coatings that increase the time necessary for the tablet to disintegrate, or layers of coatings that dissolve at different rates. In these formulations, the dosage form contains a larger amount of drug to compensate for delayed absorption and allow the blood concentration above the minimum effective concentration to be obtained. Some dosage forms contain an *enteric* coating (Figure 2-11), which does not dissolve in the acidity of the stomach and is intended to delay the release of the drug only until it reaches the small intestine. The purpose of the delay is to either protect an acid-sensitive drug from the effects of stomach acid or to protect the gastric mucosa from the irritating effects of the drug. In these situations, delayed dissolution becomes an advantage.

Because absorption rate depends on blood flow to the site of absorption, exercise decreases drug absorption from the intestinal tract as blood is shunted away from this area to increase supply to the muscles. The extent to which exercise will affect oral drug absorption depends in part on the lipid solubility; drugs that are more lipid soluble are likely to be affected to a greater extent as blood flow is the more limiting factor compared with membrane permeability. In other words, blood flow is the rate-limiting step for oral absorption of drugs that readily cross membranes, therefore reduced blood flow reduces the absorption rate.

Sublingual and Buccal

Drugs administered sublingually or buccally are placed under the tongue or against the cheek, respectively. Typically, the dosage form is tablet *triturates*, which are small tablets usually produced by placing moistened powdered formulation in a mold and allowing it to dry. These tablets are less durable than compressed tablets and thus will dissolve more rapidly when placed under the tongue or against the cheek. A rich supply of blood vessels in these areas facilitates the absorption of the drug into the blood stream despite the small surface area. Drugs administered by these routes must be relatively potent so that only a small amount of drug need be absorbed to produce the therapeutic effect. Organic nitrates such as nitroglycerin, erythrityl tetranitrate, and isosorbide dinitrate may be administered by these routes to treat angina pectoris. Nitroglycerin is available in dosage as little as 0.3 mg/tablet and provides a peak response in 3 to 5 minutes. This rapid therapeutic effect is a major advantage of these routes but the drug must be readily soluble in the mouth if administered in tablet form, yet sufficiently lipid soluble to pass quickly through membranes. In other words, a balance between lipid solubility and water solubility is advantageous. The sublingual and buccal routes also protect the drug from the first pass effect, which would render sublingual nitroglycerin tablets ineffective if swallowed.

Rectal

The rectal route of drug administration is advantageous in patients who are unconscious, vomiting, or too young to easily swallow oral dosage forms during illness. With this route, the drug is administered as a suppository that is made of a substance such as cocoa butter or polyethylene glycols, which melt at body temperature. The drug dissolves in the rectum and is absorbed into the bloodstream by the hemorrhoidal veins. A disadvantage to this route is that the extent of absorption into the bloodstream often is variable and incomplete. Some drugs in the opiate analgesic and anti-*emetic* categories are available as suppositories for use when either pain or nausea make it difficult for the patient to take these drugs orally.

Parenteral

The primary *parenteral routes* are intravenous, intramuscular, and subcutaneous. Some drugs, such as proteins administered for a systemic effect, are limited to parenteral routes because they are inactivated or poorly absorbed by the gastrointestinal tract. The parenteral routes produce the most rapid therapeutic response and are advantageous for drug administration to patients who are unable or unwilling to take drugs orally. However, as disadvantages, more skill is needed to administer drugs by these routes and the dosage forms, syringes, and needles must be handled carefully to prevent contamination.

Intravenous injections require aqueous solutions (ie, no particles visible). Intramuscularly injected dosage forms include aqueous solutions, suspensions, and emulsions. Drugs that are irritating to tissue may cause pain or necrosis at the site of subcutaneous injections but may be suitable as intramuscular injections.

Parenteral Absorption

As absorption refers to entry of the drug into the bloodstream, there is no absorption component associated with intravenous injection. The rate is only dependent on the time it takes to administer the drug. This is the preferred route for emergency administration of drugs.

Intramuscular injection provides more rapid absorption of drug than the subcutaneous route. In both routes, the drug must cross membranes and therefore lipid solubility of the drug will impact its rate of absorption. As with the oral route, if the intramuscular drug is not administered in solution form, it must dissolve at the site of injection. Consequently, drugs given as suspensions or emulsions will have a slower *onset of action*. These dosage forms can also be used for the purpose of providing a longer *duration of action*. Insulin in solution (eg, Humulin R) administered subcutaneously has an onset and duration of action of 30 minutes to 1 hour and 6 to 8 hours, respectively. This is in contrast to 1 to 2 hour onset and 18 to 24 hour duration for Humulin N, which is an insulin suspension.

As mentioned previously, blood flow plays a significant role in determining the rate of absorption. Intramuscular sites generally have better blood flow than subcutaneous sites and thus absorption can be noticeably quicker by the intramuscular route. Exercise increases blood flow to skeletal muscle and skin, which will increase drug absorption from these sites. Vasoconstriction, from use of an ice pack at the injection site for example, will reduce the absorption rate of drugs. This principle is used to an advantage for local anesthetics in which vasoconstrictors are co-administered to delay the anesthetic from being carried from the local *site of action*; epinephrine added to lidocaine for use in dentistry is an example.

Surface area can play some role in subcutaneous and intramuscular injection. As with other routes of administration, increasing the surface area for the drug to contact tissue will increase the absorption rate. Massaging the site of injection spreads the dose of drug over a larger area to increase absorption rate. Movement of the muscle after intramuscular injection can accomplish a spreading effect as well as increasing blood flow. The site of an intramuscular injection depends on the availability and size of the muscle mass, volume to be injected, degree of discomfort expected from the injection, and patient's preference.

Topical

Drugs administered by topical routes (eg, skin, eyes, nose, throat, etc) are applied to the surface for the purpose of obtaining either a systemic or a local effect. Drugs applied topically for a localized effect include anti-inflammatory agents, antimicrobial agents, skin moisturizers, sunscreens, and various other drugs for specific dermatological uses. Topically applied drugs for a systemic effect must be relatively potent so that small amounts absorbed through the skin will elicit the therapeutic effect. Drugs used in this fashion are available for estrogen replacement, angina pectoris, hypertension, motion sickness, and analgesia. The rate at which drugs are absorbed depends on the surface area over which they are applied and on their lipid solubility; the more lipid soluble, the more readily the drug will penetrate the epidermis. Using a *lipophilic* vehicle (eg, an ointment) will also increase the rate of absorption for drugs that are not very lipid soluble. The permeability of drugs through the skin is increased if the skin is moist or if the blood flow is increased at the site of application such as near areas of skin that is inflamed, abraded, or burned.

Whether intended for a local or systemic effect, drugs applied to mucous membranes are absorbed readily as there is no epidermal barrier and blood supply is typically rich. Drugs applied to the eye usually are intended for a local effect although a systemic effect may occur. For example, ophthalmic application of timolol (Timoptic), a drug used for treatment of glaucoma, has caused significant bronchial constriction with difficult breathing for patients who also have asthma.

There are many dosage forms used for topical application. The characteristics of emulsions, suspensions, and solutions have been previously discussed although for topical use sweetening and flavoring agents are obviously not needed. Instead, however, other ingredients are added as preservatives, stabilizers, and skin protectants. In addition, lotions, creams, and ointments are very common. Lotions and creams are water washable preparations for external use only; lotions have more of a liquid consistency. Ointments are semisolid preparations for external use only and although some ointments are water washable, most have an oil base. Ointments also act as excellent emollients (ie, moisturizers; soften skin by increasing moisture content).

When drugs are applied to the skin for a systemic effect, it is referred to as *transdermal delivery*. Ointments and creams for this purpose are somewhat messy and it is difficult to determine the amount of drug that will be delivered to the bloodstream. Transdermal patches use various thin layers of adhesives, polymer matrices, membranes, and drug reservoirs to control the rate of drug released for contact with the skin. Examples of drugs available by transdermal delivery are clonidine (Catapres-TTS) for hypertension, estradiol (Estraderm) for estrogen replacement therapy, nicotine (Nicoderm) as a smoking cessation aid, nitroglycerin (Transderm-Nitro) for treatment of angina, and scopolamine (Transderm Scop) for motion sickness.

Inhalation

The inhalation route is actually a topical route of administration because the drug is being applied to the surface of the membrane, but it is also considered separately because of the unique characteristics and specialized delivery mechanisms. Except for gases as general anesthetics, drugs are generally not administered by inhalation for the purpose of obtaining a systemic effect because the amount of drug delivered to the lungs by inhalation, and the amount absorbed into the bloodstream, is too variable.

Inhalation is the route of choice for the administration of some drugs used to treat asthma. The inhalation dosage forms most frequently used are aerosols and dry powders, which are administered using *metered dose inhalers* (MDI) and *dry powder inhalers* (DPI). Good inhalation technique is required to optimize the delivery of the drug to the lung. The use of MDI and DPI, along with other treatments for asthma, will be discussed more thoroughly in Chapter 9.

The rich blood supply to the lungs, permeability of the membranes, and large surface area provide for rapid absorption of drugs by inhalation. For some drugs, the *onset of action* is <5 minutes. The challenge with self-administered inhalation therapy, such with the routine treatment of asthma, is to get an adequate and consistent dose into the lungs.

Summary

Absorption is the process of the drug moving into the bloodstream; route of administration is the entry mechanism used to get the drug into the blood and dosage form is the physical form of the drug used for administration. The oral route is the most common method of administering drugs and thus many solid and liquid dosage forms (eg, tablets, capsules, syrups, suspensions) are available for oral use. Parenteral routes (eg, intravenous, intramuscular, subcutaneous) can produce a more rapid response, but they also require more skill to inject the drug. In some cases, the condition of the patient or the type of drug used will necessitate a parenteral route. Drugs administered by sublingual, buccal, and inhalation routes are absorbed quickly because of the rich blood supply at these sites. In contrast, absorption of drug from the surface of the skin for a systemic effect (transdermal) is relatively slow as the drug must penetrate the epidermis. Nonetheless, transdermal patches are a convenient means of providing slow but continuous delivery of potent drugs.

Absorption by the oral route occurs primarily from the small intestine. The drug must be dissolved in the aqueous gastrointestinal tract and then penetrate the gastrointestinal membrane to enter the blood. A balance between water solubility and lipid solubility facilitates absorption, but drugs have varying degrees of these characteristics and thus the rate of absorption varies among drugs. Food in the stomach will decrease the absorption rate because it takes longer for the drug to move into the small intestine. Strenuous physical exercise will also delay stomach emptying whereas light exercise will stimulate it.

DISTRIBUTION

Distribution refers to the movement of the drug throughout the body to the various compartments. Aside from blood, these compartments include the CNS, cells (eg, muscle, adipose, liver, kidney), excretory fluids (eg, urine, bile, sweat), and plasma fluids proteins (primarily albumin). The site of action is a component of one or more of these compartments. Drugs generally do not distribute evenly throughout these compartments. The specific compartments that a drug distributes into, and the extent to which it distributes, depend on:

- The chemical structure of the drug
- Blood flow to the tissue
- Structure of the capillaries feeding the tissue

Once a molecule is in the blood, regardless of its lipid or water *solubility*, it will eventually penetrate the endothelial cell of the capillaries because of their huge surface area and because, except for the CNS (see *blood-brain barrier*), the capillaries that feed tissues have some spaces between epithelial cells. Molecular size is a major hindrance for larger water soluble molecules such as *polypeptides* but they will eventually penetrate slowly, possibly between endothelial cells or by other mechanisms.

Blood flow to tissue will significantly impact drug distribution. Some tissues, such as the liver, kidney, and brain, have greater blood flow than fat or bone. Consequently, distribution will be faster to the sites with greater blood flow. Treating solid tumors or infections of the bone pose some therapeutic challenges because the blood flow to these sites is low. To obtain sufficient drug distribution at these sites of action, higher doses of drug, administration for longer periods, or injection directly into the tissue site are sometimes necessary.

Capillary structure varies among tissues and will affect drug distribution. For example, water soluble and ionized drugs do not readily penetrate the CNS capillaries unless there is a specific transport process for them. The structural components around the CNS capillaries provide an additional barrier and there are no spaces between the endothelial cells of the CNS capillaries. Therefore, in the CNS, passive diffusion is the major mechanism by which drugs cross the membrane; the more lipid soluble drugs will cross the membrane more readily. In addition, there are transport mechanisms that remove some drugs that gain entry into the CNS. The *blood-brain barrier* is the term used to describe these attributes of the CNS. If the site of action is not the CNS, access to the CNS is a disadvantage as additional adverse effects are likely. Consider, for example, all the OTC cold remedies that have drowsiness as an adverse effect. On the other hand, distribution into the CNS is desirable for sedatives and opiate analgesics because the *site of action* is within the CNS.

The placental barrier is somewhat similar to the blood-brain barrier in that there are mechanisms that restrict the entry of drugs from the mother to the developing baby. As with the blood-brain barrier, drugs that are more lipid soluble, such as alcohol, more readily diffuse into the baby's blood. However, the placental barrier is not as exclusionary as the blood-brain barrier, and thus most drugs will have at least some degree of entry to the unborn baby.

The chemical structure of the drug will determine the lipid solubility, degree of ionization, and chemical binding characteristics. Lipid soluble drugs will tend to distribute more readily into the CNS and into fat cells. Drugs that are ionic also will not be distributed evenly; they will move faster to one side of a cell membrane than the other if there is a pH difference on the two sides (see Figure 2-8). The chemical binding characteristics will determine to which receptors on which cells the drug will bind, and also, as discussed earlier, the extent of plasma protein binding.

Summary

Drug distribution is the movement of drug into body fluids, tissues, and attachment to albumin; the greater the distribution into these sites, the lower the concentration available to reach the site of action. The degree of lipid solubility will determine the degree of distribution into the CNS and into fat tissue. The blood-brain barrier is a term used to describe the unique membrane structure of the capillaries of the CNS that restricts entry to primarily lipid soluble drugs.

METABOLISM

Drug metabolism, also known as biotransformation, refers to the chemical alteration of the drug by one or more enzymes in the body (Figure 2-12). The liver is the primary site of this biotransformation but the kidney and intestinal cells also have a significant level of drug metabolism, and to a lesser extent, so do the lungs and brain. The drug reacting with the metabolizing enzyme is called the parent drug or substrate; the products of the reactions are called metabolites.

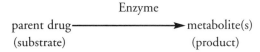

It is common for a drug to be converted to more than one metabolite. Drug metabolism usually makes the drug inactive and more water soluble, which is important in preparation of the drug for excretion as the urine is aqueous and is the primary route for excretion. Drug metabolism and excretion provide the two mechanisms by which the actions of drugs are terminated.

A multitude of drug metabolizing enzymes have been identified. Although most drug metabolism results in loss of biological activity, other scenarios also occur as shown in Figure 2-13. Sometimes the biological activity of the metabolite is more, somewhat less than, or the same as the parent drug. For example, about 10% of codeine is metabolized to the more potent morphine, aspirin is quickly metabolized to the equipotent salicyclic acid, and the major metabolite of diazepam (Valium) is less active than the parent compound. In some cases, such as diazepam (Valium), the active metabolite has a longer half-life than the parent drug and thus the observed *duration of action* is longer although *potency* is less. Sometimes the drug administered is in an inactive form, referred to as a prodrug, and the metabolizing enzymes convert the drug to the active drug. A prodrug is used when it provides an advantage over the active drug such as better oral absorption or diminished gastrointestinal irritation.

Cytochrome P450 enzymes (CYP or P450) are a large group of enzymes that metabolize many drugs. The CYP group of enzymes is divided into families, subfamilies, and individual *isoenzymes* that are designated by a series of numbers and letters. Some drugs are metabolized by more than one CYP enzyme. Aside from being metabolized by P450 enzymes, some drugs either increase (induce) or decrease (inhibit) the activity of these enzymes. The concept of inhibiting and inducing enzyme is discussed further in the next chapter regarding drug interactions.

The effect of exercise on the rate of drug metabolism is complex and research has not provided a set of useful general principles. During exercise, the blood flow to the liver is reduced and therefore it would seem that the liver metabolism rate should also decrease. However, exercise increases the metabolism for some drugs that are highly protein bound, presumably because the liver becomes more efficient at extracting protein-bound drug as blood flow decreases. Sporadic versus routine exercise may also affect the metabolism rate differently; routine exercise seems to

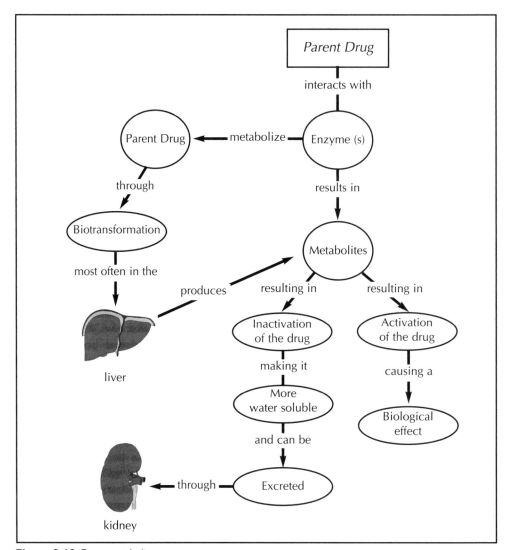

Figure 2-12. Drug metabolism.

increase liver metabolism efficiency for some drugs. Some enzymes are induced whereas others are inhibited by exercise. The therapeutic significance of these effects on specific drugs has not been established.

Summary

The parent drug is the drug administered to the patient; the metabolite is the product after a metabolism reaction. Most drug metabolism occurs in the liver. Metabolism usually inactivates the drug and prepares it for excretion by the kidney by making the drug more water soluble. In some cases, however, drug metabolism produces a metabolite that also has biological activity. The CYP450 enzymes are a group of enzymes that metabolize many drugs. The activity of some of these enzymes is increased (induced) or decreased (inhibited) by other drugs and thus can be the cause of some drug interactions.

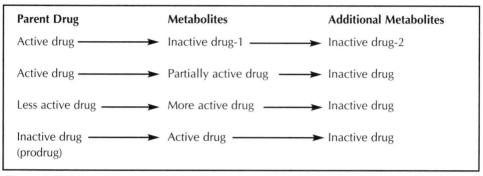

Parent Drug	Metabolites	Additional Metabolites
Active drug ⟶	Inactive drug-1 ⟶	Inactive drug-2
Active drug ⟶	Partially active drug ⟶	Inactive drug
Less active drug ⟶	More active drug ⟶	Inactive drug
Inactive drug (prodrug) ⟶	Active drug ⟶	Inactive drug

Figure 2-13. Metabolism schemes. The parent drug can be converted to a metabolite by metabolizing enzymes. Oftentimes, more than one metabolizing enzyme will react with the drug to produce additional metabolites. The metabolites of some drugs may have therapeutic activity that is less than or more than the activity of the parent drug. Sometimes the form of the drug administered is inactive (also called a prodrug) to gain an advantage, such as enhanced absorption. An enzyme converts the prodrug to the active form, which is eventually inactivated.

EXCRETION

Excretion of drugs is simply removal of the drug from the body. *Polar compounds* are more readily excreted than nonpolar compounds; therefore, at least a portion of each dose of many drugs undergoes one or more metabolic reactions to make it more polar. The kidney is the most important organ for excretion of drugs, although the bile is also a significant route. Excretion of drugs by sweat, saliva, and lungs occurs for many drugs but the quantity excreted through these routes is insignificant when exercise is not a factor. During exercise, there is an increased blood flow to the lungs and skin but sufficient data are not available regarding the excretion of drugs to conclude any practical significance. Therefore, excretion of drugs by sweat, saliva, and lungs is not discussed further.

Renal Excretion

The kidneys contain more than two million *nephrons*, each containing various components including a *glomerulus* and a *renal tubule*. The renal excretion rate of a drug is dependent on the net effect of glomerular filtration rate, tubular secretion, and tubular reabsorption. The rate of these mechanisms is dependent on rate of blood flow to the kidneys, concentration of drug in the blood, pH of the urine, and presence of other tubular-secreted acids and bases.

As shown in Figure 2-9, protein-bound substances remain in the blood and are not allowed to enter the renal tubule; *free drug*, whether *ionic, polar,* or *nonpolar*, will enter as glomerular filtrate. The renal tubule provides additional mechanisms for compounds to enter from the blood (see Figure 2-9). There is an active transport mechanism for acids and also for bases that transports these ionic drugs into the renal tubule (tubular secretion). Because these mechanisms use protein carriers, the rate of tubular secretion depends on the blood concentration of the drug but the carriers can be saturated. Sometimes drugs that use the same transport mechanism will compete for the limited transport proteins, resulting in an altered rate of drug excretion. The classic illustration of this is penicillin G and probenecid. Penicillin G is rapidly secreted into the renal tubule by the *acid secretion transporter*. As a means to decrease the excretion rate of penicillin G, probenecid was developed, which competes for the same acid transporter and thus inhibits the renal tubular secretion of penicillin G so that it has a longer duration of action.

Although glomerular filtration excludes protein-bound drugs, the extent of protein binding does not significantly affect the rate of excretion of drugs. Because the drug is reversibly bound to plasma protein, as some of the free drug enters the renal tubule by filtration or by tubular secretion, some bound drug will release from the plasma protein to become free drug to quickly maintain the constant percentage of bound drug.

As the fluid passes through the various segments of the renal tubule, compounds can be reabsorbed back into the bloodstream. Active transport mechanisms exist for polar and ionic endogenous compounds such as glucose and amino acids, although passive diffusion is the major mechanism for the reabsorption of drugs. As the degree of ionization will determine the rate of passive diffusion for ionic drugs, the pH of the tubular urine plays an important role in determining the rate of excretion of these drugs. When the urine is more acidic, drugs that are bases will be more highly ionized and thus will be excreted quicker. When the urine is more basic, acidic drugs will be more ionized and be excreted faster. The urinary pH can fluctuate from 5 to 8 as a result of diet, exercise, and presence of drugs and thus can affect the rate of excretion of ionic drugs. The excretion rate of salicyclic acid, a metabolite of aspirin, is increased by several fold if the urine pH is 8 as compared with pH 6.

Exercise can decrease blood flow to the kidney and could decrease the renal clearance rate of some drugs. However, urinary pH can also decrease during exercise, which will alter the reabsorption of ionic drugs. Decreased urine output can increase the tubular concentration, leading to faster reabsorption by passive diffusion. Other factors that could impact excretion rate but have not been thoroughly studied are the intensity of exercise, hydration status of the athlete, and the extent of excretion from sweat. The impact of exercise also varies depending on the extent of drug metabolism versus kidney excretion as a means to terminate the drug activity. For example, if exercise increases liver metabolism for a drug but clearance of that drug is primarily by urinary excretion, then the net effect of exercise may be to decrease the clearance rate.

Biliary Excretion

Some drugs pass from the liver into the bile and are eventually secreted into the small intestine. These may be either lipid soluble or the more polar metabolites. If the drug enters the small intestine, it may be excreted in the feces or reabsorbed into the blood. Once the drug is reabsorbed, it may be excreted by the kidney or resecreted by the liver and reabsorbed from the intestine again. The reabsorption-secretion process is referred to as *enterohepatic* recycling and can extend the duration of the therapeutic effect of some drugs.

Summary

The kidney is the major site of drug excretion although some drugs are also excreted in the bile. Drugs enter the renal tubule of the kidney through filtration at the glomerulus or, in the case of acids and bases, through an active transport mechanism that secretes the drug into the renal tubule. The more lipid soluble (nonpolar) the drug, the more likely it will be reabsorbed back into the blood from the renal tubule. A larger proportion of acid drugs will be reabsorbed if the urine is acidic because the acid drug will become more unionized (more lipid soluble) in the acid environment; the opposite is true of bases.

Box 2-6. Potential Effects of Exercise on Drug Pharmacokinetics

- Light exercise will decrease stomach emptying time and strenuous exercise will increase stomach emptying time.

- Oral absorption of drugs is diminished by exercise due to decreased blood flow to gastrointestinal tract.

- Absorption from skin and skeletal muscle is increased by exercise due to increased blood flow to these areas.

- Exercise increases the duration of action by drugs cleared primarily by the kidney because of diminished clearance by this route. However, this may be modified for drugs that are acids and bases since renal tubular reabsorption of acids may increase, and bases may decrease, as urinary pH decreases during exercise. Duration and intensity of exercise may determine the extent to which kidney clearance of drugs is affected.

- Exercise results in diminished blood flow to the liver and thus increased duration of action by drugs that are inactivated by the liver. This is modified, however, for drugs that are highly protein bound (eg, NSAIDs), because there is a longer time for the drug to separate from the protein bound state and then be inactivated by the liver. Routine exercise may have the opposite effect by increasing the metabolic efficiency and activity of liver enzymes.

- As fluid is lost during exercise the volume of distribution should diminish, increasing the concentration of drug reaching the site of action. However, some drugs are excreted through sweat but the impact on overall excretion is relatively unknown.

- Drugs that have a significant first pass effect may have enhanced blood concentrations when the exercise and oral administration are close together.

- A long-term exercise program may alter liver enzymes, hormone levels, and protein binding of some drugs which can affect metabolism and excretion rates.

- The impact of exercise on pharmacokinetic parameters are more likely to be significant during intensive exercise of long duration, on therapeutic response occurring from drugs that have a shorter $t\frac{1}{2}$, from drugs that have an effective dose similar to the toxic dose, and with drugs for which a continuous therapeutic effect is most critical.

EFFECTS OF EXERCISE

The effect of exercise on the rate of absorption, distribution, metabolism, and excretion is quite complex. No doubt this is a prime reason that relatively little has been studied regarding this subject. Some studies present conflicting data or results that are of uncertain practical application. In a comprehensive review by Reents,[1] every therapeutic drug category reviewed indicated that few studies had been conducted, data were not available, or results were contradictory regarding the effect of exercise on pharmacokinetics. Because exercise affects so many functions such as blood flow, respiration, fluid volume, and pH, more than one pharmacokinetic parameter may be altered at the same time.

During exercise, blood flow shifts to the muscles and skin and away from the visceral area, kidney, and liver. Blood flow can affect each of the pharmacokinetic parameters, but these have not been studied in a large number of drugs. Consequently, the effects of exercise could include more than one of the general actions listed in Box 2-6, depending on the drug, type of exercise, and the intensity and duration of the exercise.

The bottom line for the athletic trainer is to be aware that, in some situations for some drugs in some athletes, exercise could have a significant effect on the pharmacokinetic parameters. With currently available data it is difficult to predict the occurrence of an exercise-induced problem (or advantage). However, the potential for a significant impact should not be discounted as the diminished clearance of a relatively toxic drug due to exercise could elicit some adverse or toxic effects.

REFERENCE

1. Reents S. *Sport and Exercise Pharmacology.* Champaign, Ill: Human Kinetics; 2000.

BIBLIOGRAPHY

Banker GS, Rhodes CT, eds. *Modern Pharmaceutics: Third Edition, Revised and Expanded.* New York, NY: Marcel Dekker; 1996.

Gennaro AR, ed. *Remington, The Science and Practice of Pharmacy.* 20th ed. Baltimore, Md: Lippincott Williams & Wilkins; 2000.

Shargel L, Yu A. *Applied Biopharmaceutics and Pharmacokinetics.* 4th edition. Stamford, Conn: Appleton & Lange; 1999.

Somani SM. *Pharmacology in Exercise and Sports.* Boca Raton, Fla: CRC Press; 1996.

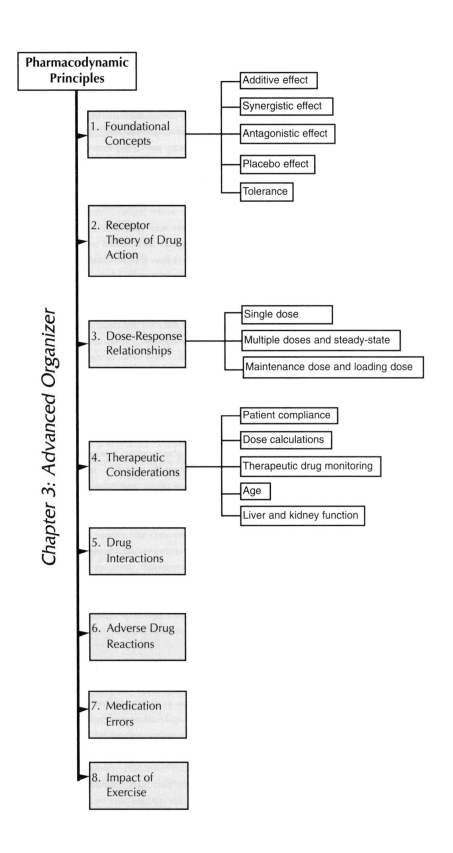

Chapter 3: Advanced Organizer

Pharmacodynamic Principles

1. Foundational Concepts
   - Additive effect
   - Synergistic effect
   - Antagonistic effect
   - Placebo effect
   - Tolerance

2. Receptor Theory of Drug Action

3. Dose-Response Relationships
   - Single dose
   - Multiple doses and steady-state
   - Maintenance dose and loading dose

4. Therapeutic Considerations
   - Patient compliance
   - Dose calculations
   - Therapeutic drug monitoring
   - Age
   - Liver and kidney function

5. Drug Interactions

6. Adverse Drug Reactions

7. Medication Errors

8. Impact of Exercise

PHARMACODYNAMIC PRINCIPLES
Mechanism of Drug Action
and Therapeutic Considerations

CHAPTER OBJECTIVES

At the end of this chapter, the reader will be able to:
- Explain the concept of pharmacodynamics and how it is applied to explaining the biological effects of drugs.
- Differentiate between pharmacokinetics, pharmacodynamics, and therapeutics.
- Explain the two major ways by which pharmacological tolerance occurs.
- Summarize the receptor theory of drug action.
- Explain the dose-response principle and how it is related to achieving a maximum dose response.
- Explain the concept of potency and how it relates to producing a biological effect.
- Explain how the relative safety of a drug is determined.
- Explain how multiple doses of a drug reach a steady-state of blood concentration to produce a biological effect.
- Differentiate between a maintenance dose and a loading dose of a drug.
- List variables that affect patient compliance with drug therapy and ways to improve compliance with the drug regimen.
- Summarize the concept of therapeutic drug monitoring.
- Explain why individuals respond differently to a drug regimen based on their age.
- Describe how liver and kidney function can be used to determine appropriate drug dosage.
- Define a drug interaction.
- List and describe seven mechanisms by which a drug interaction can occur.
- Define an adverse drug reaction.
- List and describe eight categories of adverse drug reactions.
- Identify several ways medication errors can occur and how they may be prevented.
- Explain the potential impact that exercise has on pharmacodynamics.

Pharmacodynamics is the study of the impact of drugs on the body. The primary focus of pharmacodynamics is on the molecular mechanism by which drugs exert their therapeutic and adverse effects. The molecular mechanism encompasses biochemical mechanisms and physiological responses. As the dose changes, the degree and type of response may also change as the drug occupies more receptors in a particular tissue and additional receptors in other tissues. Consequently, the dosage regimen required to optimize therapeutic effects and minimize adverse effects can be determined, at least in part, by the molecular mechanism of action. Stated another way, pharmacodynamics centers primarily on the mechanism of drug action.

Box 3-1. Areas of Study

	Definition	Focus
Pharmacokinetics	The study of the impact of the body on drugs.	On the rate and extent to which drugs are absorbed into the bloodstream, distributed throughout the body, metabolized, and finally excreted.
Pharmacodynamics	The study of the impact of drugs on the body.	On the molecular mechanism by which drugs exert their therapeutic and adverse effects.
Therapeutics	The study of the parameters that determine the most appropriate therapy for a patient.	Considers the parameters necessary to individualize treatment for the specific patient, including all of the patient's diseases, all of the drugs the patient may be using, the dosage regimen of each drug, and the impact of potential adverse effects.

Therapeutics is the study of the parameters that determine the most appropriate therapy for a patient. It considers the parameters necessary to individualize treatment for the specific patient, including all of the patient's diseases, all of the drugs the patient may be using, the dosage regimen of each drug, and the impact of potential adverse effects. Therefore, knowledge of the pharmacodynamic and pharmacokinetic principles is a necessary component of therapeutics (ie, to determine the most appropriate therapy for the patient). The lines separating pharmacokinetics, pharmacodynamics, and therapeutics are not always clear (Box 3-1). For example, the *dose-response effect* of a drug occurs as a result of the absorption, distribution, metabolism, and excretion characteristics of the drug, but the specific dose-response effects are also a result of the *mechanism of action*; all of which will determine the therapeutic use of the drug.

In this chapter, we will discuss the theoretical basis for the mechanism of drug action, the dose-response relationships, the mechanisms for common adverse effects, and therapeutic considerations that may affect the treatment regimen for some patients.

FOUNDATIONAL CONCEPTS

Some of the foundational concepts discussed in the previous chapter will be used in this chapter; others are unique to pharmacodynamics and therapeutics. It is important to see the relationship among some of these principles to truly understand the significance of the concept. To realize that protein binding discussed in Chapter 2 (eg, has an effect on the amount of drug reaching the receptor, or that the response from a drug may be altered due to the effect of other drugs on liver metabolizing enzymes).

Additive Effect

The term *additive effects* is self-explanatory: the response obtained from two or more drugs is equal to the sum of the responses obtained when the drugs are used individually. The therapeutic responses being measured usually are the same response (eg, pain relief or skeletal muscle relaxation). For example, the concurrent use of ibuprofen (Motrin) and naproxen (Naprosyn), two nonsteroidal anti-inflammatory drugs (NSAIDs), provides additive analgesic effects but no redeeming therapeutic benefit and thus is generally discouraged (see Chapter 7). As in this example, concurrent use of two or more drugs should be avoided if no therapeutic advantage is obtained. Sometimes, however, there is an advantage of using a combination of drugs that give additive effects, such as reducing the adverse effects of a drug by using a lower dose but yet obtaining the same net therapeutic effect with the addition of the second drug. For example, if a moderate dose of inhaled corticosteroid as long-term therapy does not adequately control asthma, the addition of another long-term drug (noncorticosteroid) is recommended rather than increasing the corticosteroid dose, thereby decreasing the potential of adverse effects from a higher dose of corticosteroid but yet controlling the asthma (see Chapter 9).

Synergistic Effect

When drugs exhibit *synergistic effects* it means that the use of two drugs together produces a response greater than what would be expected by adding the response observed from using each drug alone. To put it mathematically, if drug A and B each produce "X" amount of response when used alone, but used together they produce >2X response, they are synergistic. An example is the use of probenecid along with penicillin G as discussed in Chapter 2. Probenecid alone does not have antibacterial activity, but it inhibits the renal tubular secretion of penicillin G and thus significantly increases the duration of action of penicillin G. Another example is the synergistic effect of any NSAID added to codeine for pain relief (see Chapter 7).

Antagonistic Effect

When the use of a second drug reduces the effect of another drug, the second drug has an *antagonistic effect* to the first. If one drug binds to a certain receptor as an *agonist*, it will initiate a certain response. If a second drug binds to the same receptor, thus preventing the agonist response, the second drug is an antagonist, also known as a *competitive antagonist, receptor antagonist,* or *blocker.* An antagonistic effect may be due to a receptor antagonist or to an unrelated mechanism (ie, the antagonist does not bind to the agonist's receptor). For example, the use of an antacid with a tetracycline antibiotic will have an antagonistic effect on the tetracycline by binding the tetracycline and preventing it from being absorbed. Drugs that have an antagonistic effect can sometimes be an advantage if it is desirable to reverse the effect of a drug. Naloxone (Narcan), for example, is an opioid receptor antagonist that is used to reverse the potentially fatal respiratory depression effects from an overdose of opioids such as heroin or morphine. Many over-the-counter (OTC) cold preparations combine a nasal decongestant with an antihistamine to gain an additive therapeutic effect (ie, improved air flow) but the decongestant also causes some central nervous system (CNS) stimulation, which has an antagonistic effect on the drowsiness side effect from the antihistamine.

Placebo Effect

It is important to differentiate between a *placebo* and a *placebo effect.* A placebo effect is either a therapeutic or adverse response that cannot be attributed to the pharmacological effect of the drug. A placebo is a dosage form that contains no active ingredient; capsules filled with lactose are an example. The most common, but not exclusive, source of the placebo effect occurs when treating symptoms associated with subjective responses. A variety of other symptoms have been shown to respond to placebo in as much as 35% of the population. These responses from placebo include relief of fever, headache, anxiety, nausea, and pain from many sources including angina and ulcers. The placebo effect is not imaginary. It may be due in part to the release of hormones or neurotransmitters, not as a consequence of pharmacological activity of any drug, but as a result of the patient anticipating a response from what he or she believes is the drug. The use of a placebo is uncommon except in research and clinical drug studies, which use a placebo group of subjects to determine therapeutic efficacy.

Although the use of a placebo is rare for therapy, the placebo effect is a common phenomenon and can be used as a therapeutic advantage. Because the expectations of the patient can contribute to the placebo effect, this portion of the response can be fostered by the attending health care professional if he or she provides encouragement and an optimistic outlook regarding expected therapeutic outcomes. If a patient is convinced that pain relief is imminent upon administration of an analgesic, a placebo effect may bring greater or quicker relief than what would be expected from the drug alone.

Tolerance

Tolerance is the diminished response to a drug as a result of continued use. In other words, to get the same effect from the drug as previously obtained, the dose of the drug must be increased. Not all drugs produce tolerance. For those drugs known to produce tolerance, however, the effectiveness of the drug should be monitored so that the dose can be adjusted appropriately. Tolerance is especially prevalent among the opioid analgesics, CNS stimulants, benzodiazepines, barbiturates, and ethanol.

When tolerance develops to one drug in a pharmacological category (eg, CNS depressants, CNS stimulants), there is usually cross tolerance to other drugs within that category. If a patient develops tolerance to morphine, the patient will also have a degree of tolerance to the other morphine-like drugs such as codeine and meperidine (Demerol). Tolerance is a relatively slow process, taking at least days to weeks to develop depending on the drug. Rate of tolerance can also vary for different effects from the same drug. For example, tolerance to the appetite suppressant effects of cocaine and amphetamines develops more quickly than tolerance to the euphoric effects.

The benzodiazepines are a group of CNS depressant drugs with muscle relaxant and anti-anxiety effects. Examples include diazepam (Valium) and clorazepate (Tranxene). Barbiturates are another group of CNS depressants with several uses including inducing sedation or sleep. Examples include phenobarbital (Luminal) and secobarbital (Seconal).

There are two major mechanisms that cause pharmacological tolerance: liver enzyme *induction* and receptor effects. Using alcohol as an example, chronic alcohol use causes the liver to produce more molecules of *drug metabolizing* enzymes (see Chapter 2). Because there are more molecules of enzymes, the rate of drug metabolism (alcohol in this case) by these enzymes will be increased. This results in a decreased level of drug in the blood. Consequently, the chronic alcohol user gradually requires more drinks to reach the same level of intoxication. As discussed later in this chapter, drugs that *induce* liver enzymes also have the potential to cause drug interactions by affecting the metabolism rate of other drugs.

Another mechanism for tolerance is a change in either the number of receptors or the affinity of the receptors for the drug. (As discussed later in this chapter, the affinity is the strength of the chemical bonding interaction between the drug and the receptor.) In this situation, the blood level of the drug is not being reduced, but rather the responsiveness at the receptor. Examples are the opioid analgesics, CNS stimulants, and benzodiazepines. Because drugs of the same drug category typically bind to the same receptor, it is easy to see why a cross-tolerance is common with-

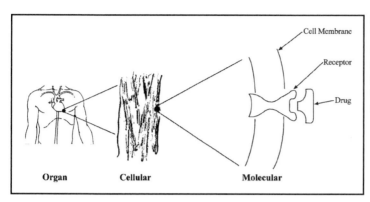

Figure 3-1. Site of action. The site of action is in specific tissues at the cellular and molecular level, often at a receptor on the cell membrane to which the drug chemically fits.

in a category. Also, if different effects from a drug are caused from the drug binding to different types of receptors, it is not surprising that the tolerance develops more rapidly to one effect than another. Tolerance to the pain relief from morphine is more rapid than to the constipation side effect. Barbiturates are a group of CNS depressants to which tolerance develops due to both mechanisms, enzyme induction and changes in receptor activity. Regardless of mechanism, pharmacologic tolerance is reversible in that it eventually disappears after the drug is discontinued. In addition to the pharmacologically-based tolerance discussed in this section, there is also learned tolerance in which the person learns from experience to change his or her behavior while under the influence as a means to compensate for the CNS effects (eg, making a conscious effort to walk in such a way so as not to appear to be intoxicated).

Summary

Pharmacodynamics is a study of the impact that drugs have on the cells of the body, with a focus on the mechanism by which all the effects occur. Sometimes the magnitude of the observed effects is modified by the presence of other drugs. If the presence of more than one drug leads to a reduced total response, the drugs are antagonistic; if the total combined response is what would be expected by adding the individual responses, the drugs are additive; if the total is more than would be expected from adding the individual responses, the drugs are synergistic. If a "drug" is given that has no active ingredient, the "drug" is called a placebo and any perceived response by the patient is called a placebo effect. If the response of a drug diminishes after continued use, the reduced response is a result of tolerance. Drugs that are CNS stimulants and depressants are particularly known for the tolerance they produce. Cross tolerance occurs among drugs in the same drug category, such that if tolerance exists to morphine, it will also exist with codeine.

RECEPTOR THEORY OF DRUG ACTION

In a broad sense, any macromolecule to which a drug binds and initiates a biological response can be called a *receptor*. This would include enzymes, DNA, RNA, transport proteins, as well as receptors on membranes that bind *endogenous* hormones and neurotransmitters. Almost all drugs act by binding with these macromolecules. There are some exceptions, such as antacids, which directly neutralize stomach acid. In any case, the principle is that most drugs interact with some component of the cell, and this interaction causes a biochemical change. The point of interaction with the receptor is also called the *site of action* (see Chapter 2) for the drug (Figure 3-1).

Figure 3-2. Drug-receptor activity. Drugs bind to the same receptors used by hormones and neurotransmitters. When agonists (Drugs A and C) bind to their respective receptor they initiate a transduction mechanism, which causes a specific biological response. When an antagonist (Drug B) binds, it prevents initiation of the transduction mechanism. The ability of the drug to chemically bind (fit) with the receptor is its affinity. The ability of the drug to either initiate or prevent the transduction mechanism is its intrinsic efficacy. Only tissues that have a receptor for the drug will be affected by the drug. Drug A mimics hormone A; Drug B does not initiate transduction mechanisms and thus is a blocker of the response by neurotransmitter B; Drug C mimics hormone C; Drug D has no receptor on this cell, thus neither initiates nor inhibits any response from the cell.

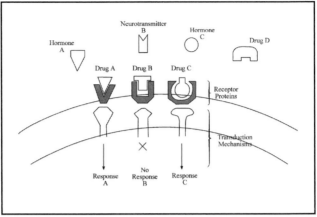

When discussing receptors, it is most useful to focus on the receptors located on the surface of membranes as they are the most important type of receptor for a wide range of drugs. An understanding of the mechanism of drug action at these receptors also helps to understand other concepts. These cell surface receptors are the binding sites of many endogenous hormones and neurotransmitters. In fact, as shown in Figure 3-2, a drug that binds to a receptor is merely mimicking (agonist) or blocking (antagonist) the effect of endogenous compounds. The receptor only exists so that a biological response can be regulated through the binding of an endogenous compound.

Every cell has many different types of receptors imbedded within the membrane and there are multiple copies of each receptor that the cell produces. One means by which the cell self-regulates the amount of chemical signal that it receives through the receptors is to increase or decrease the number of receptors it makes. For example, a diminished concentration of cholesterol in the blood will cause an increased synthesis of low density lipoprotein (LDL) receptors on the surface of the cell so that more cholesterol will bind to the receptor and be taken into the cell. A constant exposure of cells to morphine-like drugs will cause cells to decrease the production of morphine receptors and, as previously discussed, will cause tolerance to the morphine. Therefore, the number of receptors on the cell's surface is in flux.

Cells contain the specific receptors that are responsible for regulating the metabolic functions of that cell. In other words, every cell does not contain every type of receptor. From a pharmacological standpoint, this cellular selectivity of receptors limits the adverse effects from drugs as the effects of each drug are limited to the cells that have the type of receptor for that particular drug. In other words, if drug A only binds to receptor type A, drug A will only have an effect on cells that have receptor A. There are various classes of receptors, such as alpha- (α) and beta- (β) *adrenergic*, but there are also subtypes that are designated by subscripts, such as α_1, α_2, β_1, and β_2. Subtypes are also selective for tissues, and thus drugs that are selective for certain subtypes will be more selective for a particular tissue. Drugs that are β_1-adrenergic agonists will increase the heart rate but will not cause bronchial dilation because β_1-receptors are located on the surface of heart muscle cells whereas β_2-receptors are located on bronchial muscle cells.

The interaction between a receptor and drug exists because the chemical structure of the drug corresponds (or matches), to some degree, with the chemical structure of the receptor (see Figure 3-2). This means that chemical bonds can form between the drug and the receptor. These bonds usually are reversible and thus the drug binds to the receptor and then releases, back and forth.

Drug + Receptor ⟷ Drug-Receptor ⟶ Biological response
　　　　　affinity　　　　　　　　efficacy
　　　　component　　　　　　component

The strength of this bonding interaction is called the affinity of the drug for the receptor. The greater the affinity, the greater the chemical interaction, or chemical fit, of the drug for the receptor.

Affinity and efficacy are the two components of the drug's interaction with the receptor that determine the type and extent of biological response. The intrinsic efficacy is the ability of the drug to cause the receptor to initiate a domino effect of chemical reactions (*transduction mechanism*) that ultimately causes the biological response (see Figure 3-2), such as increased heart rate. There are several types of transduction mechanisms. One well-documented transduction mechanism involves the activation of the membrane protein called G-protein, which leads to the activation of the enzyme adenyl cyclase inside the cell. This, in turn, produces cyclic AMP, which continues the domino effect through several more steps. Cyclic AMP (cAMP) is one of many compounds called second messengers because they continue the signal (message) intracellularly from the first messenger (the hormone) located outside the cell. Regardless of whether the drug or the endogenous hormone combines with the receptor, the same chain of events is initiated beginning with the transduction mechanism and ending with the biological response:

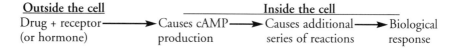

Outside the cell　　　　　　　　　　　**Inside the cell**
Drug + receptor ⟶ Causes cAMP ⟶ Causes additional ⟶ Biological
(or hormone)　　　　production　　　series of reactions　　response

The receptor theory of drug action explains how an agonist and antagonist can bind to the same receptor but have opposite effects (Figure 3-3). Drugs that bind to the same receptor as an endogenous compound and initiate the transduction mechanism will mimic the effects of the endogenous compound and are agonists. Drugs that bind to the same receptor as the endogenous compound but are unable to initiate the transduction mechanism will block the effects of the endogenous compound and are antagonists.

To some extent, the receptor mechanism of drug action can be thought of as a lock (receptor) and key (drug) system in which more than one key will fit into the lock but only the keys that are able to turn the tumblers in the lock will unlock the door (agonist); when the other keys (antagonist) are in the lock they prevent the correct key from unlocking the door. To be able to unlock the door, the first criterion is that the key must fit into the keyhole (ie, the affinity). The second criterion is whether the key is able to turn the locking mechanism to unlock the door (ie, the efficacy). If both agonist and antagonist are present, the effect that will predominate is dependent on the relative agonist/antagonist concentration at the site of action, affinity for the receptor, and efficacy.

Summary

The mechanism of action of most drugs, for both therapeutic and adverse effects, is that the drug chemically combines with a component of the cell referred to as the receptor. A receptor is

Figure 3-3. Receptor theory of drug action. When an agonist binds to the receptor, a transduction mechanism is initiated and ultimately a response increases. The antagonist can also bind to the same receptor, which prevents the biological response. This theory explains how an agonist and antagonist can bind to the same receptor and have opposite effects.

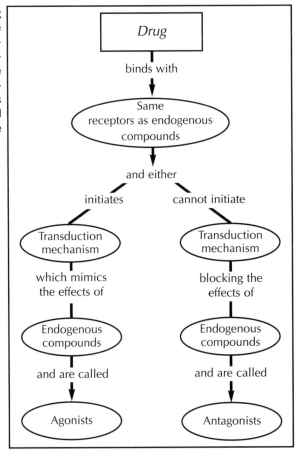

generally a large molecule, typically a protein that has specific chemical characteristics that only allow it to bind to molecules (eg, hormones and drugs) with corresponding chemical characteristics (similar to a lock and key). When the drug binds to the receptor to initiate a sequence of events inside the cell, the drug is called an agonist; when the drug binds to the receptor to inhibit the sequence of events, the drug is an antagonist. The strength of the binding of the drug for the receptor is called the affinity of the drug for the receptor; like the "fit" of the key into the lock. The ability of the drug to produce the biological response is called the efficacy of the drug; like the ability of the key to turn the lock.

DOSE-RESPONSE RELATIONSHIPS

Aside from *affinity* and *intrinsic efficacy* contributing to the biological response, the receptor theory of drug action also assumes that the extent of drug response is directly and linearly dependent on the number of receptor sites occupied by the drug. As more drug is given, the concentration of drug at the *site of action* (ie, at the receptor) also increases. Once a drug molecule is in the vicinity of the receptor, the likelihood of the drug coming in contact with the receptor is a by-chance occurrence and therefore the frequency that this event occurs is a matter of statistical probability based on the concentration of the drug and receptors; the more drug and/or

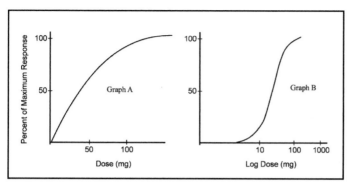

Figure 3-4. Dose-response principle. As the dose of the drug is increased, drug molecules will occupy a larger percentage of receptors and cause a larger biological response. If the observed response is plotted against the dose on a linear scale (Graph A), a hyperbolic curve results in which the response increases gradually until a maximum response is obtained when all of the receptors are occupied. If the same data are plotted using a logarithmic scale (Graph B) for the dose, a sigmoid curve results but the data show a linear relationship between dose and response for a significant portion of the dosage range.

receptor molecules, the greater the chances of the drug being in contact with the receptor. Drug-receptor interaction is generally a reversible process, with the drug response being initiated only when the drug and receptor are chemically interacting (drug-receptor).

$$\text{Drug + Receptor} \longleftrightarrow \text{Drug-Receptor} \longrightarrow \text{Drug response}$$

Therefore, as the concentration of the drug increases, more drug molecules will occupy more receptors, which will then produce a greater response. This is the basis for the *dose-response* principle and is shown in Graph A of Figure 3-4. As more receptors are occupied by drug molecules, the chances of a drug finding a free receptor becomes less until the dose is high enough that all of the receptors are occupied by drug and therefore additional drug does not produce additional effect; maximal response is achieved. Once all of the receptors are occupied, there are no other variables to affect the magnitude of response by that drug. Therefore, increasing the dose further will not increase the response. If the same data are plotted using logarithmic scale for the dose (Graph B of Figure 3-4), a sigmoid curve results but provides a significant segment that is linear (between approximately 20% and 80% of maximal response). The logarithmic dose plot not only provides a more conveniently usable linear portion, but also, as shown in Figure 3-5, allows a broader dose range to be represented on the same graph.

Single Dose

A typical dose-response curve for a single dose of three hypothetical drugs is shown in Figure 3-5. If pain relief is the response being measured, note that the maximal effect obtained by drug C is lower than for drug A and drug B. In this example, drugs A and B could represent the opioid analgesics morphine and codeine, and drug C could represent aspirin, which relieves pain by a different mechanism compared with opioids.

The *ED50* (effective dose) is the dose of drug that is effective in producing 50% of a specified response. The ED50 could represent the average dose needed to produce 50% of a maximal response in a group of people or the dose that will produce a specific effect in 50% of the patients. For example, it could be the dose of codeine that reduced the frequency of coughing by 50%, or the dose of codeine that eliminated the cough in 50% of the patients. The ED50 allows a comparison of effective drug dosages (see potency on page 60) among drugs being used for the same therapeutic effect. Also as described, the ED50 can be used to calculate the *therapeutic index*, which is an indicator of the relative safety of the drug.

Figure 3-5. Dose-response and potency. The dose-response curve is shown for three hypothetical pain relievers, Drugs A, B, and C. As the dose increases, more receptors are occupied by the drug and thus the percent of maximal pain relief increases until all the receptors are occupied and no additional relief is obtained. The dose that produces 50% of maximal response (ED50) is shown for each. Drug A is the most potent because the dose to reach the same ED50 is lowest for Drug A. Drug C is the least potent but also does not have the intrinsic activity to produce the same maximal response as Drugs A and B.

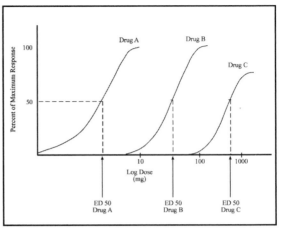

Potency is a term used to compare the dose of a drug required to produce a particular effect relative to the dose of another drug that acts by a similar mechanism to produce that same effect. The position of the dose-response curve along the X axis is indicative of potency. In the case of Figure 3-5, drug A is more potent than drug B as it takes considerably lower dose of drug A to produce the same ED50 response compared to the dose for drug B. Potency is determined by affinity, efficacy, and pharmacokinetic parameters, but is of little therapeutic importance because drug dosages are adjusted to compensate for differences in potency. An *equipotent* dose is used when comparing the efficacy of similar drugs (ie, doses are adjusted to give the same response). Consequently, although ibuprofen is more potent than either aspirin or acetaminophen for minor pain relief, 200 mg of ibuprofen is considered equipotent as an analgesic as 650 mg of either aspirin or acetaminophen. Potency, however, does impact the feasibility of using a drug by some routes of administration, such as sublingual and transdermal, because it is physically very difficult to get large quantities of drug to quickly dissolve under the tongue or to diffuse through the skin. Therefore, potent drugs, such as nitroglycerin with an effective dose of <1 mg, are the most practical for these dosage forms.

The dose-response curve is also useful for estimating the relative safety of a drug. The *LD50* (lethal dose) is the dose that will cause death in 50% of the population as extrapolated from animal data (Figure 3-6). The ratio of the LD50/ED50 is the *therapeutic index* (TI). The larger the TI, the greater the margin of safety. Notice in Figure 3-6 that the dose required to produce pain relief in 100% of the population does not overlap the dose that will kill any of the population. However, from a practical standpoint, we may not want to use death as the determination point for relative safety. The *TD50* (toxic dose) is the dose that will produce a specific toxic effect in 50% of the population. Generally, a specific toxic effect is used to determine the therapeutic index using the ratio TD50/ED50. In Figure 3-6, some patients receiving a dose at the higher end of the normal range will experience the toxic symptom and thus will require a change in therapy. Obviously, use of the normal dosage range of a drug with a TI of 10 will be less likely to cause death or toxicity than a drug with a TI <5. Examples of drugs with a low therapeutic index are aminoglycoside antibiotics, warfarin (Coumadin), some cardiac drugs, and some anticonvulsants used to treat epileptic seizures; these drugs require closer therapeutic drug monitoring.

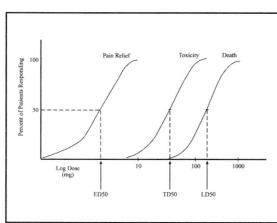

Figure 3-6. Dose response and therapeutic index. The dose-response curve is shown for three responses from a hypothetical pain reliever. Response A is pain relief, response B is a toxic symptom, and response C is death. The therapeutic index is an indication of relative safety of the drug as determined by the ratio of either LD50/ED50 or TD50/ED50. The greater the ratio, the greater the safety as a larger dose can be given without occurrence of toxic effects. In this example, the dose required to achieve pain relief in 100% of the patients overlaps a portion of the toxicity curve. Therefore, for a small percentage of patients, a dose of drug necessary to relieve pain will also cause some of the toxic symptoms. However, there is no overlap between the curve representing pain relief and the curve representing death.

The significance of the TI is relative to the responses being used to calculate it. For example, if a drug has a TI of 3 when using ringing in the ears as the toxic effect, it would be considered safer than a drug with TI of 3 for which the lethal dose was used for the calculation. The TI provides an impression of the degree of safety associated with the drug but the specific value does not provide much clinically relevant information except as means of noting that additional caution is necessary when using drugs that have a low TI. In fact, these drugs are likely to require additional clinical monitoring, such as a periodic check for changes in liver or kidney function as a result of drug toxicity.

> *An example of TI calculations is shown. If in a test group of animals, half go to sleep with 100 mg of the sedative phenobarbital, and half die at a dose of 260 mg, then TI = LD50/ED50 = 260/ 100 = 2.6 = a low therapeutic index.*

Another type of monitoring for drugs with a low TI is therapeutic drug monitoring (see below). This monitoring is used to check the blood (or serum) concentration of the drug and then to alter the drug dosage based on that blood concentration. This type of dosage adjustment is used to keep the drug concentration within a certain range (or window). When the drug concentration is kept within this therapeutic window, the incidence of toxicity is minimized. The width of the therapeutic drug concentration is a more clinically useful indicator of safety than the TI; examples are given in Table 3-1. All of the drugs in Table 3-1 have a relatively narrow therapeutic window, which also means they are relatively more toxic (hence the need to monitor the blood concentration). The athletic trainer is not likely to encounter many athletes taking drugs with a narrow therapeutic window, but understanding the concept is beneficial to the understanding of the relative safety of drugs. The blood concentrations of drugs that have a relatively wide therapeutic range are typically not monitored because they are safer.

Multiple Doses and Steady-State

When multiple doses of a drug are administered (Figure 3-7), the blood concentration increases beyond the concentration obtained by a single dose and eventually levels off when the rate of drug becoming *bioavailable* equals the rate of drug being removed through metabolism and/or excretion (ie, clearance). This leveling effect is the *steady-state concentration.* Once steady-state is reached, continued therapy at the same dose and *dosing interval* will not increase the peak

Table 3-1. Therapeutic Range of Serum Drug Concentration for Selected Drugs

Generic Name	Trade Name	Drug Category	Therapeutic Concentration[1]
amikacin	Amikin	aminoglycoside antibiotic	20 to 30 mg/L[2]
digoxin	Lanoxin	antiarrhythmic, congestive heart failure	0.8 to 2.5 µg/L
phenobarbital	Luminal	anticonvulsant	10 to 30 mg/L
phenytoin	Dilantin	anticonvulsant	10 to 20 mg/L
procainamide	Pronestyl	antiarrhythmic	4 to 8 mg/L
theophylline	Theo-Dur	antiasthmatic	10 to 20 mg/L
valproic acid	Depakene	anticonvulsant	50 to 100 mg/L

[1]Represents serum concentration appropriate for most patients.

[2]Represents peak concentration range for amikacin.

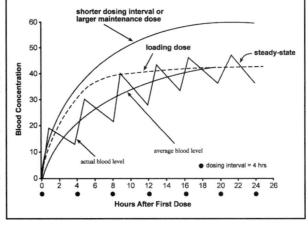

Figure 3-7. Multiple dose effect. A drug with a half-life (t½) of about 5 hours is given every 4 hours (●) beginning with time zero. After each dose the blood concentration increases to a peak and then decreases to the lowest concentration just prior to the next dose. The blood concentration increases until steady-state is reached beyond 4 half lives (>20 hours). A higher steady-state concentration is reached by either increasing the dose or decreasing the dosing interval. Giving a loading dose will increase the blood concentration quicker.

blood concentration. If a drug is given at a regular dosing interval, four times each day for example, at some point the rate of drug clearance will equal the rate of drug absorbed. The mathematics of this principle establishes that if the same dose is administered at a regular dosing interval, the amount of drug in the body will be 87.5% of steady-state after dosing has been continued beyond three half-lives, approximately 94% after four half-lives, 97% after five half-lives, and 98.4% after six half-lives; this principle is shown in Figure 3-8. So, for therapeutically relevant purposes, steady-state can be considered attained after dosing has continued for a time beyond four to five half-lives of the drug. Using this principle, if 250 mg of naproxen (t½ 14 hours) is administered every 12 hours, the peak blood concentration will continue to increase after each 12-hour interval, reaching 94% of steady state after absorption of the sixth dose at 60 hours (first dose at time zero). Continued therapy at this dosage regimen for naproxen will not increase the peak blood concentration beyond another 6%.

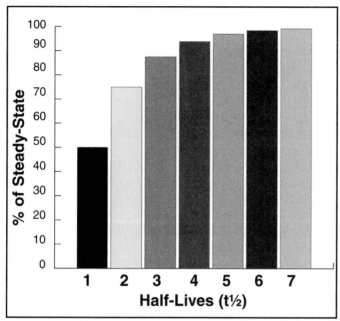

Figure 3-8. Achieving steady-state. As a general principle, when dosing of a drug is at a regular interval (eg, every 12 hours), the blood level after each half-life reaches a concentration equal to ½ of the concentration remaining to reach steady-state. Therefore, if t½ is 14 hours: 1.) 14 hours (1 t½) after the first dose, the blood concentration is 50% of steady state; 2.) 28 hours (2 t½) after the first dose, the blood concentration is 50% + ½ (50%) = 75% of steady-state; 3.) 42 hours (3 t½) after the first dose, the blood concentration is 75% + ½ (25%) = 87.5% of steady-state; 4.) 56 hours (4 t½) after the first dose, the blood concentration is 87.5% + ½ (12.5%) = 93.8% of steady-state; and 5.) 70 hours (5 t½) after the first dose, the blood concentration is 93.8% + ½ (6.25%) = 96.9% of steady-state. When the sixth dose is given at 60 hours (the first dose being at zero hours), steady-state is reached (approximately), which is after 4 t½.

The steady-state level obtained can be altered by either of two methods: changing the dosing interval or changing the dose. Figure 3-7 illustrates an increase in the blood concentration when the dosing interval is shortened (eg, from 4 hours to 3 hours), or if the maintenance dose is increased but the dosing interval is not changed. In either situation, the amount of drug that is bioavailable increases. If the dosing interval is made longer (eg, from 4 to 6 hours), or if the dose is reduced, the steady-state concentration will decrease.

Maintenance Dose and Loading Dose

A dose administered at a regular dosing interval on a repetitive basis is called a *maintenance dose*. This maintenance therapy could be a 10-day course of antibiotic therapy or 10 years (ie, long-term or chronic) of antihypertensive therapy. In Figure 3-7, the dosing interval is 4 hours and the t½ is about 5 hours. The blood concentration attained after the dose at 20 hours (after 4 half lives) approximates the steady-state level. However, if it is important to more quickly reach a blood level approximating steady-state, to treat an infection or a cardiac dysrhythmia, a loading dose can be given. The *loading dose* is one or more doses that are higher than the maintenance dose and administered at the beginning of therapy for the purpose of achieving the desirable therapeutic concentration quicker. The steady-state level obtained after the loading dose(s) is the same as it would be without the loading dose, assuming no change in the maintenance dose and dosing interval.

Summary

The larger the dose, the larger the number of receptors that will be occupied by the drug, and thus a larger response. When the dose reaches a certain concentration so that most of the receptors are occupied by drug, it is statistically less likely that the drug will find an available receptor, thus the response tapers off. These principles are the basis for the typical dose-response relationship in which the response increases with increasing dose, up to a point. The ED50 is the dose that produces the therapeutic effect in 50% of the population; the LD50 is the dose that is lethal to 50% of the population; and the TD50 is the dose that causes a specified toxic symptom in 50% of the population. One indicator of relative safety of a drug is the TI, which can be calculated based on the ratio of LD50/ED50 or TD50/ED50; in either case, the larger the number, the greater the difference between the dose that is effective and the dose that causes significant problems. The therapeutic window is a target range of drug concentration in the blood that produces the best therapeutic effect while minimizing toxic effects.

When doses of a drug are given at a regular dosing interval, eventually the blood concentration will level-off regardless of how much longer the dosing interval is maintained. This level of drug is called the steady-state blood concentration and occurs after the dosing has occurred for a time beyond approximately four to five half-lives (t½) of the drug. For a drug with a t½ of 5 hours, steady-state is approximately reached when dosing at regular intervals goes beyond 20 hours. The amount of drug given at regular intervals is called the maintenance dose. As a means of attaining steady state quicker than 4 t½, a loading dose can be given, which is an initial dose that is larger than the maintenance dose.

THERAPEUTIC CONSIDERATIONS

From the dose-response relationships it is evident that a standard dose used in a population of patients will not produce the same response in each patient. Some patients will experience maximum therapeutic effect with minimal adverse or toxic effects, whereas the response of other patients will fall elsewhere on the dose-response curve. The latter group of patients may require an increase or decrease in dose to obtain the necessary balance between therapeutic effectiveness and adverse effects. Each patient's response to a particular therapy will be dictated by his or her specific pharmacokinetic and pharmacodynamic parameters, which are affected by genetics, age, gender, body size, and drug interactions from concurrent therapy.

Patient Compliance

Patient compliance refers to the extent to which the patient is taking the medication as prescribed. Obviously, medications will only produce the desired therapeutic outcome if the proper dosage regimen is maintained. Nonetheless, poor patient compliance is a major cause of poor therapeutic outcomes. Some of the reasons for patients not adhering to the prescribed dosage regimen are:
- Cost of the medication is too high
- Forgetting to take the medication
- It is inconvenient to take the medication (eg, inhalation asthma medications)
- Poor patient education regarding the necessity to take medications as prescribed

Patient compliance improves if the patient does not have to take the medication as frequently each day; thus once per day dosing significantly improves patient compliance compared with a three times per day dosing regimen.

The athletic trainer can have an impact on improving patient compliance by educating the patient as to the importance of adhering to the prescribed dosing regimen. An understanding of the mechanism of action of the drug, drug dosing principles, and proper drug administration techniques can be useful. With this information, the athletic trainer can provide appropriate education to assist the patient in maintaining therapeutic outcomes from the use of chronic medications. For example, a patient taking half the prescribed dose to obtain half the benefit may in fact be obtaining no benefit as the minimum *effective dose* may not be reached. A patient using a corticosteroid inhaler prior to exercise rather than for daily, long-term therapy does not understand the proper dosing principle or *mechanism of action* of the drug and is obtaining little or no benefit from the inhaler. The patient should understand the purpose for each drug, the necessity for adhering to the prescribed dosage regimen, and the proper technique for drug administration.

Dose Calculations

The standard dose for drugs with a high *therapeutic index* is often set at two or three levels—children, adults, and elderly. The dose for children is sometimes refined according to age (eg, one dose for ages 2 to 5 and another dose for children 6 to 11). The basis for these divisions is to compensate for the increased *volume of distribution* that accompanies increased size. As the likelihood for toxicity or significant adverse effects increases (ie, lower therapeutic index), the calculation of the dose becomes more specific. The dose can be calculated on the basis of weight (mg/kg) or body surface area (mg/m^2) of the patient. Body surface area correlates more closely with renal and metabolic capacity than does body weight, assuming normal kidney and liver function. Charts are available to determine the body surface area based on the patient's height and weight. As an example, a patient that is 6 feet and 170 pounds has a surface area of 2 m^2.

Therapeutic Drug Monitoring

Because there can be significant variability of response from one patient to another, drugs that have a low therapeutic index are sometimes monitored by measuring the blood (or plasma or serum) concentration of the drug. As mentioned above, this is referred to as *therapeutic drug monitoring*. Measuring the blood concentration leaves no question regarding the extent to which age, genetics, disease, patient compliance, or other parameters have affected bioavailability. The blood level is determined after the patient is at steady-state. For some drugs, a normal range of blood concentration has been established; above this level the incidence of toxic effects greatly increases, and below this level there is a greater likelihood the drug is subtherapeutic (ie, below the minimum effective concentration). The range between the low and high desired concentration is referred to as the *therapeutic range* or *therapeutic window.* Theophylline (Theo-Dur), as an example, is used for the treatment of asthma (see Chapter 9) and has a therapeutic range of 10 to 20 mg/L. As the concentration of theophylline moves above 20 mg/L, the incidence of adverse effects increases; whereas concentrations below 10 mg/L are less likely to be therapeutically effective. Drugs with a small therapeutic index will have a narrow therapeutic window. Besides theophylline, other examples of drugs that are frequently monitored include some antidysrhythmic drugs, anticonvulsants, and aminoglycoside antibiotics, examples of which are shown in Table 3-1. Dosage adjustments are made based on the blood concentration after the drug has reached steady-state. By keeping the concentration within the therapeutic window, toxic effects and ineffective dosage regimens can be avoided.

Box 3-2. Pharmacokinetic and Pharmacodynamic Parameters That are Altered in the Elderly

- Diminished function of liver metabolizing enzymes and reduced blood flow that decreases biotransformation rate of drugs and increases the duration of action.
- Reduced kidney function decreases the excretion rate of drugs and increases the duration of action.
- Reduced blood flow to the gastrointestinal tract reduces the extent of oral absorption.
- Reduced gastric emptying and gastrointestinal motility can alter drug absorption rates.
- Increased proportion of body fat as muscle mass decreases can increase the volume of distribution of lipid soluble drugs and thus decrease the concentration at the site of action.
- Diminished albumin concentration, primarily as a consequence of reduced liver function, can decrease the extent of protein binding and increase the response from drugs that are highly protein bound.
- Increased number of diseases in a given patient will increase the number of drugs being used and thus increase the likelihood of drug interactions.
- Change in level of exercise may alter pharmacokinetic parameters as discussed in Chapter 2.

Age

Although the athletic trainer may not be working with infants, a discussion of some therapeutic problems from infants to the elderly illustrates the type of potential problems that may occur. Although dose adjustment based on size is an obvious necessity for therapy to newborns and infants, the capability for drug clearance by the liver and kidney is also reduced through the first year or so. Consequently, it is necessary to closely monitor the effects of drugs administered to newborns and infants, especially for drugs with a low *therapeutic index*. A reduced dosage range for children is established for drugs suitable for use in children. The adult oral dose for ampicillin to treat certain infections is 1 to 4 g/day whereas for children it is 50 to 100 mg/kg/day. However, not all drugs have been approved for use in children, even at reduced doses. Other drugs, such as the asthma medication zafirlukast (Accolate), were first approved for use in adults and then approved later for use in young children.

Besides dose, there are other important issues related to drug administration in children. Some drugs should not be used in children due to adverse or toxic effects that are unique to children. Tetracycline antibiotics bind to developing teeth and will cause a permanent staining. There is concern regarding the extent to which chronic use of corticosteroids for treatment of asthma in children may delay growth. Sometimes it is preferable to have special drug dosage forms and formulations for children. Liquids are easier for some children to swallow than solid dosage forms as long as the liquids are adequately sweetened and flavored. Because elixirs contain alcohol, they are often avoided in children.

The elderly may also require adjustments in dosing for some drugs. The percentage of the population aged >60 years is increasing and many elderly patients maintain an exercise routine as part of their lifestyle. As a person ages, several pharmacokinetic and pharmacodynamic parameters are altered, which may warrant an adjustment in drug dose, especially for drugs with a smaller therapeutic index (Box 3-2).

It is important to note that these changes occur gradually as a person ages, and thus the impact varies among patients. In addition, the picture is complicated by the fact that there are multiple changes occurring simultaneously in the same patient. Finally, it is not only the altered therapeutic effect that is of concern in the elderly, but also the adverse effects. Elderly patients tend to have an enhanced response to many adverse effects, such as the central and autonomic effects of drowsiness, confusion, urinary retention, constipation, and hypotension. It is very difficult to predict the extent of change on all of the pharmacokinetic parameters. Consequently, the best therapy is attained through therapeutic drug monitoring or by monitoring the outcomes of initial therapy, the occurrence of adverse effects, and the concurrent administration of other drugs to determine the need for therapy adjustments. If the therapeutic outcome or adverse effects are not acceptable, age-related factors should be considered in the young and the elderly.

Liver and Kidney Function

Because the clearance of drugs occurs primarily by the liver and kidney, a reduction in the efficiency of these organs through disease or the aging process may necessitate a dosage adjustment to attain the proper therapeutic response but avoid adverse effects. The key question is how much dosage adjustment is needed? Sometimes the liver and kidney function must be monitored to determine the extent to which dosage adjustment is necessary. Evaluation of liver function can be done by measuring the blood level of aspartate aminotransferase, also known as serum glutamic oxaloacetic transaminase, and alanine aminotransaminase, also known as serum glutamic pyruvate transaminase. Although elevated concentration of these enzymes in the blood are indicative of acute liver cell damage, they cannot be directly correlated with loss of drug metabolizing activity. Other indicators of diminished liver function are elevated bilirubin concentration, decreased albumin, and prolonged blood clotting time; the liver is key in the metabolism of bilirubin, albumin, and blood clotting factors. Again, although the levels of these compounds are indicators of liver function, they do not provide a quantitative determination of the loss of drug metabolizing capability.

In contrast to liver function, the extent of kidney function can be calculated. One measure of kidney function is creatinine clearance. Creatinine is a waste product of muscle metabolism that is produced at a relatively constant rate per day based on the amount of muscle mass. It is filtered at the glomerulus and is not reabsorbed, thus creatinine excretion rate is a good measure of kidney function. Creatinine clearance refers to the rate (mL/min) at which the kidney clears the blood of creatinine; normal is 100 to 120 mL/min. If kidney function is diminished, less blood will be cleared of creatinine per minute. Dosage adjustment calculations of some drugs that are cleared primarily by the kidney have been established based on creatinine clearance. Aminoglycoside antibiotics and digoxin (Lanoxin) are among these drugs.

Summary

The optimal drug therapy is one that provides the right drug at a dose that produces the most effective therapeutic effect with the least adverse effects. Many factors affect the ability to reach optimal drug therapy. Lack of patient compliance (ie, the patient does not take the drug properly) is a major hindrance to optimal drug therapy. Poor compliance often occurs because the patient does not understand the proper use of the drug or the importance of adhering to the dosage regimen.

Proper dosage is obviously important if optimal effectiveness is to be attained. The dosage calculation may be based on the patient's age, weight, or body surface area, depending typically on the degree of toxicity associated with the drug. To fine-tune the dose, the response of the patient to the drug may be monitored so that the dosage regiment can be modified based on the patient's response. Alternatively, the blood concentration of the drug can be measured and used as the gauge for dosage adjustment. Infants, young children, and the elderly sometimes respond differently than the rest of the population, resulting in less than optimal response to therapy. Special monitoring and adjustments in therapy are often necessary for these populations.

Because the liver and kidneys are responsible for clearance of drugs, the level of efficiency of these two organs impacts the response to drug therapy. Sometimes these organs must be evaluated to determine the extent to which they are functioning. The measure of liver enzymes and creatinine clearance can be useful to assess whether the liver and kidneys, respectively, are functioning properly. Adjustment of drug dosage may be necessary if either of these organs are functionally deficient. There are obviously a multitude of factors that can hinder the ability to achieve optimal drug therapy.

DRUG INTERACTIONS

A *drug interaction* occurs when the addition of another drug increases or decreases the effect obtained from the therapy. Some drug-drug interactions are beneficial and are incorporated into the therapeutic plan. For example, the use of multiple drugs to treat asthma and hypertension. In other situations, interactions between drugs are detrimental because they reduce therapeutic effectiveness, increase the incidence of adverse effects, or increase toxicity. For example, alcohol can increase the likelihood of toxicity of acetaminophen (see Chapter 7) and also increases the CNS depressant effects of all other CNS depressants (see Chapter 8). Some foods and herbs can cause drug–food and drug–herbal interactions, respectively, but these interactions are not generally incorporated into the therapeutic plan and thus they are viewed as adverse drug reactions and are discussed later in this chapter. There are thousands of interactions of drugs with other drugs, food, and herbal remedies. Many drug handbooks (see Table 1-8) list some drug interactions for each drug and some books focus exclusively on drug interactions (eg, *Drug Interactions Handbook*). Internet sites also provide drug interaction information; an example with search capability for >5000 drugs and herbs is www.drugdigest.org/DD/Interaction/ChooseDrugs (note: case sensitive). It is beyond the scope and intent of this text to mention all of these interactions but a few examples are provided in Table 3-2. *As a general rule, drugs with a low therapeutic index and drugs for which a diminished response may have critical consequences must be particularly monitored for potential interactions.* Obviously, the likelihood of drug interactions increases as the number of drugs being taken by the patient increases.

There are many mechanisms that cause drug interactions. Some are a result of changes in pharmacokinetic parameters and others are due to pharmacodynamic changes. These mechanisms are described below and summarized in Table 3-3.

- Receptor antagonist. When two drugs have an affinity for the same receptor, one drug will displace the other and thus diminish the response of the other, especially if one is an agonist and the other an antagonist. Propranolol (Inderal) is a β-adrenergic antagonist (ie, a β-blocker); pirbuterol (Maxair) is a β-adrenergic agonist used for the treatment of asthma. If propranolol was being used to reduce hypertension, it could diminish the effectiveness of pirbuterol at a time when the patient needs it to treat an acute asthma attack.
- Enzyme induction. This occurs when a drug (the inducer drug) increases the synthesis of one or more metabolizing enzymes.

Often the inducer drug increases the amount of metabolizing enzyme that is responsible for metabolizing a second drug. Consequently, enzyme induction will diminish the response from the second drug. Occasionally, the metabolites are more active, in which case the inducer drug

Table 3-2. Examples of Drug Interactions With Other Drugs, Food, and Herbs

Drug	*Interacting Substance*	*Potential Consequence* (tables that provide examples of drugs)
ACE inhibitors	NSAIDs	Decreases antihypertensive effect (Tables 6-4, 12-8)
acetaminophen	alcohol	Increases toxicity
ampicillin	sulbactam	Increases effectiveness of ampicillin (Table 5-2)
antifungal agents, oral	proton pump inhibitors	Decreases absorption (Table 11-1)
antifungal agents, oral	H_2-blockers	Decreases absorption (Table 11-2)
antifungal agents, oral	grapefruit juice	Decreases effectiveness of oral antifungal drugs
antihistamines	alcohol	Increases sedation, particularly with first generation antihistamines (Table 10-3)
antihypertensive drugs	nasal decongestant	Decreases physiological effectiveness (Tables 10-2, 12-6, 12-7, 12-8, 12-9)
antihypertensive drugs	herbs	Some herbs (eg, black cohosh, California poppy, golden seal, coleus, quinine) may increase antihypertensive effect excessively
antihypertensive drugs	herbs	Some herbs (eg, ginger, ginseng, kola, bayberry, blue cohosh, cayenne, licorice) may decrease antihypertensive effect
caffeine	grapefruit juice	Increases CNS stimulation of caffeine
calcium channel blockers	grapefruit juice	Increases occurrence of adverse effects (Table 12-9)
CNS depressants	alcohol	Increases CNS depression effects (Table 8-2)
corticosteroids, systemic	antifungal drugs	Decreases metabolism and may increase toxic effects (Table 6-6)
corticosteroids, systemic	NSAIDs	Increases incidence of ulceration and bleeding
diazepam (Valium)	alcohol	Enhances CNS depression; potential toxicity
fluoroquinolones	dairy products and antacids	Diminishes absorption (Table 5-5)
nasal decongestants	caffeine	Increases cardiovascular adverse effects and CNS stimulation (Table 10-2)
opioid analgesics	acetaminophen, aspirin, ibuprofen	Synergistic analgesic effect (Table 7-2)
oral contraceptives	many drugs	Diminishes the effectiveness of oral contraceptive (Table 3-5)

continued

Table 3-2. Examples of Drug Interactions With Other Drugs, Food, and Herbals (continued)

Drug	Interacting Substance	Potential Consequence (tables that provide examples of drugs)
oral contraceptives	St. John's Wort	Diminishes the effectiveness of progestin contraceptives
tetracyclines	dairy products and antacids	Diminishes absorption (Table 5-4)
warfarin (Coumadin)	aspirin, other NSAIDs	Increases anticoagulant effect; potentially spontaneous bleeding
warfarin (Coumadin)	broccoli, cabbage	Vitamin K-rich foods decrease anticoagulant effect
warfarin (Coumadin), aspirin, other NSAIDs	herbs	Herbs that have anticoagulant or antiplatelet effects (eg, garlic, ginkgo biloba, ginseng, green tea, grape seed) may increase bleeding/bruising
β-agonist	β-blocker	Physiologically oppose each other; diminishes asthma therapy effectiveness (Tables 9-5, 12-6)
β-blockers	NSAIDs	Decreases antihypertensive effect

CNS=central nervous system

Table 3-3. Types of Drug Interactions Summarized

Drug Interaction Type	Description
Receptor antagonist	When two drugs have an affinity for the same receptor, one drug will displace the other and thus diminish the response of the other; one is an agonist and the other an antagonist.
Enzyme induction	This occurs when a drug (the inducer drug) increases the synthesis of one or more metabolizing enzymes.
Enzyme inhibition	Occurs when two drugs bind to the same metabolizing enzyme, but one drug is the substrate for the enzyme whereas the other is an inhibitor.
Physiologic antagonism	The physiological effect of two drugs given concurrently oppose each other without either drug directly interfering with the mechanism of action or pharmacokinetic parameters of the other.
Physiologic agonists	Two or more drugs when used concurrently result in an increase in physiological effects, either additive or synergistic, but the drugs do not have the same mechanism of action or affect the pharmacokinetic parameters of the other.
Absorption effects	The use of one drug inhibits the absorption of another drug if given concurrently.
Excretion effects	One drug increases or decreases the excretion rate of another drug.
Protein binding	One drug binds to the same site on plasma albumin as another drug, thus preventing it from binding and resulting in more free (active) drug.

will increase the response from the second drug because the more active metabolite is produced faster. Enzyme induction is a relatively slow process requiring the inducer drug to be present for days to weeks to demonstrate a maximum effect. Cytochrome P450 enzymes (see Chapter 2) are particularly affected by inducers, although other enzymes can be too.

> *Recall from Chapter 2 that liver enzymes metabolize drugs and typically inactivate the drug. The more enzyme molecules present, the faster the rate of metabolism and the faster the inactivation of the drug. A faster inactivation results in a diminished effect from the drug.*

Drug A = Inducer of enzyme B

Enzyme B
Drug B—————————————➤ Metabolite of Drug B

Drug A increases the synthesis of Enzyme B.
When Drug A and B are used concurrently,
the induction of Enzyme B by Drug A increases
the metabolism rate of Drug B.

Some anticonvulsants and alcohol are examples of liver enzyme inducers. Examples of drugs that are significantly affected by enzyme inducers are oral anticoagulants, estrogen contraceptives, antidepressants, and theophylline for asthma therapy; the therapy may need to be adjusted for these drugs to compensate for enzyme induction.

- *Enzyme inhibition.* This drug interaction occurs when two drugs bind to the same metabolizing enzyme, but one drug is the *substrate* for the enzyme whereas the other is an inhibitor. As inhibition of a metabolizing enzyme will decrease the activity of that metabolizing enzyme, the bioavailability of the substrate drug (Drug B) will increase.

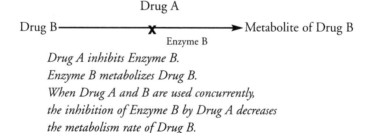

Drug A
Drug B—————————✗—————————➤ Metabolite of Drug B
Enzyme B

Drug A inhibits Enzyme B.
Enzyme B metabolizes Drug B.
When Drug A and B are used concurrently,
the inhibition of Enzyme B by Drug A decreases
the metabolism rate of Drug B.

When the substrate drug and inhibitor drug are used concurrently, the substrate drug will have a longer duration, increased blood concentration, and greater biological response than expected. This enhanced response may include adverse effects and toxicity. Examples of inhibitors of metabolizing enzymes that are known to impact the level of other drugs include erythromycin (Erythrocin), cimetidine (Tagamet), some antifungal agents such as fluconazole (Diflucan), antidepressants referred to as selective serotonin reuptake inhibitors such as fluoxetine (Prozac), and grapefruit juice.

- *Physiologic antagonism.* In this situation, the physiological effect of the two drugs given concurrently oppose each other without either drug directly interfering with the mechanism of action or pharmacokinetic parameters of the other. One drug decreases blood pressure whereas the second drug increases blood pressure, for example. This type of interaction is particularly important in treatment of diseases such as hypertension, diabetes, hypercholesterolemia, and asthma because there are many prescription as well as OTC products that have physiological effects that exacerbate these diseases. Nasal decongestants used to treat symptoms of the common cold can increase blood pressure and blood glucose and thus act as physiologic antagonists of therapy for hypertension and diabetes.

- *Physiological agonists.* Similar to physiological antagonism in that two or more drugs used concurrently do not have the same mechanism of action, but in this case the result is an increase in physiological effects, either additive or synergistic. An example is the use of the anticoagulant warfarin (Coumadin) with aspirin, which also prolongs blood clotting; the result may be excessive anticoagulation. Sometimes the physiological agonistic response is desirable

> *As an example of enzyme inhibition, if cimetidine (Tagamet), a drug used to treat gastrointestinal problems (see Chapter 11) is added to therapy that includes a β-blocker such as propranolol (Inderal) for treatment of hypertension (see Chapter 12), within a day the cimetidine will begin to inhibit the enzyme that had been metabolizing propranolol. As less enzyme is available to metabolize propranolol, the blood level of propranolol will increase and may cause adverse effects. In this scenario, if the cimetidine is to remain as part of the therapy, the dose of propranolol should be reduced to decrease the incidence of adverse effects.*

and is the basis for using two or more drugs with different mechanisms of action to treat the same disease, such as for treatment of cancer or hyptertension (see Chapter 12).

- *Absorption effects.* The use of one drug could inhibit the absorption of another drug if given concurrently. Laxatives, such as milk of magnesia, which contain divalent cations (ie, metal ions that have a charge of +2, such as Ca^{++}, Mg^{++}, Al^{++}), will bind to tetracycline and fluoroquinolone antibiotics and inhibit their absorption (see Chapter 5). Typically, dosing of the interfering drug (eg, milk of magnesia) should be about 2 hours before or 1 hour after the other drug.
- *Excretion effects.* One drug could increase the excretion rate of another drug, for example by changing the pH of the urine or by competing for the tubular secretion sites as in the case for the concurrent use of probenecid with penicillin G (see Chapter 2).
- *Protein binding.* For drugs that are highly bound (see Table 2-2) to plasma protein (ie, albumin), only a small amount of any dose is available to reach the *site of action* at any given time. Sometimes the drug binding site on the protein is the same for several drugs. As drug B occupies the site, drug A cannot. If drug A used alone is 99% protein bound (1% free), and the dosage regimen is established on that basis, and then drug B is added to therapy and displaces 2% of drug A from the protein, the amount of free drug A is increased to 3%. Because it is only the free drug that reaches the site of action to cause a response, the effective drug is now 3% of the total drug A rather than the original 1%; a three-fold increase.

It is impossible to remember all of the potential drug interactions associated with every drug. Even with the availability of drug handbooks and computer-based information it is difficult to assess the practical significance of the interaction. Drugs with a wide *therapeutic window* are less likely to pose a noticeable difference in response as a result of a drug interaction. Nonetheless, it is important for the athletic trainer to understand the principles of drug interaction; if an unexpected drug effect is observed, a drug–drug, drug–herbal, or drug–food interaction should be considered and steps taken to refer the patient. The physician and pharmacist can determine whether a potential interaction exists so that appropriate modification of therapy can be made.

Summary

Drug interactions have a significant impact on the effectiveness of drug therapy in many patients. The more drugs that are used concurrently in a patient, the greater the probability for drug interactions. There are many mechanisms that can be responsible for these drug interactions. It is obviously counterproductive to use two drugs that produce the opposite effects, such as an *agonist* and *antagonist*. Less obvious are the many instances in which groups of drugs share the same metabolizing enzymes. When one of these drugs increases the level of the metabolizing enzymes (ie, enzyme induction), it causes other drugs to be metabolized quicker by that same enzyme, thus reducing the duration of action of the other drugs. Inhibition of drug metabolizing enzymes can also be the cause of drug interactions. When a new drug is added to existing therapy and the new drug inhibits the metabolizing enzyme that inactivates the initial drug, the initial drug will be metabolized slower and thus the duration of action will be extended. If adding a drug to therapy inhibits the absorption or increases the renal excretion of another drug, the effectiveness of drug therapy will be affected and an adjustment in dosage regimen may be necessary. Protein-bound drug molecules are inactive but if a drug is added to therapy that releases more free drug from the protein binding sites, the number of active molecules of drug will increase; again an adjustment of the dosage regimen may be necessary. In all cases of drug interactions, the need for dosage adjustment is dependent on whether the change in drug response is significant. The clinical significance of these interactions varies with the magnitude to which the drug response is altered and the degree of toxicity of the drugs affected.

ADVERSE DRUG REACTIONS

An *adverse drug reaction* (ADR) is any undesirable response from a drug. These reactions can range from dry mouth to life-threatening organ damage. The incidence of clinically significant ADR is reflected in the fact that approximately 5% of hospitalizations are a result of an ADR. In addition, >10% of hospitalized patients experience at least one ADR. Some ADRs may occur after just one dose of the drug whereas others occur only after continued use of the drug. Sometimes a drug is removed from the market because a severe ADR is identified after the drug has been used in a large number of patients (ie, postmarketing monitoring). Adverse drug reaction can be subdivided into the following categories, which are summarized in Table 3-4.

- *Side effects.* These are expected responses based on the pharmacologic action of the drug. They are also dose related so that larger doses will increase the frequency of side effects. Because of differences among patients in the pharmacokinetic and pharmacodynamic parameters, not every patient will experience each side effect associated with a drug, but the percentage of the population that will experience any give side effect is predictable based on previous observations. Side effects are usually less severe compared with most other ADRs. Examples of side effects are dry mouth, constipation, increased heart rate, hypotension, gastrointestinal upset, and drowsiness. In some cases, the dose of the drug may have to be decreased to diminish the severity of the side effect. As discussed earlier, elderly patients are susceptible to diminished clearance of drugs and may require a lower dose to decrease the occurrence and intensity of side effects.
- *Allergic reactions.* Allergic reactions from drugs occur in approximately 5% of the population. Some patients have been misidentified as having a drug allergy due to the inaccurate identification of other ADRs as an allergy. The intensity of drug-induced allergic reactions is usually independent of dose. An initial sensitization exposure to the drug is required to

Table 3-4. Categories of Adverse Drug Reactions

Category	Description
Side effects	Expected responses based on the pharmacologic action of the drug.
Allergic reactions	Exaggerated immune response initiated by the exposure to certain drugs or other chemicals.
Organ cytotoxic effects	Adverse effects on organs.
Idiosyncratic reactions	Reaction that is peculiar to an individual or a defined group of people.
Drug-drug interactions	Interaction of two or more drugs that results in a disadvantage to the patient.
Drug-food interactions	Interaction of a drug with food that results in an adverse patient reaction.
Drug-herb interactions	Interaction of a drug with herbal products that results in an adverse patient reaction.
Drug use during pregnancy	It is assumed that most drugs cross the placenta barrier to some extent, and thus pose the potential for adverse reactions in this selected population for whom the drug was not intended.

initiate the allergic response. Allergic reactions are immune responses with symptoms that can vary considerably among patients, but the drug should be discontinued regardless of the severity of the allergic response. Symptoms can be as mild as urticaria or as severe as a life-threatening bronchoconstriction and hypotension associated with anaphylactic reaction. Dermatologic reactions are the most common type of allergic response, but these usually are mild and disappear after discontinuation of the drug. If a drug causes anaphylaxis, symptoms will usually occur within 30 minutes after exposure to the drug. The drug of choice for the initial treatment of anaphylaxis is epinephrine administered subcutaneously or intramuscularly. Generally, the most common device used to self-deliver the epinephrine intramuscularly is an EpiPen (Figure 3-9). Although the athletic trainer may help prepare the device for use, the patient must self-administer the medication. The procedure for self-administering an EpiPen is listed in Box 3-3. Because anaphylaxis is a medical emergency, the emergency medical plan should be activated upon its recognition. Even if an EpiPen is used, the patient needs to be seen by a physician immediately as additional medical treatment may be necessary.

About 80% of all allergic drug reactions are caused from β-lactams antibiotics, NSAIDs, and sulfonamides (ie, certain sulfur-containing compounds). The β-lactam antibiotics consist of two groups of antibiotics with similar chemical structure: the penicillins and the cephalosporins (see Chapter 5). Allergic reactions occur more often with this group of drugs than with any others but yet the incidence is <10%. Although allergic reactions to the β-lactams are usually mild, anaphylaxis can occur.

Aspirin and other NSAIDs cause urticaria in approximately 1% of the general population; other patients may experience symptoms from rhinitis to anaphylaxis. Aspirin and other NSAIDs can also induce asthma attacks in 3% to 39% of patients with chronic asthma, depending on the subpopulation of asthma patients.

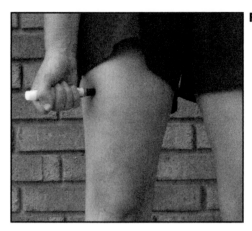

Figure 3-9. Epi-Pen administration.

Box 3-3. Procedure for Administering the EpiPen Auto-Injector

To Administer...

Step	Action
1	Grasp the unit, with the black tip pointing downward.
2	Form a fist around the unit (black tip down).
3	With other hand, pull off the gray activation cap.
4	Hold black tip near outer thigh.
5	Swing and jab firmly into outer thigh so that unit is perpendicular (at a 90 degree angle) to the thigh.
6	Hold firmly in thigh for several seconds.
7	Remove unit, massage injection area for several seconds.
8	Check black tip: If needle is exposed, dose was delivered. If not, repeat steps 4 to 7.

Note: Most of the liquid (about 90%) stays in the unit and cannot be reused.

After Usage...

9	Bend the needle back against a hard surface.
10	Carefully put the unit (needle first) back into the carrying tube (without the gray activation cap).
11	Recap the carrying tube.
12	Take unit to hospital so that the physician can inspect it and it can be disposed of properly.

Adapted from www.epipen.com.

Sulfonamides include drugs in the categories of antibiotics, diuretics, and oral hypo-glycemic agents used to treat type 2 diabetes. Allergic reactions to sulfonamide antibiotics occur in approximately 3% of the general population and with a lower frequency in the other sulfonamides categories. The most common manifestations from sulfonamides are dermatologic and may include fever.

- *Organ cytotoxic effects.* Some drugs have adverse effects on organs, particularly the liver, kidney, and pancreas. Drugs such as acetaminophen, NSAIDs, and sulfonamide antibiotics can cause hepatotoxicity and susceptibility is increased if the liver function is already compromised by chronic alcohol use or disease. Most of the time hepatotoxicity is due to a metabolite, which either initiates an immune reaction or has direct toxicity on the liver cells. Nausea, anorexia, and jaundice are symptoms common to hepatotoxicity. Many drugs such as NSAIDs (ibuprofen, Chapter 6) and aminoglycoside antibiotics (Amikin, Chapter 5) have the potential to cause nephrotoxicity. Toxicity is usually dose-related. Pancreatitis can also result from administration of some drugs such as estrogens, sulfonamides, and tetracyclines. Organ function tests are sometimes part of the standard protocol for use of some drugs to monitor for potential organ cytotoxicity. These ADRs typically require a reduction of drug dosage or discontinuation of the drug depending on the severity of the adverse response.

- *Idiosyncratic reactions.* An idiosyncrasy is a reaction that is peculiar to an individual or a defined group of people. As a result of genetic makeup that is different than the general population, a patient may be very sensitive to small doses of a drug or highly insensitive to high doses of a drug. The gene that codes for a specific drug metabolizing enzyme, for example, may code for an abnormal structure for the enzyme so that it metabolizes the drug much slower than the normal enzyme. Consequently, the drug may have an unusually long duration of action. Alterations of the receptor structure through a change in the structure of the gene that codes for the receptor could increase or decrease the affinity or efficacy related to that receptor.

- *Drug–drug interactions.* As discussed previously, as the number of drugs used concurrently in the same patient increases, there is an increased likelihood of drug interactions. When the drug interaction results in a disadvantage to the patient, the drug interaction is an ADR. These drug interactions may result from the use of prescription, OTC, or herbal medicines or alcohol. Oral contraceptives are examples of drugs that interact with several other drugs, resulting in either a decreased effectiveness of the oral contraceptive or an altered effect from the other drug. Table 3-5 lists some examples of drug interactions with oral contraceptives.

- *Drug–food interactions.* Because each patient's diet changes daily, it is difficult to incorporate the impact of drug–food interactions into the dosage regimen of the patient. Consequently, most significant drug–food interactions are considered ADRs. Warfarin (Coumadin), for example, is an anticoagulant for which many drug–food interactions have been reported; all vitamin K containing foods (eg, broccoli, cabbage, lettuce, green tea) are physiologic antagonists to warfarin activity. Dairy products are rich in calcium and can prevent the absorption of tetracycline antibiotics. Aged cheeses and meats should be avoided in patients being treated with monoamine oxidase inhibitors (MAOIs), a class of antidepressants, because they may enhance the effect of these drugs. Examples of monoamine oxidase inhibitors are tranylcypromine (Parnate) and phenelzine (Nardil).

- *Drug–herbal medicine interactions.* As with drug–food interactions, drug–herbal medicine interactions are generally considered ADRs because it is difficult to predict the extent of the interaction. Contributing significantly in this regard is the lack of established standards of quality for these products. Nonetheless, many drug–herbal medicine interactions have been reported. For example, St. John's wort, which has been used to treat many conditions including depression, may increase the activity of MAOIs used concurrently to treat depression. Ginkgo has been used to treat conditions that include peripheral vascular disease and dementia and may increase the effects of anticoagulant drugs being used concurrently. Athletic trainers should be aware that herbal medicines contain compounds that have the potential to cause interactions and thus should be considered along with prescription and OTC drugs when considering a patient's total drug usage.

Table 3-5. Examples of Drug Interactions with Oral Contraceptives

Generic Name	Trade Name	Result of Interaction/Comments
phenobarbital	Luminal	Diminishes effectiveness of oral contraceptives. Other barbiturates may have same effect.
carbamazepine	Tegretol	Diminishes effectiveness of oral contraceptive. Other anticonvulsants such as phenytoin (Dilantin) and felbamate (Felbatol) have a similar effect.
ampicillin	Omnipen	Anecdotal reports of diminished oral contraceptive effect. Other penicillins may have a similar effect.
griseofulvin	Fulvicin	Diminishes effectiveness of oral contraceptive. Other antifungal drugs may have a similar effect.
pioglitazone	Actos	Possibility that oral contraceptive decreases the oral hypoglycemic effect of this and other hypoglycemic drugs such as tolazamide (Tolinase).
rifampin	Rifadin	Diminishes effectiveness of oral contraceptive by this antibiotic.
St John's Wart		May diminish effectiveness of oral contraceptive.
doxycycline	Vibramycin	Anecdotal reports of diminished oral contraceptive effect. Other tetracyclines may have a similar effect.
warfarin	Coumadin	Decreases the anticoagulant effect of warfarin.

- *Use during pregnancy.* Because the placenta does not exclude molecules to the same extent as the *blood-brain barrier*, it is assumed that most drugs cross the placental barrier to some extent. This poses the potential for adverse reactions in a selected population for whom the drug is not intended. The Food and Drug Administration (FDA) has a use-in-pregnancy rating system (Table 3-6), which considers the extent to which information about the drug has ruled out the drug as a risk factor for the developing baby against the potential benefit of the drug to the patient. No effort is made in this textbook to specify the pregnancy risk of the drugs discussed. Such information is available, however, in many drug information handbooks. Online sources are also available that provide information about use of drugs in pregnancy and during breastfeeding. For example, www.perinatology.com/exposures/druglist.htm provides such information for an extensive list of drugs along with search capability.

Summary

Adverse drug reactions is a broad term that refers to any undesirable response from a drug. Side effects are predictable, dose-related adverse effects. Allergic reactions range from relatively minor rash to life-threatening anaphylaxis. Most allergic drug reactions are caused by penicillins

Table 3-6. Food and Drug Administration Ratings for Drug Use-in-Pregnancy Safety

Category A	Controlled studies show no risk. Controlled studies in pregnant women have failed to demonstrate a risk to the developing baby in any trimester of pregnancy.
Category B	No evidence of risk in humans. Controlled studies in pregnant women have not shown increased risk of abnormalities to the developing baby despite adverse findings in animals, or, in the absence of adequate human studies, animal studies show no risk. The chance of harm to the developing baby is remote, but remains a possibility.
Category C	Risk cannot be ruled out. Controlled human studies are lacking, and animal studies have shown a risk or are lacking also. There is a chance of harm to the developing baby if the drug is administered during pregnancy; however, the potential benefits may outweigh the potential risk.
Category D	Positive evidence of risk. Studies in humans, or investigational or postmarketing data, have demonstrated risk to the developing baby. Nevertheless, potential benefits from the use of the drug may outweigh the potential risk (eg, in a life-threatening situation or serious disease).
Category X	Contraindicated in pregnancy. Studies in animals or humans, or investigational or post-marketing reports, have demonstrated positive evidence of abnormalities or risk in the developing baby, which clearly outweighs any benefit to the patient.

and cephalosporin antibiotics, NSAIDs, and sulfonamides (eg, certain diuretics, oral hypoglycemic drugs, and sulf-containing antibiotics). Some drugs produce toxicity to selective organs and thus therapy with these drugs require periodic monitoring of organ function. Other drugs cause unusual and unpredictable adverse reactions to a small population of people due to some specific genetic make-up of that group of people. Interactions with food, herbal medicines, or other drugs also pose the potential for initiating ADRs. Use of drugs during pregnancy must be with caution because of the potential harm to the developing baby. An FDA classification of use-in-pregnancy risk categories is a useful guide regarding the relative risk-to-benefit of using any drug during pregnancy.

MEDICATION ERRORS

Medication errors result in the wrong dose or the wrong drug being administered to the patient. The consequences of these errors range from having relatively little effect to being fatal. These errors are often caused from miscommunication of oral or written instructions from one health care professional to another or to the patient. For example, a pharmacist who fails to repeat the verbal order back to the physician, or notorious is the poor handwriting of physicians that results in the misinterpretation of the prescription by the pharmacist. Contributing significantly to the problem is the fact that there are an increasing number of drugs that have similar spellings or pronunciations with another drug. For example, Levatol (penbutolol) and Lipitor (atorvastatin) are close in spelling but quite different in terms of their effects. Although this pair of drugs has only three letters in common, coupled with poor handwriting or misspelling, they can be confused. These type of look-alike or sound-alike drugs account for approximately 15% to 25% of reported medication errors. Table 3-7 lists some of the many examples of drug pairs that look or sound alike. The problem is compounded when the dosage unit is the same for the

Table 3-7. Examples of Drugs With Similar Names

aspirin	Asendin	Darvocet-N	Darvon-N
aspirin	Afrin	Demerol	Demulen
albuterol	atenolol	Demerol	Dymelor
albuterol	Albutein	Demerol	Temaril
Aldomet	Aldoril	digoxin	Desoxyn
Aldomet	Anzemet	digoxin	digitoxin
Aleve	Alesse	digoxin	doxepin
Amicar	Amikin	Ecotrin	Edecrin
Amicar	amikacin	Ecotrin	Akineton
ampicillin	aminophylline	ephedrine	epinephrine
Atrovent	Alupent	ethanol	Ethyol
bacitracin	Bactrim	Femara	Femhrt
bacitracin	Bactroban	Maalox	Maolate
baclofen	Bactroban	Maalox	Marax
baclofen	Beclovent	Mylanta	Milontin
Benadryl	Bentyl	Nicobid	Nitro-Bid
Benadryl	Benylin	Nicoderm	Nitro-Derm
Benadryl	benazepril	penicillamine	penicillin
Bicillin	V-Cillin	Percogesic	paregoric
Bicillin	Wycillin	PhosLo	PhosChol
Brethaire	Brethine	prednisolone	prednisone
Brethine	Banthine	Prozac	Prilosec
Brethine	Brethaire	Reminyl	Robinul
cefamandole	cefmetazole	rimantadine	ranitidine
cefazolin	cefprozil	Septra	Sectral
Cefobid	cefonicid	Septra	Septa
Cefotan	Ceftin	sulfasalazine	sulfisoxazole
cefoxitin	Cytoxan	sulfasalazine	Salsalate
cefoxitin	cefotaxime	sulfasalazine	sulfadiazine
cefoxitin	cefotetan	Ticlid	Tequin
cefizoxime	ceftazidime	Triaminic	TriHemic
cefizoxime	cefotaxime	Triaminic	Triaminicin
cefizoxime	cefuroxime	Tylenol	Tylox
Celebrex	Cerebyx	Tylenol	Tuinal
codeine	Cardene	Verelan	Vivarin
codeine	Lodine	Verelan	Voltaren
Cytoxan	Cytotec	Verelan	Ferralyn
Cytoxan	Cytosar U	Verelan	Virilon
Cytoxan	CytoGam	Vicodin	Hycodan
Cytoxan	cefoxitin	Volmax	Flomax
Cytoxan	Ciloxan	Zyrtec	Zyprexa

Note: Trade names are capitalized.
Adapted from Davis NM. Drug names that look and sound alike. *Hospital Pharmacy*. 1999;34:1160-1178.

two drugs, such as Lanoxin (digoxin) 0.125 mg tablets and Levoxine (levothyroxine) 0.125 mg tablets.

Besides wrong drug, administering the wrong dose is another type of error. Misplaced decimal points have resulted in toxic symptoms or death. For doses that are less than one unit, use of a decimal without a zero to the left of the decimal (ie, .5 rather than 0.5) has resulted in 10-fold error; a decimal point should never be used without a digit to the left (leading zero) when writing a dose. The lack of a leading zero can also cause a misinterpretation of the desired drug (eg, Flomax .4 mg mistaken for Volmax 4 mg).

Misinterpretation of oral instructions to the patient is also a significant contributor to medication errors. The health care professional cannot assume that the patient understands the directions exactly as they were intended. The best way to ensure that the patient understands when and how to take medications is to have him or her repeat back his or her interpretation of the instructions. In some cases, such as use of asthma inhalers, the patient should demonstrate the use of the medication so that there is no confusion as to proper technique. Because misinterpretation of instructions to the patient is a significant problem, the athletic trainer can play a role in reducing medication errors. As a check-point beyond the physician and pharmacist, the athletic trainer can ensure that the athlete clearly understands medication-use instructions.

IMPACT OF EXERCISE

The effect of exercise on the pharmacodynamics is primarily due to the pharmacokinetics discussed in Chapter 2. In other words, the dose-response effects, as a result of getting the drug to the site of action, depend on the absorption, metabolism, distribution, and excretion parameters. The effect of exercise directly on the pharmacodynamics (ie, the effect on the response from the drug once it is at the site of action) has not been extensively studied in humans. Exercise can affect the number and intrinsic efficacy of some receptors, such as β-adrenergic receptors, but the varied impact on the pharmacokinetic parameters deters any conclusive statement regarding therapeutically significant changes in the pharmacodynamics as a result of exercise.

Exercise is a component of nondrug therapy for treatment of some conditions such as diabetes, hypertension, cardiovascular disease, and arthritis. Theoretically, therefore, exercise should contribute to the effectiveness of the drugs used to treat these diseases. Yet, again, due to a change in multiple parameters, there is little evidence that exercise alone will improve the disease to the extent that a reduction in drug therapy is predictable. Complicating the picture of exercise effects on pharmacodynamics is that exercise alters the release of some endogenous hormone and neurotransmitters, which may alter the pharmacokinetics and pharmacodynamics of some drugs.

BIBLIOGRAPHY

Bachmann KA, Lewis JD, Fuller MA, Bonfiglio MF, eds. *Drug Interactions Handbook*. Hudson, Ohio: Lexi-Comp Inc; 2003.

Brody TM, Larner J, Minneman KP. *Human Pharmacology, Molecular to Clinical*. 3rd ed. St Louis, Mo: Mosby; 1998.

Claxton AJ, Cramer J, Pierce C. Systematic review of the associations between dose regimens and medication compliance. *Clin Ther*. 2001;23:1296-1310.

Davis NM. Drug names that look and sound alike. *Hospital Pharmacist*. 1999;34:1160-1178.

Maize DF, Culhane JM. Tools for evaluating drug action. *US Pharmacist*. 2001;26:42-47.s

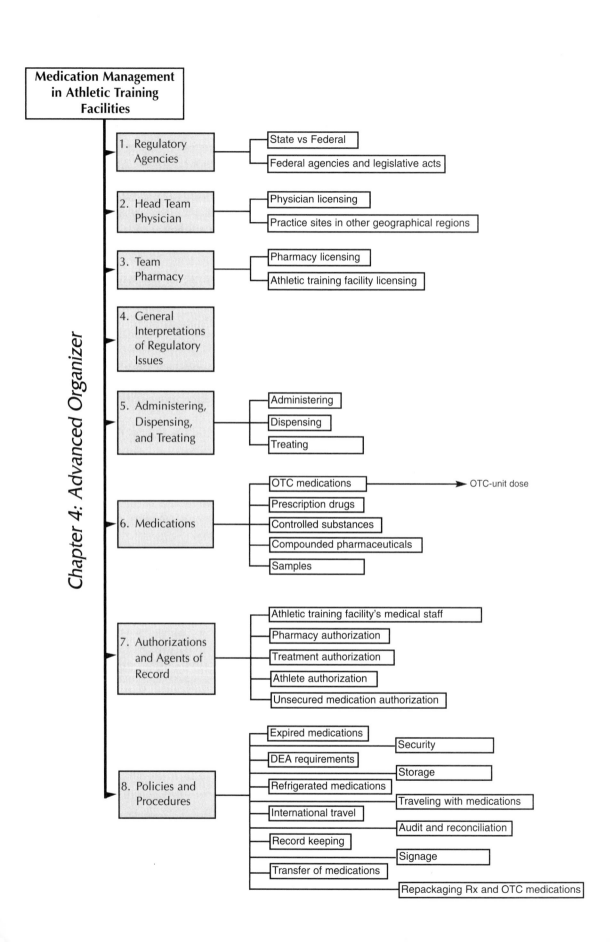

MEDICATION MANAGEMENT IN ATHLETIC TRAINING FACILITIES

Robert Nickell, RPh, FACA, FAPO

CHAPTER OBJECTIVES

At the end of this chapter, the reader will be able to:
- Explain the role of state and federal regulations regarding prescription medications.
- Explain the role of various federal agencies in the regulation of medications.
- Locate federal regulations that are pertinent to the dispensing, administering, storing, packaging, labeling, and transporting medications.
- Explain the role of the head team physician and team pharmacy regarding licensing in regards to multiple sites and travel.
- Differentiate between discretionary and nondiscretionary decisions.
- Differentiate between an administered dose, dispensed dose, and treatment.
- Differentiate between over-the-counter (OTC) medications, prescription drugs, controlled substances, compounded pharmaceuticals, and drug samples and explain pertinent regulations regarding each.
- Explain the concepts of authorizations and agents of record and describe how to meet these two standards.
- Write policies and procedures to meet state and federal laws regarding dispensing, administering, storing, packaging, labeling, and transporting of medications.

Medications and athletes have been intertwined since the first Olympic Games were held centuries ago. Athletes are competitive by nature and therefore seek access to top-of-the-line physicians, treatment programs, and medications. Quick rehabilitation is critical to the success of the athlete and the team. In many cases, initiating treatment for an athlete can greatly affect the outcome of a contest, game, or championship.

Within the past 20 years, government agencies and the media have taken an interest in the process of drug delivery in athletic training facilities. Major universities and professional teams have experienced significant legal, financial, and regulatory setbacks due to improper management of prescription drugs. Federal and state citations and grievances have been filed against team physicians, athletic directors, certified athletic trainers, and professional teams and organizations.

Within the past few years, not only have athletes been seriously injured because of medication mismanagement, but some cases have led to fatalities. As more drug-related errors are discovered and reported, the interest and involvement from government agencies regarding the management of prescription medications in athletic training facilities will increase significantly. If an athletic training facility is audited, the investigation will involve the review of record keeping; drug labeling, packaging, dispensing, administration, storage, and security; facility licensure; and much more. Ignorance, long-term practice, or denial are no excuses for violating the law. Athletic training facilities must implement the proper medication management practices to comply with federal drug laws.[1]

Imagine if a federal law carried a minimum citation of $5000 and up to 1 year in jail for each violation. Violations are counted by the number of actual and potential incidences. If there were 100 small containers of samples in the athletic training room in an unlocked, unsupervised environment, the inspector or medical board could actually make a charge of >100 individual violations against the organization, athletic department, head athletic trainer, and the team physician.

REGULATORY AGENCIES

The purpose of regulatory agencies is to protect the consumer and the public. Their concerns include issues relating to drug diversion, negligence, licensure, and wrongful medical practice. Through the enforcement of regulations written by legislatures and consumer boards, regulatory agencies ensure the provision of health care by qualified practitioners.

In many cases, there is no specific language addressing regulatory issues either at the state or federal level with regard to athletic training as a medical industry. When a law does not exist concerning a certain practice, the inspector must attempt to interpret the code from other laws affecting similar practices of medicine. National and state bodies governing athletic training must be proactive and establish internal policies and standards of practice.

State Versus Federal

In general, state and federal regulations for prescription medications are closely aligned. The rule of thumb is if state and federal laws are in conflict, the licensed entity should follow the stricter of the two codes. Most state laws are directed toward physicians who are dispensing for profit to the general population which may create a conflict of interest, or competition with local pharmacies. Only a few states, including Ohio, South Carolina, Virginia, California, and Florida, have acknowledged that medical practice exists in athletic training facilities. Federal and state laws are consistent when the physician is dispensing or administering directly to his or her patients in a closed environment. Table 4-1 summarizes state pharmacy practice acts and drug laws as well as the role of the athletic trainer in dispensing and administering medications. It is illegal for an athletic trainer to dispense medication, although there is some variability in state laws regarding the administration of nonprescription mediation by licensed health providers in a single dose pack.[1] For the purposes of this chapter, we will focus on federal laws that specifically relate to the dispensing of medications by physicians directly to their own athletes.

Federal Agencies and Legislative Acts (Also See Chapter 1)

Several federal agencies are responsible for different functions related to the regulation of medications. These include the Food and Drug Administration (FDA), Drug Enforcement Administration (DEA), Occupational Safety and Health Administration (OSHA), and the Federal Trade Commission (FTC). The function of each of these organizations is outlined in Box 4-1.

Additionally, there are also numerous federal legislative acts designed to regulate medication control and distribution. Box 4-2 shows a chronological time line of creation and implementation based on changes in society and in the practice of medicine. Box 4-3 highlights specific federal regulations pertinent to athletic training facilities.

Table 4-1. State Pharmacy Practice Acts and Drug Laws

State	Dispense	Administer	Certified Athletic Trainer Dispense	Certified Athletic Trainer Administer
AL	#	*	No	*, †
AK	‡	IIII	No	*, †
AZ	¶	¶¶	No	*, †
AR	**	*	No	*, †
CA	¶	IIII	No	*, †
CO	‡,II	IIII	No	*, †
CT	¶	IIII	No	*, †
DE	#	*	No	*, †
FL	††, ‡‡	***	No	*, †
GA	¶	¶¶***	No	*, †
HI	‡	¶¶	No	*, †
ID	#	*	No	*, †
IL	‡	*	No	*, †
IN	¶	*	No	*, †
IA	§	IIII	No	*, †
KS	§	IIII	No	*, †
KY	II	¶, IIII	No	*, †
LA	‡	IIII	No	*, †
ME	¶	*	No	*, †
MD	¶	*	No	*, †
MA	¶,**	*	No	*, †
MI	‡	*	No	*, †
MN	¶	*	No	*, †
MS	§§	IIII	No	*, †
MO	§	IIII	No	*, †
MT	§	IIII	No	*, †
NE	‡	¶¶	No	No
NV	‡	*	No	*, †
NH	II,**	***	No	*, †
NJ	‡	¶¶	No	*, †
NM	‡	¶¶		
NY	*	*	No	*, †
NC	#,§§	IIII	No	*, †
ND	¶	##	No	No
OH	¶	*	No	*, †
OK	**	IIII	No	*, †
OR	¶	*	No	*, †
PA	**	IIII	No	*, †
RI	**	¶¶	No	No
SC	II,¶,**	IIII	No	*, †
SD	¶¶	IIII	No	*, †
TN	‡	IIII	No	*, †
TX	#	IIII	No	*, †

continued

Table 4-1. State Pharmacy Practice Acts and Drug Laws (continued)

State	Dispense	Administer	Certified Athletic Trainer Dispense	Certified Athletic Trainer Administer
UT	¶	IIII	No	*, †
VT	#	*	No	*, †
VA	¶	¶ ¶	No	No
WA	*, §§	IIII	No	*, †
WV	¶	IIII	No	*, †
WI	¶	¶ ¶	No	*, †
WY	‡	IIII	No	No

* Not included in the definition of "practice of pharmacy."

† Not included in Medical Practice Act.

‡ Dispense means to deliver a controlled dangerous substance or controlled substance analog to an ultimate user of research subject pursuant to the lawful order of a practitioner, including the prescribing, administering, packaging, labeling, or compounding necessary to prepare the substance for that delivery.

§ Substitute prescription drug for controlled substance in footnote ‡.

II Dispense or dispensing means to deliver one or more doses of a prescription drug in a suitable container, appropriately labeled for subsequent administration to or use by a patient or other individual entitled to receive the prescription drug.

¶ Dispense or dispensing means the preparation and delivery of a drug or device to a patient or patient's agent under a lawful order of a practitioner in a suitable container appropriately labeled for subsequent administration to, or use by, a patient.

Dispense means preparing and packaging a prescription drug or device in a container and labeling the container with information required by state and federal law; filling or refilling drug-container prescription drugs for subsequent use by a patient; or providing quantities for unit-dose prescription drugs for subsequent administration.

** Dispense means to sell, distribute, leave with, give away, dispose or deliver, or supply.

†† Dispense is not considered administration.

‡‡ Dispensing is done by a pharmacist.

§§ Dispense is interpreted as delivery of a prescription drug by a practitioner of drug or device for administration to a patient.

IIII Administer means the direct application of a drug to a patient or research subject by injection, inhalation, or ingestion, whether topically or by any other means.

¶ ¶ Administer means the direct application of a controlled dangerous substance or controlled substance analog, whether by injection, inhalation, ingestion, or any other means, to the body of a patient or research subject by (1) a practitioner (or in his presence by a his lawfully authorized agent) or (2) the patient or research subject at the lawful direction and in the presence of the practitioner.

Administration is the delivery of prescription medication to the user under the lawful order of a practitioner or midlevel practitioner.

*** Administer or administration means the provision of a unit dose of medication to an individual patient as a result of the order of an authorized practitioner of the healing arts.

Reprinted with permission from Kahavov L, Furst D, Johnson S, Roberts J. Adherence to drug-dispensation and drug-administration laws and guidelines in collegiate athletic training rooms. *Journal of Athletic Training.* 2003;38(3):252-258.

Box 4-1. Function of Federal Agencies in Regulating Medications

Agency	Function
Food and Drug Administration (FDA)	Responsible for overseeing and regulating the manufacturing, repackaging, and relabeling of prescription drugs. The FDA also regulates sample medications and is responsible for the enforcement of regulation resulting from food, dietary supplement injuries, or complaints.
Drug Enforcement Administration (DEA)	Oversees licensure and certification of all locations where controlled substances are ordered, received, stored, administered, or dispensed.
Occupational Safety and Health Administration (OSHA)	Responsible for contamination, storage, disposal, and public exposure to medication risks.
Federal Trade Commission (FTC)	Responsible for regulating medications transported over state lines that have not yet been prescribed and/or dispensed to the patient.

Box 4-2. Federal Acts Related to Medication Control and Distribution

Date	Act	Purpose
1938	Federal Food, Drug and Cosmetic Act (FDCA) (52 Stat, 1040; 21 USC 301 et al)	This law was established to regulate the safety, quality, purity, strength, and labeling of drugs.
1951	Humphrey Amendment	Was enacted in 1951 and took effect in 1952. This amendment established two classes of drugs by differentiating between prescription and nonprescription or over-the-counter medications.
1962	Good Manufacturing Practice (GMP) Regulations	Were established by the Kefauver-Harris Amendment, which required all repackaging operations to meet minimum standards for the repackaging of medications.
1970	Federal Comprehensive Drug Abuse Prevention and Control Act	Regulated the manufacture, distribution, and dispensing of drugs that have a potential of abuse. Registration with the DEA is required to legally assume any of these responsibilities.
1970	Poison Prevention Act	Passed to regulate the packaging of prescription and nonprescription drugs in child-resistant safety containers.
1983	Federal Anti-Tampering Act	Established to mandate tamper resistant packaging on all nonprescription drugs.
1983	Fair Packaging and Labeling Act	Mandated labeling of contents of nonprescription drugs to assist consumers in identifying similar products.
1987	Prescription Drug Marketing Act	Mandated the accountability of sample drugs from the manufacturer to the physician to the end user.

continued

Box 4-2. Federal Acts Related to Medication Control and Distribution (continued)

Date	Act	Purpose
1988	Anti-Drug Abuse Act	Reclassified anabolic steroids as controlled substances.
1990	Omnibus Reconciliation Act (OBRA 90)	Mandated drug review, patient medication records, and verbal patient education as part of the dispensing of prescription medications.
2003	Health Insurance Portability and Accountability Act (HIPAA)	Mandated the protection of patient information and confidentiality by all health practitioners involved with protected health information (PHI).

Box 4-3. Federal Regulations Specific to the Management of Prescription Medications in the Athletic Training Facility

Prescription Drug Marketing Act

21 CFR 5.115 - Sample medication control
21 CFR 1301.23(1) - DEA certificate required for separate locations
21 C.F.R. 1301.75 - Storage of controlled substances
21 C.F.R. 1301.44 - DEA certificate readily retrievable
21 C.F.R. 1301.90 - Security of personnel for handling of controlled substances
21 C.F.R. 1304.4 - Record-keeping requirements for controlled substances
21 C.F.R. 1304.02(d) - Defines a physician who prescribes, administers, and dispenses controlled substances
21 C.F.R. 1304.11-12(b) - Inventory requirements for controlled substances
21 C.F.R. 1304.13 - Reconciliation requirements for controlled substances
21 C.F.R. 1305.12 - Reporting a theft of a controlled substance
21 C.F.R. 1301.92 - Responsibility to report drug diversion

Food, Drug, and Cosmetic Act

21 U.S.C. 360(g) - Requirement to utilize a FDA licensed pharmacy repackager
21 U.S.C. 353(b)(2) - Labeling of prescription medications

Poison Prevention Packaging Act

15 U.S.C. 1471 - Packaging of controlled substances and prescription medications
15 U.S.C. 1473 (b) - Exception to PPPA for prescriber dispensing of nonchild safety container

Federal Controlled Substance Act

21 U.S.C., 824(a)(f) - DEA certificate required
21 U.S.C. 802(10) - Prescriber dispensing
21 U.S.C. 823 (f) - DEA certificate required for separate locations
21 U.S.C. 802(10) - Defines a dispensing physician vs an individual practitioner
21 U.S.C. 827(c) (1) (A) (B) - Acquisition and Disposition record-keeping requirements for individual practitioners dispensing controlled substances.

HEAD TEAM PHYSICIAN

Anytime there are medications stored at an athletic training facility, there must be a licensed physician who accepts responsibility for the medications. This is required if there is only one medication such as an inhaler or EpiPen for emergencies or an entire dispensary. All medications ordered, received, stored, dispensed, and/or administered to the athlete are the legal responsibility of the licensure of the head team physician.

Physician Licensing

Most physicians maintain a DEA certificate to prescribe controlled substances. However, the DEA requires an additional and separate DEA certificate for any and all locations where controlled substances are ordered, received, stored, administered, and dispensed. In some cases, a team physician will maintain up to five or six separate DEA certificates, depending on the number of teams and organizations they are representing. In some states (eg, New York, Illinois, Ohio, and Florida), a state-controlled substance license is required in addition to the DEA certificate.

Practice Sites in Other Geographic Locations

It is not unusual for an organization to operate a summer or spring practice camp in another state. Even if this camp is used for only 1 month, the licensure laws must be followed. According to most state and federal agencies, if a physician sets up practice for >5 days (this is an average, the amount of time is arbitrary and can be anywhere from 2 days to 1 week depending on the agency and the inspector answering the question) at any one location and stores, dispenses, administers, or receives medications of any kind, he or she is required to license the additional athletic training facility and to maintain a personal license to practice medicine in that state. For example, if an organization is located in New York and has a summer practice camp in Philadelphia, the team physicians must obtain a license to practice in Pennsylvania, or the organization must affiliate with a local physician licensed to practice medicine in that state. Additionally, a large university may have more than one athletic training facility on campus. If each athletic training facility receives, stores, administers, or dispenses medications, then each would require separate and distinct licensing.

TEAM PHARMACY

In a best-practice situation, each athletic training facility should have a designated team pharmacy. It is ideal to have one pharmacy service the entire organization. This allows for consistency in packaging, consultation, site inspections, and audit control. This pharmacy should be on call and ready to service the athletes, athletic trainers, and team physicians with all of their medication questions, prescription supplies, special compounds, and regulatory affairs. The team pharmacy should be an integrated element of the sports medicine practice within the athletic training facility.

Pharmacy Licensing

The team pharmacy is required to be licensed by the state in which it is located and by the DEA to handle controlled substances. If an athletic team is traveling, or has a summer or spring practice camp in another state, the team pharmacy may also have to be licensed to practice pharmacy in that state to ship medications across state lines. The team pharmacy must be licensed by

Producers of drugs or devices, or "manufacturers," include the activity of "repackaging," defined as, "changing the container, wrapper, or labeling of any drug package to further the distribution of the drug from the original place of manufacture to the person who makes final delivery or sale to the ultimate consumer." Repackaging of drugs by a pharmacy is considered to be a manufacturing activity, and is therefore under FDA jurisdiction (21 USC§360 Federal Food, Drug, and Cosmetic Act: Drugs and Devices).

the FDA if it is prepackaging medications that are not yet designated for an individual athlete but will be dispensed or administered by the team physician in the athletic training facility.

Athletic Training Facility Licensing

On behalf of the team physician, the athletic trainer should maintain a copy of the team pharmacy licenses from the state board of pharmacy and DEA and an FDA repackaging permit. If the athletic training facility is contracted with a waste disposal company and medications are placed there, the waste disposal company must be licensed to destroy prescription medications and a copy of the license should also be kept on file.

GENERAL INTERPRETATIONS OF REGULATORY ISSUES

When a regulatory agency is investigating an alleged drug-related mismanagement complaint, it will need to determine who has made discretionary vs nondiscretionary decisions. The persons making discretionary decisions must be licensed to do so. Within the athletic training facility, discretionary decisions such as diagnosing, prescribing, dispensing, and administering can ONLY be made by the physician and may not be delegated to unlicensed personnel. An illustration of the discretionary decision process is as follows:

1. The diagnosis of the athlete is considered a discretionary decision. In some cases, the team physician may contact the athletic trainer and discuss the condition of the athlete. The physician may want to review previous medications the athlete has used and may rely on the athletic trainer for evaluation. However, the team physician must make the final assessment for the medical diagnosis.

2. After making the medical diagnosis, the physician may make the discretionary decision of prescribing. The physician may ask the athletic trainer which medications the athlete has taken in the past (OTC/prescription). The athletic trainer may help identify possible allergies, but the choice of which medication to be administered or dispensed must be made by the team physician. When team physicians are dispensing or administering medications from their own office or practice location, they are not required to write a prescription, although they must keep an accurate record of the transaction. A written prescription is required when a licensed entity other than the team physician is dispensing the medication. Part of the definition of dispensing is the interpretation of a prescription order.

3. The dispensation or administration of medications is considered a discretionary decision. Only a physician or other duly licensed authorized person, such as a pharmacist, nurse practitioner, or physician assistant, is allowed to dispense or administer medications. The athletic trainer may assist in nondiscretionary roles such as record keeping and the labeling process.

A physician may use assistants or medical staff to assist in the "process" of dispensing under supervision. Record keeping, delivery, and minor labeling are among several nondiscretionary decisions appropriate for the athletic trainer to perform. Only the physician can make the final decision and authorize the medication to the athlete.

Box 4-4. Difference Between Administered Dose, Dispensed Dose, and Treatment

Administered dose	A medication given to a patient that is consumed within 24 hours.
Dispensed dose	An amount of medication to be consumed by the patient over a period of time >24 hours.
Treatment	Medications applied or injected within the athletic training facility.

ADMINISTERING, DISPENSING, AND TREATING

There are three ways in which medications can be delivered by the physician. Each way has a clear regulatory definition (Box 4-4). Medications can be administered, dispensed, or applied as a treatment within licensed athletic training facilities.

Administering

An "administered" dose is defined by law as a medication given to the patient that is consumed within 24 hours. The labeling requirements for an administered dose are quite different from a dispensed dose. According to the FDA, a dose administered by the licensed entity has minimal labeling requirements, such as directions for use and patient's name, but still must adhere to the same record-keeping requirements such as inventory, reconciliation, and drug usage logs.

Have you ever wondered why manufacturer samples come in such small quantities? A frequent question is, "Why all this packaging for two pills in one small container?" The reason is because a "sample" is designed by law to serve as an administered dose. However, if the physician grabs a handful of sample containers, the medication now becomes a dispensed dose and must be labeled and recorded according to state and federal dispensing laws.

Dispensing

A "dispensed" dose is an amount of medication to be consumed by the patient over a period of time >24 hours. The best method of delivery for a dispensed dose in athletic training facilities is a "therapeutic dose pack," which is prepackaged by a licensed FDA repackager in an appropriate course of therapy. The FDA requires that any entity that packages medications in advance for anyone other than the patient must obtain licensure to do so. An athletic training facility, student health center, local pharmacy, or hospital should not package their own therapeutic dose packs for physician dispensing unless they are licensed by the FDA to repackage.

All dispensed doses are subject to state and federal laws for packaging, labeling, and record-keeping requirements. They must contain the following on the label as well as on the dispensing log:

- Patient name
- Date of service
- Physician name
- Medication name
- Strength
- Dosage form
- Quantity

- Expiration date
- Lot number
- Initials of medical assistant recording data as well as initials of the dispensing physician
- Address of the athletic training facility where the medications were dispensed

Treating

Finally, a medication can be administered as a treatment. Because the treatment is applied or injected within the athletic training facility, there are no labeling requirements; however, all records must still be maintained. Treatments are either injections used during a surgical or medical procedure or medications applied according to the physician's orders via iontophoresis or phonophoresis as part of on-going rehabilitation.

MEDICATIONS

Over-the-Counter Medications

OTC medications are products that can be purchased without a prescription and are not considered a food or dietary supplement. OTC medications are regulated by the FDA. If the athletic trainer is asked by the athlete for a recommendation of an OTC medication and the athletic trainer has listened to the athlete and made a recommendation, the athletic trainer could be illegally making a medical diagnosis. Athletic training facilities should maintain protocols for the recommendations of OTC medications, and implement a drug usage log containing the athlete's name, date of service, name of medication, strength, dosage form, quantity, purpose, the initials of the athletic trainer, and the initials of the athlete. The athletic trainer should act within the scope of practice for athletic training at all times. The scope of practice is determined by the laws governing the practice of athletic training in a particular state as well as the Role Delineation Study published by the National Athletic Trainers' Association Board of Certification Inc. If the practice falls outside these parameters, in some cases, comparing the practice of peers in a similar situation would suffice. It is important to note athletic training students do not have a legally defined scope of practice, and therefore these types of responsibilities should not be delegated by the athletic trainer.

OTC—Unit Dose

OTC medications should not be left on the athletic training facility counters in bulk containers for the athletes to simply "scoop up" what they desire. In addition to creating record-keeping and potential therapy problems, this can lead to contamination from athletes pouring medications into their hands and then re-pouring them back into the container. Almost 90% of all OTCs are available as unit dose packs. A unit dose pack is designed as an administered dose and is pre-labeled to meet the requirements of the FDA and OSHA. If bulk drug medications such as sucrose tablets, vitamins, or calcium supplements are required for the athletes, the medications should be sent to a licensed FDA repackager to be placed in unit dose containers, or individual smaller containers should be purchased for individual athletes as deemed appropriate by the medical staff.

Prescription Drugs

All medications requiring a prescription are considered dangerous drugs. The FDA stipulates that any container for prescription medications prior to dispensing must carry the designation,

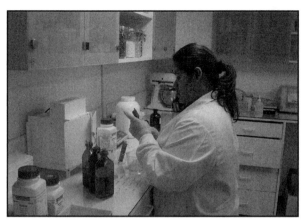

Figure 4-1. Compounded pharmaceutical. All pharmacists are licensed to compound; however, it has become such a specialty that training and experience can make quite a difference in the effectiveness and quality of the compounded product.

"Rx ONLY" (see Figure 1-2) on the label. Even it has been used in the athletic training room for years, if it bears the mark "Rx ONLY" it must be considered a prescription drug and treated as such according to state and federal laws.

Controlled Substances

Controlled substances are prescription drugs the DEA has determined to be "drugs of abuse" or "drugs of potential abuse." The medications are placed into five separate schedules (see Table 1-7).

Compounded Pharmaceuticals

A compounded pharmaceutical is prepared from raw chemicals in the team pharmacy (Figure 4-1). Although all pharmacists are licensed to compound, it has become such a specialty that training and experience can make quite a difference in the effectiveness and quality of the compounded product. The athletic trainer should check the qualifications of the team pharmacy if the team physician wishes to use compounded products.

Never accept unsolicited compounded products that are mailed by any pharmacies directly to your athletic training facility. According to the FDA, any compounded product is a prescription drug and all regulations must be followed. There is no such thing as a "sample" compounded pharmaceutical.

Compounded products may be extremely helpful in sports medicine and are used by many organizations.

Samples

Sample medications are sometimes considered trivial or not as regulated as prescription drugs. However, they are prescription and are governed by state and federal laws and enforced by the FDA. Sample medications are placed in small packages because they are designed to be "administered" doses. There are very specific guidelines that must be followed whenever sample medications are dispensed or administered by the physician (Box 4-5).

Box 4-5. Guidelines for Dispensing or Administering Sample Medications by a Physician

1. A pedigree or chain of custody must exist.

A pedigree is a receipt that must be supplied by the licensed entity or person delivering the sample medications to the receiving entity or person. The receipt must include the name of physician or manufacturer representative delivering and receiving, the name of the medication, the strength, the dosage form, the quantity, the lot number, the expiration date, the date of transfer, and the signatures of the physicians. The concept behind a pedigree is that the FDA inspector should be able to follow the trail of the sample medication from the manufacturer to the end user.

2. A separate audit and reconciliation must be maintained.

The FDA requires a separate audit and reconciliation for all sample medications, which shall account for each and every dose and dosage form being received and administered or dispensed by the physician's office or athletic training facility.

3. Samples must be stored separately from other prescription drugs.

Samples must be stored in a locked and secured cabinet separate from all other prescription drugs and controlled substances as they are not labeled in advance and can only be administered directly by the physician.

Adapted from 21 CFR 5.115 - Sample medication control

AUTHORIZATIONS AND AGENTS OF RECORD

Athletic Training Facility's Medical Staff

In many instances, the head team physician is not employed by the university or professional team. Likewise, the athletic training staff is not employed by the physician.

In addition, in most cases the organization pays for the medications and medical supplies that are used by the physician within the athletic training facility. Therefore, the physician must implement a strict agency of authorization for all individuals working within the facility. The agency statements should reflect the nondiscretionary decisions and actions to be performed by the athletic training staff and should include the following:

1. Authorization to forward prescription orders on behalf of the team physician.
2. Authorization to access the medication cabinet for purposes of inventory control and record keeping.
3. Authorization to assist the physician with nondiscretionary decisions.
4. A statement to the fact that this agency is created in the best medical interest of the athletes according to the head team physician.

The agency statement should be signed annually and updated as necessary by all practicing team physicians and all athletic trainers acting as agents for the physicians.

Pharmacy Authorization

The team physician must sign a separate annual acknowledgment directed to the pharmacy designating which members of the medical staff are authorized to forward prescription orders on

Name and strength of medication	Amount used in treatment	Type of modality	Date of treatment	Name of ATC	Name of physician	Time variable of treatment

Figure 4-2. An example of a form with necessary information that must be completed when any iontophoresis or phonophoresis treatment is given.

the physician's behalf. The document must also contain the exact physical address of the athletic training facility where the medications will be sent.

Treatment Authorization

In most athletic training facilities, the athletic trainer decides when to use iontophoresis or phonophoresis according to the standing orders and protocols of the athletic health care team. Because these treatments involve the use of prescription medications, state and federal regulations must be followed.

Prior to using any prescription medication for iontophoresis or phonophoresis, the athletic trainer must have written authorization from the team physician licensed to practice medicine in the athletic training facility. This authorization under protocol and according to the practice of medicine must be in the best medical interest of the athlete as determined by the physician. A record (Figure 4-2) must be maintained of the:

- Amount of medication used
- Type of modality
- Date of treatment
- Name of the athletic trainer
- Name of the authorizing physician
- Amount of time for the treatment

In some states, these treatments have been recognized specifically in law and every individual treatment prescription for an athlete must be prescribed in the athlete's name and dispensed in advance and used only for that particular athlete. Because iontophoresis and phonophoresis involve the use of prescription medications, these forms of treatment should be implemented by the athletic trainer and not delegated to a student.

Athlete Authorization

It is prohibited by law for anyone to pick up a prescription for someone other than immediate family unless they have been granted permission in writing. The pharmacy is responsible for ensuring this procedure. In many cases, the athletic training facility staff will act on behalf of the athlete by either picking up medications at the local pharmacy or signing for deliveries of medications. Each year the athlete should sign an authorization granting permission to specific members of the athletic training facilities staff to forward prescription orders, receive, pick up, secure, store, travel, and/or administer medications that have been prescribed and dispensed for him or her.

Unsecured Medication Authorization

Under certain circumstances there may be a need for prescription medication to be left in an unsecured location of the athletic training facility. Federal law specifically states that all medications are to be locked and secured. However, in the practice of medicine, the physician may want certain medications available for emergency reasons or treatments and may therefore choose to store them in an unsecured area. If this situation arises in the athletic training facility, it is a discretionary decision of the physician that is documented in writing. This documentation must list the medication to be left unsecured and the reason for the request; it should be signed by the head team physician, maintained on file, and renewed annually. Some of the medications most commonly stored in this way are: ethyl chloride, silver sulfadiazine, albuterol (inhaler), sodium chloride (for irrigation), Bactroban, EpiPen, and dexamethasone.

POLICIES AND PROCEDURES

A policy and procedure manual should be kept current and on file. This manual should be reviewed and revised annually by a committee consisting of the head team physician, the athletic trainer, and the team pharmacist. The purpose of this manual is to clearly define all aspects of the practice and operations of the athletic training facility. Policy and procedure statements reflecting more or less than the actual operation would suggest a need to change either the manual or the practice of operation. Every athletic training facility will have its own separate and unique policies and procedures. However, the general concepts mentioned in this chapter should be included in the manual.

Expired Medications

There is no justification for expired medications being stored in a facility or being administered or dispensed to an athlete. Expired medications must be removed from the active supplies. The medication name, strength, dosage form, quantity, lot number, expiration date, and the initials of the staff person doing the recording should be logged. A copy of the log should accompany the prescription medications to the outside agency contracted to handle their destruction. OTC medications that are expired should be disposed in a biohazard waste container. Flushing expired prescription and OTC medications is inappropriate.

Security

According to state and federal laws, all medications must be stored in a locked and secured cabinet or container. There are no specific laws to define "secure"; it is left up to the licensed professional to determine what is considered reasonable. Accordingly, "Rx Only" medications should not be found unsecured on an athletic training room counter.

> The term agency is used to define a "transfer of authority," similar to a power of attorney, except used as a definition for custodian or trustee to hold the key and have access to a licensed area belonging to the physician.

If the athletic training facility maintains medications that must be refrigerated, the refrigerator must have a lock. All access to keys or combination locks to the medical cabinet or locations where medications are stored and secured must be part of the policy and procedure manual. The head team physician must specifically identify and authorize by signature on agency statements those individuals being granted access. This authorization should be kept on file and maintained in a readily retrievable format for at least 3 years. There are some states, such as Ohio, that prohibit the granting of agency for keys. In some cases, some investigation may need to be done to determine whether a general manager, athletic director, or custodian may have a universal key that is not accounted for.

Drug Enforcement Agency Requirements

1. The DEA has a few specific regulations for controlled substances that are different than those for prescription drugs.
2. The DEA requires that controlled substances be stored securely and separately from all other prescription drugs.
3. The DEA requires a biannual inventory of all controlled substances. The inventory must be kept on file in a readily retrievable format.
4. The DEA requires any nonlicensed personnel who have been previously convicted of a crime relating to controlled substances to notify the professional licensed by the DEA maintaining responsibility for the controlled substances of this conviction in writing.
5. The DEA requires a separate certificate for every physical location where controlled substances are received, stored, administered, or dispensed.
6. The DEA requires separate records for acquisition and disposition of controlled substances.

Storage

Most medications must be stored at room temperature and in a dry environment. They should be stored in containers that allow for easy identification of the labeling. Controlled substances must be stored separately from all other prescription drugs. Medications should be stored in a secured and locked location within the athletic training facility.

Refrigerated Medications

All medications, including medications that require refrigeration, must be locked and secured. If there are vaccines or injections that require refrigeration, the refrigerator must be located in the licensed area at all times. It is a violation of federal and state law to store food or other nonpharmaceutical items in the same refrigerator as medications.

Traveling With Medications

Medications that have not been dispensed and labeled for the end user must be transported by a licensed individual or become the responsibility of the licensed individual upon reaching the intended destination. Some states have allowed the athletic trainer to transport medications under the conditions the he or she has access to a local physician or the team physician who is traveling separately. In other states, such as Ohio, it is prohibited by law for anyone other then the physician to transport medications that are not designated for the end user. In all cases, the medications must be locked and secured at all times. These drugs are the responsibility of the head team physician and must be tracked according to established policy and procedures of the athletic training facility.

Box 4-6. Considerations When Traveling Internationally With Medications

1. Have on hand at all times an inventory list of all medications being transported on behalf of the team. Include the name of the medication, strength, dosage form, and quantity. This may be requested or required for customs inspection.

2. An international travel policy and procedure manual should be carried with the medications.

3. A copy of the license for the team physician traveling and a signed permission slip for any medical staff who may be transporting medications on their behalf in between events or locations.

4. A list of all authorized athletes and staff traveling with the team should be maintained on file.

5. A signature file by the athlete or the legal guardian should be kept on file authorizing the physician and medical staff to treat the athletes during domestic and international travel.

6. Medication records should be reconciled immediately upon return to the states.

International Travel

State and federal laws do not specifically address international travel and therefore every effort must be made to follow the policies and procedures of the athletic training facility. Sometimes the team physician desires to bring medications manufactured in the United States. In many international events, avoiding banned substances is essential. The physician and medical staff must be able to read and comprehend the labeling on the medications dispensed or administered to the athletes. As in all situations, medications must be tracked and recorded. Some ideas to consider when traveling internationally are listed in Box 4-6.

Audit and Reconciliation

All medications should be completely audited and reconciled every year. This includes every dose and dosage form dispensed or administered. The audit should balance and the data maintained on file in a readily retrievable format for a period of 3 years.

Record Keeping

An assistant and/or medical staff may assist the physician with record keeping relating to the dispensing or administration of medications. The team physician is required by law to maintain all prescription data in a readily retrievable location for 3 years. These data should include the athlete's name, date of service, Rx number, physician name, medication name, strength, dosage form, quantity, expiration date, lot number, initials of assistant, and initials of physician. The records must also show a complete audit and reconciliation of all medications used within the athletic training facility. Auditing and reconciling should be done on an annual basis.

Basic records should include copies of all licenses for physicians, pharmacies, and waste disposal companies. Inventory records should include invoices, drug usage logs, reconciliation reports, separate controlled substance inventories, return drug reports, sample receipt logs and usage, and copies of any agency statements made by the physician. Records must be kept in storage for a minimum of 3 years and must be readily retrievable at all times.

Signage

Each athletic training facility should have an area or room specifically designated for the team physicians for examination of athletes and practice of medicine. That room should have proper signage signifying the space as a licensed medical office or clinic. This designated room should also be the site for medication storage.

Transfer of Medications

All medications are required by law to be labeled, except for sample medications when they are given in an administered dose. In some cases, the team physician has written a prescription in the name of the athletic trainer who provides the medication for athletes during treatments or travel. This is illegal in every state. It is against federal law for anyone to transfer medication prescribed and dispensed to them to someone else.

Repackaging Prescription and Over-the-Counter Medications in the Athletic Training Facility

Almost every athletic trainer uses a kit for practice and competition. When the athletic trainer is acting as the caregiver on behalf of the athlete, all regulations come into play. Taking bulk OTC medications and placing them into smaller plastic bottles for transport is repackaging and would be in violation of law. The bottles must be properly labeled by a licensed FDA repackager, and the original container may never be used again. Regulations regarding the storage and security of medications are not negated when the medications are packed in an athletic training kit. The athletic trainer should ensure that all medications contained in his or her kit are secure and are accessed only by the appropriate personnel.

Summary

There are many state and federal laws that govern the use, storage, record keeping, and transportation of OTC and prescription medication used in an athletic training facility. Athletic trainers should know federal laws as well as the pertinent state laws of the state in which they practice. Federal agencies responsible for different functions related to medications are the Food and Drug Administration (FDA), The Drug Enforcement Administration (DEA), and the Occupational Safety and Health Administration (OSHA). If the federal and state laws conflict, the stricter of the two laws should be followed.

The team physician has the legal responsibility of all medications and all discretionary decisions related to diagnosing, prescribing, dispensing, and administering drugs. The physician must have proper licensure in the state in which the team practices, including summer or spring practice camps.

Additionally, it is illegal for an athletic trainer to dispense medication, or to use prescription drugs for iontophoresis or phonophoresis without written authorization. Responsibilities of the athletic training staff relative to medications include: to assist the physician, conduct inventory control, participate in the development of policy and procedures manual, and maintain appropriate records. Basic records should include a copy of the licenses for the physicians, pharmacies, and waste disposal companies, drug use logs, annual medication audit reports, policies and procedures manual, record of athletes receiving or being administered medications, controlled substance inventories, and documentation to authorize drugs to be in an unsecured area.

All drugs must be stored in a locked and secured cabinet or container, whether they are OTC, prescription, controlled substances, compounded pharmaceuticals, or samples. Refrigerated items must also be locked. Controlled substances must be stored separately from other prescription drugs. Repackaging of medication must also be according to FDA regulations. Storage, security, and repackaging regulations also apply to drugs in the athletic trainer's kit.

Following state and federal regulations is important for the safety of the athletes as well as the integrity of the program. Therefore it is important for athletic trainers to be aware of and comply with these regulations.

REFERENCE

1. Kahanov L, Furst D, Roberts J. Adherence to drug-dispensation and drug-administration laws and guidelines in collegiate athletic training rooms. *Journal of Athletic Training.* 2003;38:252-258.

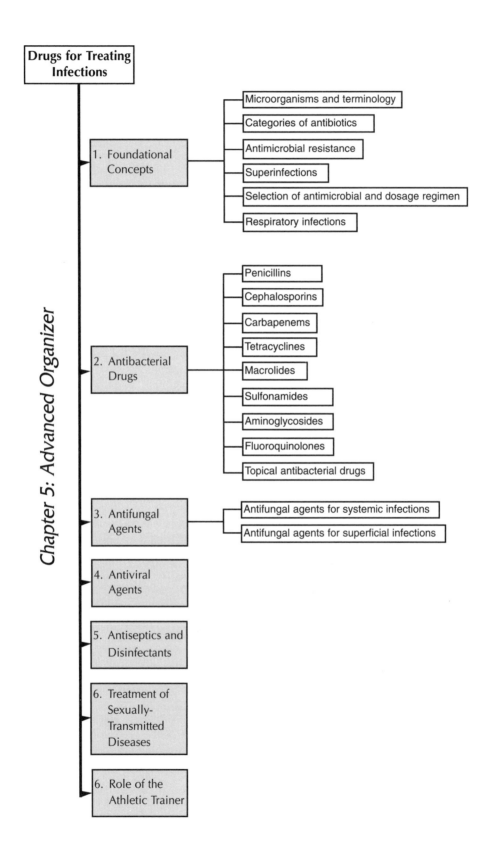

Chapter 5: Advanced Organizer

Drugs for Treating Infections

1. Foundational Concepts
   - Microorganisms and terminology
   - Categories of antibiotics
   - Antimicrobial resistance
   - Superinfections
   - Selection of antimicrobial and dosage regimen
   - Respiratory infections

2. Antibacterial Drugs
   - Penicillins
   - Cephalosporins
   - Carbapenems
   - Tetracyclines
   - Macrolides
   - Sulfonamides
   - Aminoglycosides
   - Fluoroquinolones
   - Topical antibacterial drugs

3. Antifungal Agents
   - Antifungal agents for systemic infections
   - Antifungal agents for superficial infections

4. Antiviral Agents

5. Antiseptics and Disinfectants

6. Treatment of Sexually-Transmitted Diseases

6. Role of the Athletic Trainer

DRUGS FOR TREATING INFECTIONS

CHAPTER OBJECTIVES

At the end of this chapter, the reader will be able to:
- Explain the differences between infections caused by bacteria, fungi, or viruses.
- Explain the mechanism(s) of action for antimicrobial, antifungal, and antiviral medications.
- List and describe the categories of antibiotics.
- Describe the process that results in a microorganism becoming resistant to an antibiotic drug(s).
- Explain how superinfections result from antibiotic therapy.
- List three considerations in prescribing an antibiotic medication.
- Discuss the role that antibiotics have in treating upper and lower respiratory infections.
- Differentiate between nine categories of antibiotic drugs.
- Explain the differences between superficial and systemic fungal infections.
- Summarize the causes, characteristics, and drug regimen for various types of fungal infections.
- Indicate the use of antiseptics and disinfectants.
- Summarize the role of the athletic trainer for patients who are taking antibiotic medication(s).

This chapter discusses basic information regarding infections and their treatment. Although the focus is on bacterial infections, fungal and viral infections are also discussed. *Antimicrobial* agents are among the most frequently prescribed drugs and thus it is important for the athletic trainer to have a clear understanding of the appropriate use of these drugs. Obviously, infections such as bacterial respiratory infections or systemic fungal infections have the potential to impact an athlete's performance. Use of the most effective antimicrobial agent at the most effective dosage will allow the athlete to return to optimal performance more quickly.

FOUNDATIONAL CONCEPTS

Antimicrobial refers to any drug used to treat any microorganism (eg, bacteria, fungi, or viruses). Some principles will be referred to throughout the discussion of antimicrobial agents. These include the terminology related to the infecting microorganism, microbial resistance, superinfections, selection of antimicrobial drug, and categorization of antimicrobial drugs.

Microorganisms and Terminology

Bacteria are single-cell organisms that, unlike human cells, contain a rigid outer cell wall in addition to a cell membrane. Although much of the cellular metabolism is similar to human cells, there are significant differences, which are the target of drug therapy. For example, in bacteria, the enzymes and *ribosomes* required for replication, transcription, and protein synthesis are somewhat different than in human cells. The term *antibiotic* usually refers to a drug used to treat bacterial infections although the origin of the term is broader and sometimes refers to any antimicrobial agent. *Antibacterial* specifically applies to treatment of bacterial infections. Fungi also contain metabolic processes that are unique from human cells but some of the differences that exist with bacteria do not exist with fungi. Consequently, it is often more difficult to treat fungal infections without also affecting similar processes in human cells. Viruses can only propagate by using the enzymes and genetic replicating system of the host cell, and thus drugs that target these processes also affect human cells. Because there are fewer biochemical processes that are unique to viruses, there are fewer antiviral drugs to treat these infections.

Categories of Antibiotics

As will be discussed later, the most frequently used method of grouping antibiotics is by the chemical structure. Penicillins, tetracyclines, and sulfonamides ("sulfa drugs") are examples of three classes of antibacterial agents that are based on chemical structure. Another classification is by *mechanism of action*, such as drugs that inhibit the synthesis of the bacterial cell wall, alter the integrity of the cell membrane, inhibit protein synthesis, inhibit *nucleic acid* synthesis, and inhibit utilization of nutritional compounds.

A broader categorization classifies the drug as bactericidal or bacteriostatic. *Bactericidal* refers to a drug that kills bacteria whereas *bacteriostatic* drugs will slow the normal growth rate of the bacteria so that the patient's immune system has a better opportunity to eliminate the infecting organisms. If the patient's immune system is not functioning optimally due to a disease (eg, acquired immunodeficiency syndrome [AIDS]) or use of another drug (eg, an immunosuppressive drug to treat cancer), a bacteriostatic drug may not be effective in treating the infection. Although occasionally the concentration of drug at the *site of action* will determine whether an antibiotic is bactericidal or bacteriostatic, usually the mechanism of action is the determining factor. For example, antibiotics that inhibit cell wall synthesis are bactericidal whereas those that act solely by inhibiting protein synthesis are bacteriostatic.

Another means of grouping antibiotics is according to their spectrum of activity, narrow- vs broad-spectrum. Narrow-spectrum drugs are effective against a smaller number of similar organisms; broad-spectrum drugs are effective against a larger number of organisms of a more varied grouping. For example, narrow-spectrum antibacterial drugs may be effective against a few *gram-positive* organisms, whereas a broad-spectrum antibacterial drug may be effective against several *gram-negative* and gram-positive bacteria.

A Gram stain (named after Christian Gram) is a relatively simple laboratory test to determine whether the bacteria being tested will retain a certain dye. Whether the bacteria retains the dye (gram-positive) or not (gram-negative) is dependent on the chemical structure of the bacterial cell wall. The Gram stain test quickly eliminates many bacteria as the cause of the infection and narrows the choices of potentially effective antibiotics. For example, a test result confirming the presence of gram-negative bacteria eliminates all antibiotics that are not effective against gram-negative bacteria.

Table 5-1. Classification of Antibiotics

Example (generic name)	Chemical Structure	Mechanism of Action	Bactericidal or Bacteriostatic	Spectrum
amikacin	aminoglycoside	Inhibit protein synthesis and other mechanisms	Bactericidal	Narrow
cephalexin	cephalosporin	Inhibit cell wall mechanisms	Bactericidal	Narrow
ciprofloxacin	fluoroquinolone	Inhibit DNA synthesis	Bactericidal	Broad
doxycycline	tetracycline	Inhibit protein synthesis	Bacteriostatic	Broad
erythromycin	macrolide	Inhibit protein synthesis	Bacteriostatic	Narrow
imipenem	carbapenem	Inhibit cell wall synthesis	Bactericidal	Broad
penicillin G	penicillin	Inhibit cell wall synthesis	Bactericidal	Narrow
sulfamethoxazole	sulfonamide	Metabolic inhibitor	Bacteriostatic	Broad

Table 5-1 illustrates various means of categorizing antimicrobial drugs. It should be noted that not even broad-spectrum antibacterial drugs are effective against fungi or viruses; antifungal agents are generally only effective against fungi, and antiviral agents are only effective against viruses. Consequently, it is ineffective to use antibacterial drugs, such as penicillin, to treat viral infections such as the common cold or flu.

Antimicrobial Resistance

If a microorganism is sensitive (ie, susceptible) to an antimicrobial drug, the drug is effective in treating infections caused by that microorganism. If a microorganism that was sensitive to an antimicrobial agent becomes less sensitive or loses its sensitivity, the organism has become resistant to the drug. The terms sensitive, resistant, and susceptible are referring to the response of the microorganism to the drug; these terms are not referring to the patient and should not be confused, for example, with reference to a patient being sensitive (ie, allergic) to a drug.

Drug resistance develops because of a change in the genetic makeup of microorganisms (Figure 5-1). This change can occur by spontaneous, random mutation, which results in an advantage for the organism. The altered genetics are then passed on to successive generations of the organism. Although mutations are an important cause of resistance in bacteria, it is less common than the transfer of genetic material from a resistant bacterium to a susceptible bacterium. This transfer of genetic material can occur by any one of several mechanisms, including through a physical connector that links the organisms or through a virus that copies the DNA from one bacteria and transfers it to another. Regardless of the mechanism, the genetic material that is transferred contains the genetic code for the protein(s) that confer resistance, thus making a formerly susceptible organism resistant. Because resistance by this mechanism results in the transfer of multiple genes, susceptible bacteria can become resistant to several classes of drugs at the same time.

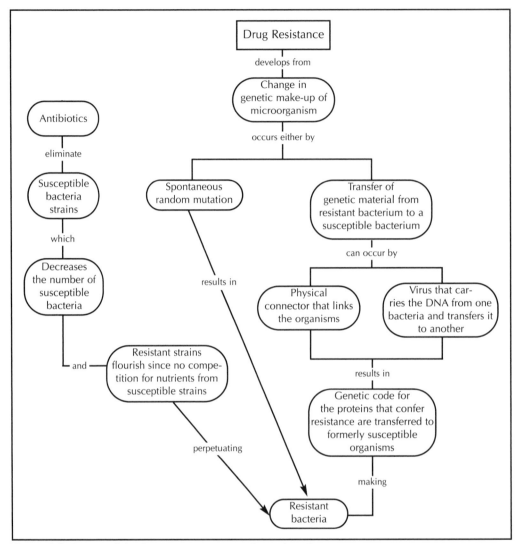

Figure 5-1. Process of developing resistance to antibiotic drug therapy.

Overuse of antibiotics promotes the development of resistant strains of microorganisms. As susceptible strains are eliminated by exposure to antibiotics, the resistant strains flourish without the competition for nutrients from the susceptible strains. The existence of more resistant strains increases the likelihood of these strains passing their drug resistance genetic characteristics to other susceptible strains. Overuse of broad-spectrum antibiotics are particularly problematic because they diminish the population of several strains of competing organisms at the same time.

The change in genetic make-up results in resistance by any one of several mechanisms. More than one mechanism may be the cause of resistance to a particular antibiotic.

- Production of an enzyme that inactivates the drug. The β-lactamases are a group of enzymes that inactivate some penicillins and cephalosporins by breaking apart a key chemical structure of these antibiotics. These enzymes are also referred to as penicillinases and cephalosporinases. Other antibiotics, such as the aminoglycosides, are also inactivated by bacterial enzymatic action on the antibiotic.

- Altered structure of the protein binding site of the antibiotic. If the DNA of the bacteria codes for an altered structure for the protein binding site, the drug will no longer bind as effectively and thus the activity of the drug will be diminished. Antibiotics such as the macrolides, penicillins, cephalosporins, and fluoroquinolones can be inactivated by this mechanism.
- Altered mechanism for entry of the drug into the microorganism. Some antibiotics enter the microorganism through transport mechanisms such as membrane channels and protein carriers. If the microorganism obtains DNA that codes for altered proteins responsible for the transport process, the rate of entry of the antibiotic into the microorganism will be diminished. Aminoglycosides and tetracyclines are examples of antibiotics to which resistance can develop by this method.

A topic related to antimicrobial resistance is nosocomial infections, also called hospital-acquired infections. These are infections that a patient contracts while in the hospital, from the hospital (or other institution such as a nursing home). Often these infections are acquired from equipment or supplies associated with intravenous infusions, dialysis, catheters, and mechanical ventilators. Because hospitals frequently use antibacterial drugs, the bacteria that survive in the hospital environment are often resistant organisms. Additionally, patients in the hospital setting are typically more severely ill and may have compromised immune responses. Nosocomial infections sometimes pose a serious treatment challenge and may markedly hinder, or even prevent, the patient's recovery.

Superinfections

Superinfections are sometimes also referred to as suprainfections. These are infections that develop during the treatment of an initial infection. If the antibiotic used to treat a specific infection also kills a sufficient number of normal *flora* in the gastrointestinal, respiratory, or urinary tract for example, the growth of resistant microorganisms will increase. The growth of the resistant strains is normally held in check by the large number of normal flora. The resistant microorganisms may be fungi or bacteria, which are not susceptible to commonly used antimicrobial agents. Broad-spectrum antimicrobials and longer duration of therapy are more likely to cause superinfections because these factors will have a larger impact on the normal flora. For the purpose of minimizing the development of drug resistance and occurrence of superinfections, it is best that the antibiotic selected has the narrowest spectrum possible while simultaneously being effective against the invading microorganism, and that the drug therapy not be continued beyond the time necessary to eradicate the microorganism.

Aside from suprainfections, another adverse effect that can develop as a result of the disruption of the normal gastrointestinal flora is diarrhea. Antibiotics with a broad-spectrum of activity have a greater propensity for affecting gastrointestinal flora and thus causing diarrhea, but also antibiotics that are absorbed poorly from the gastrointestinal tract will have a greater impact on the normal flora. An example is the comparison in the incidence of diarrhea between amoxicillin (Amoxil) and ampicillin (Omnipen). These are two penicillins with almost identical antimicrobial activity but amoxicillin is absorbed more completely after oral administration and also has a lower incidence of diarrhea. It should be noted that there are other causes of antibiotic-induced diarrhea other than disruption of normal flora (eg, direct irritation of the intestine by the tetracyclines).

Selection of Antimicrobial and Dosage Regimen

Selection of an antibiotic should take into consideration the microorganism, the site of the infection, and the patient. Although all of these factors are important, effectiveness of the antibiotic against the infecting organism is the first consideration; if the drug cannot kill or inhibit the growth of the infecting microorganism, it is futile to give the drug to treat that infection.

Ideally, the appropriate antibiotic is determined by identifying the infecting organism and determining to which antibiotic the organism is most susceptible. However, it may be necessary to begin therapy prior to the availability of the identification and susceptibility lab results, especially in cases of severe infection. The patient's symptoms will often provide sufficient information for the physician to select an antibiotic that is likely to be effective. For example, most acute ear infections are caused by *Streptococcus pneumoniae, Haemophilus influenzae,* or *Moraxella catarrhalis*, and amoxicillin is effective against many strains of all three of these organisms. In other situations, the antibiotic can be changed, if necessary, to optimize therapy based on the susceptibility lab results.

The site of the infection may limit the selection of antibiotics available because some of the drugs that are effective against the microorganism may not be able to penetrate to the site of the infection. If the cerebrospinal fluid (CSF) is infected, the antibiotic must cross the *blood-brain barrier* and thus nonpolar and unionized (see Chapter 2) antibiotics will penetrate more effectively than polar antibiotics. Note, however, that inflammation from bacterial infections does increase the penetration of some drugs into the CSF. Similarly, some drugs penetrate lower respiratory tract infections better than others. Again, drugs that are nonpolar and unionized penetrate these infected sites more effectively, and thus more readily reach the effective concentration for treating lower respiratory tract infections. Penetration of the antibiotic into the tissue can also be an issue for treating infections of various other tissues such as the heart, urinary tract, or prostate.

Factors regarding the patient must also be considered (eg, drug allergies, pregnancy, age, and existence of other diseases). Although amoxicillin is effective in the treatment of most acute ear infections, an alternative antibiotic must be selected for the penicillin-allergic patient. Some antimicrobial agents cause an increased risk of significant adverse effects to the mother or the unborn child and should be avoided. Tetracyclines can affect developing bones and teeth in young children and should be avoided. Neurological disorders can occur in newborns from the use of sulfonamides, which release bilirubin from protein binding sites on albumin, thus increasing the concentration of free bilirubin to toxic levels. Antibiotics that are excreted by the kidney or metabolized by the liver must be used with greater caution in patients who also have kidney or liver disease, respectively. Patients being treated for an infection but who also have a compromised immune system, such as patients undergoing cancer chemotherapy or patients with human immunodeficiency virus (HIV)/AIDS, may require bactericidal rather than bacteriostatic antimicrobial agents to eliminate the infecting organism.

The proper dosage regimen is also important for successful eradication of the infecting organism. The dosage and duration of therapy depends on several factors. Higher doses are required if the infected site is difficult for the antibacterial drug to penetrate. Dosage can also vary because all bacteria do not have the same degree of susceptibility to a particular antibacterial drug. The immune defense of some patients is not as effective against some bacteria, and thus a longer duration of therapy may be necessary for them. As with the treatment of other diseases, poor compliance with the appropriate duration of therapy is a common cause of treatment failure. The patient should clearly understand that all of the doses of the antimicrobial drug should be taken as prescribed. Too often patients discontinue using the drug when they begin to feel better, but unfortunately the infection may exist although the symptoms are gone. Discontinuation of the antimicrobial is a common cause of a recurrent infection.

Respiratory Infections

Respiratory tract infections are among the most common reasons patients seek medical attention and are also one of the most common groups of illnesses associated with inappropriate drug therapy. Consequently, it is worthwhile to tie together some previously mentioned foundational principles with respect to these infections. Pharyngitis is the most common upper respiratory tract infection. Most cases of pharyngitis are viral infections, and it is also often associated with the common cold. Treatment of these viral infections with an antibiotic is a scenario that contributes to the over-prescribing of antibiotics. A significant percentage of the antibiotic prescriptions written for patients outside the hospital are unnecessary. Such use of antibiotics is a potential cause of resistant strains and unnecessary adverse drug reactions. Laboratory tests of throat cultures can identify whether the infection is bacterial.

The other two most common upper respiratory tract infections, otitis media and sinusitis, are typically bacterial infections, but inappropriate use of antibiotics also occurs when infections at these sites are viral. Sometimes, however, sinusitis may be difficult to differentiate from allergies or symptoms of the common cold. Sinusitis infections are sometimes caused by bacterial strains that have developed resistance to the first choice antibiotics (from the penicillin category). This necessitates the use of an alternative therapy specific for the resistant organism. Some sinusitis infections become difficult to eradicate and require treatment beyond the usual 10 to 14 days.

The two most frequent lower respiratory tract infections are acute bronchitis and pneumonia. Acute bronchitis is usually viral, but bacterial infections do also occur. Bacteria are typically the infecting causative organism of pneumonia in adults, whereas viruses are the predominant cause in children. Pneumonia can be life threatening and therefore appropriate treatment is critical. Because numerous pathogens can be the cause, a broad-spectrum antibiotic is typically used initially until the results of cultures can identify the most effective therapy. As described above, regardless of whether the infection is of the lower or upper respiratory tract, the specific site of the infection, the ability of the drug to penetrate to the site of action, and the patient's medical history must be considered in addition to the susceptibility of the organism to the drug.

Summary

There are several means of categorizing antibacterial drugs but grouping them by chemical structure is very common. *Drug resistance* refers to a change in the susceptibility of the organism to a particular drug or group of drug; therefore, drugs that were once effective against the microorganism are no longer effective. This resistance can occur by several mechanisms but always results from a change in the genetic makeup of the microorganism. The development of resistance is a significant problem that hinders effective antimicrobial therapy.

Another problem related to antimicrobial therapy is the development of *superinfections*. These are secondary infections that occur as a result of the treatment of the primary infection. Often superinfections result from bacteria or fungi that exist in the body at low levels because of the much larger number of nonpathogenic microorganisms (normal flora) that prevent their growth. As antibiotic therapy reduces the normal flora along with the primary infection, it provides an opportunity for other pathogenic microorganisms to flourish as a superinfection. The potential for superinfections and development of resistant organisms adds to the importance of selecting the appropriate antimicrobial agent for the infection; use of broader spectrum drugs for longer time periods enhances the potential for these problems. Therefore, the goal of therapy is to select an antibiotic that most selectively targets the infecting bacteria and at the same time minimizes adverse effects.

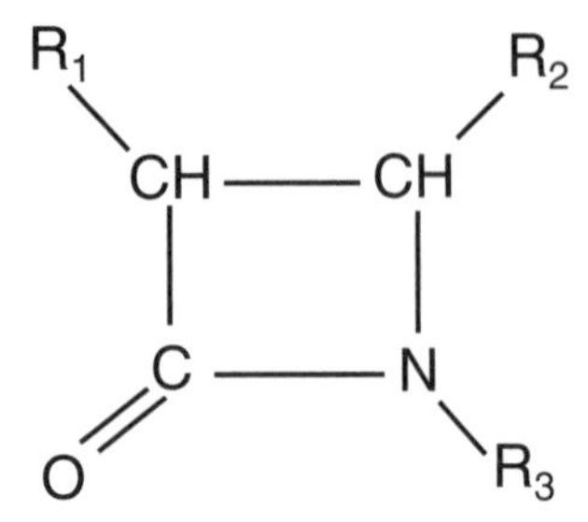

Figure 5-2. The β-lactam ring. The β-lactam ring is a structure common to the penicillins, cephalosporins, and carbapenems. Specific drugs in each of these categories differ from one another by the various chemical groups, designated by R_1, R_2, and R_3, that are attached around the β-lactam ring.

ANTIBACTERIAL DRUGS

As would be expected, antibiotics with similar chemical structure are placed in the same category, and the drugs in that category will have some pharmacological and therapeutic similarities. Discussion in this section focuses on these similarities although some important differences are also mentioned. Discussion is also limited to drugs that are members of antibiotic categories as they encompass the majority of available antibacterial drugs. It is noteworthy, however, that there are several other antibiotics that do not fall into these categories and are not discussed.

Penicillins

A drug is categorized as a penicillin if it has certain chemical structural components including a component referred to as a β-lactam ring (Figure 5-2). It is the β-lactam ring that is key to the binding of the penicillin molecule to the active site of the bacteria. However, it is also this ring that makes these antibiotics potentially vulnerable to β-lactamases (penicillinases); enzymes produced by some bacteria that break apart the β-lactam ring, thus imparting resistance to the bacteria. Penicillin G was the first of this group to be discovered when in 1928 it was observed that a mold produced a substance that killed bacteria. After clinical trials, penicillin G became available to the US military in the early 1940s. Although penicillin G was a tremendous discovery, it has some limitations. For example, most of an oral dose is inactivated by stomach acid, it has a narrow spectrum of activity, and it is inactivated by penicillinase. Consequently, chemically modified penicillins have been produced to alleviate these limitations. There are now more than a dozen penicillins available and their properties are typically compared with the characteristics of penicillin G (Table 5-2). Some penicillins are more stable to stomach acid (eg, acid-stable), are resistant to penicillinase, or have a broader spectrum of activity. Note the terms resistant and sensitive are also used to describe the susceptibility of the drug to penicillinase just as they are used to describe the susceptibility of the microorganism to the drug. Thus, a bacteria that is penicillinase-producing bacteria will be resistant to a penicillinase-sensitive drug (eg, penicillin G), whereas a penicillinase-producing bacteria will be sensitive to a penicillinase-resistant drug (eg, nafcillin).

A few penicillins are available in combination with drugs that have little antibacterial activity but are inhibitors of β-lactamases. Sulbactam, clavulanic acid, and tazobactam are β-lactamase inhibitors, which are available together in the same dosage with some penicillins, such as ampicillin and amoxicillin, that are not β-lactamase resistant. The combination of one of these agents with a penicillin gives the penicillin greater effectiveness against otherwise resistant bacteria.

Table 5-2. Selected Characteristics of Penicillins

Generic Name	Trade Name	Oral	Penicillinase	Spectrum
amoxicillin	Amoxil	Yes	Sensitive	Broad
amoxicillin plus clavulanate	Augmentin	Yes	Resistant	Broad
ampicillin	Omnipen	Yes	Sensitive	Broad
ampicillin plus sulbactam	Unasyn	Yes	Resistant	Broad
bacampicillin	Spectrobid	Yes	Sensitive	Broad
cloxacillin	Tegopen	Yes	Resistant	Narrow
dicloxacillin	Dynapen	Yes	Resistant	Narrow
methicillin	Staphcillin	No	Resistant	Narrow
mezlocillin	Mezlin	No	Sensitive	Extended
nafcillin	Unipen	Yes	Resistant	Narrow
oxacillin	Bactocill	Yes	Resistant	Narrow
penicillin G	generic	Yes	Sensitive	Narrow
penicillin V	Pen-Vee K	Yes	Sensitive	Narrow
piperacillin	Pipracil	No	Sensitive	Extended
Piperacillin plus tazobactam	Zosyn	No	Resistant	Extended
ticarcillin	Ticar	no	sensitive	extended

Penicillin G is the only natural penicillin used therapeutically. It was an impure product when it was first used and therefore the dose was based on units (U) of biological activity rather than a weight basis. Although penicillin G is now available in pure form, units are often used to designate dose. The approximate conversion is 400,000 U = 250 mg of penicillin G.

The penicillins that are acid-stable are more effectively absorbed by the oral route than penicillin G. Amoxicillin, for example, is more acid-stable than either penicillin G or ampicillin, and therefore a larger percentage of an oral dose of amoxicillin is absorbed. The penicillins are excreted rapidly by the kidney through glomerular filtration and tubular secretion. Consequently, concentrations of penicillin are high in the urine.

Penicillins have a high therapeutic index. The most notable adverse effect is the potential for allergic reactions, which occurs in up to 10% of patients, depending on the specific study. Symptoms range from skin rash to life-threatening anaphylaxis. Any of the penicillins can elicit a response in susceptible patients, and thus if a patient is allergic to one penicillin, all of them should be avoided. Prior exposure to a penicillin is necessary for an allergic reaction to occur, although exposure may not be from therapeutic use of a penicillin but through food, from animals that have been given penicillin, or through exposure to fungi that produce penicillin.

Penicillins are bactericidal drugs. Unlike mammalian cells, bacteria have a high osmotic pressure within the cell and thus they have a rigid cell wall that prevents the cell from bursting. Penicillins inhibit the activity of various enzymes that are responsible for the synthesis of the cell wall, thus causing gaps in the cell wall and lysis of the bacteria. These antibiotics are more effective when the bacteria are actively growing and undergoing cell division.

The specific susceptible bacteria vary with each penicillin and therefore it is advantageous to identify the infecting organism and conduct susceptibility testing. In general, however, peni-

Box 5-1. Facts About Penicillins

- Contain a β-lactam structure.
- Mechanism of action: Inhibit cell wall synthesis.
- Bactericidal.
- Spectrum of activity: Narrow to broad; contain subcategories based on increasing spectrum of activity; in general, effective against gram-positive and gram-negative bacteria.
- Adverse effects: Cause allergic reactions in up to 10% of patients.
- Primary uses: Infections of urinary tract, respiratory tract, and heart, as well as treating syphilis.
- Excretion: Primarily urine.
- Other notes: Inactivated by β-lactamases (penicillinases).

cillins are effective against more gram-positive than gram-negative bacteria. Penicillins generally distribute into most tissue and thus are used to treat susceptible microorganisms that cause infections of various tissue, including the urinary tract, respiratory tract, heart (endocarditis), and middle ear (otitis media) as well as syphilis. Penicillin is also used to prevent recurrences of rheumatic fever and to prevent bacterial endocarditis prior to certain dental and surgical procedures in patients with prosthetic cardiac valves, mitral valve prolapse, history of previous bacterial endocarditis, or rheumatic heart disease. Amoxicillin (Amoxil) is effective for postexposure prophylaxis to anthrax (see also doxycycline and ciprofloxacin) (Box 5-1).

Cephalosporins

There are over two dozen cephalosporins available, about twice the number of penicillins. Less than half are effective by the oral route. Cephalosporins are similar to penicillins in that they:

- Contain a β-lactam structure
- Inhibit cell wall synthesis
- Are bactericidal
- Have a high therapeutic index
- Are inactivated by β-lactamases (cephalosporinases)
- Cause allergic reactions
- Are excreted primarily by glomerular filtration and tubular secretion
- Contain subcategories based on increasing spectrum of activity

Allergic reactions to cephalosporins occur less frequently than with penicillins and anaphylaxis is rare. Some cross-reactivity exists between these two categories of antibiotics; if a patient is allergic to either the penicillins or cephalosporins, there is an increased likelihood that the patient will also be allergic to the other category. *Cross-reactivity* occurs in up to 10% of patients allergic to penicillins. Mild allergic reaction to penicillin should not hinder the use of cephalosporins in that patient, but patients who have a severe allergic reaction to penicillins should not be given cephalosporins.

Cephalosporins are grouped as first-generation through fourth-generation drugs. First-generation drugs are effective primarily against gram-positive bacteria. Second-generation drugs are more effective against some gram-negative bacteria and are more likely to be resistant to

Table 5-3. Selected Cephalosporins

Generic Name	Trade Name	Grouping	Administration*
cefaclor	Ceclor	Second generation	PO
cefadroxil	Duricef	First generation	PO
cefazolin	Ancef	First generation	IM, IV
cefdinir	Omnicef	Third generation	PO
cefditoren	Spectracef	Third generation	PO
cefepime	Maxipime	Fourth generation	IM, IV
cefixime	Suprax	Third generation	PO
cefotaxime	Claforan	Third generation	IM, IV
cefotetan	Cefotan	Second generation	IM, IV
cefoxitin	Mefoxin	Second generation	IM, IV
cefprozil	Cefzil	Second generation	PO
ceftazidime	Fortaz	Third generation	IM, IV
ceftibuten	Cedax	Third generation	PO
ceftriaxone	Rocephin	Third generation	IM, IV
cefuroxime	Ceftin	Second generation	IM, IV, PO
cephalexin	Keflex	First generation	PO
cephalothin	Keflin	First generation	IM, IV

*IM=intramuscular; IV=intravenous; PO=oral

Box 5-2. Facts About Cephalosporins

- Contain a β-lactam structure.
- Mechanism of action: Inhibit cell wall synthesis.
- Bactericidal.
- Spectrum of activity: Narrow to broad; contain subcategories based on increasing spectrum of activity.
- Adverse effects: Cause allergic reactions; cross-reactivity with penicillins (up to 10%).
- Primary uses: Respiratory tract, urinary tract, bacteremia, skin, and soft tissue infections.
- Excretion: Primarily urine.
- Other notes: Inactivated by β-lactamases (cephalosporinases).

cephalosporinases. Third-generation cephalosporins are broader spectrum and have increased resistance to cephalosporinases. The fourth-generation continues this trend with broader spectrum of activity and/or better resistance to cephalosporinases. Examples of these drugs are included in Table 5-3 (see also Box 5-2).

Carbapenems

Like the penicillins and cephalosporins, the carbapenems are β-lactam antibiotics that also inhibit cell wall synthesis and are bactericidal. These newest β-lactams are relatively resistant to β-lactamases. These drugs, imipenem (Primaxin), meropenem (Merrem), and ertapenem

Box 5-3. Facts About Carbapenems

- Contain a β-lactam structure.
- Mechanism of action: Inhibit cell wall synthesis.
- Bactericidal.
- Spectrum of activity: Broad.
- Adverse effects: Cross-reactivity may exist in patients allergic to other β-lactams.
- Primary uses: Infections of the skin and urinary tract, pneumonia, and intra-abdominal and pelvic infections.
- Excretion: Primarily urine.
- Other notes: Newer β-lactams are relatively resistant to β-lactamases.

(Invanz), are used parenterally primarily to treat gram-negative bacteria that are resistant to other antibiotics. They are useful to treat infections of the skin, urinary tract, lower respiratory tract, intra-abdominal, and pelvis. The carbapenems are usually well-tolerated but adverse effects include diarrhea, nausea, and vomiting. Cross-reactivity may exist in patients allergic to the other β-lactam antibiotics (Box 5-3).

Tetracyclines

The tetracyclines have been on the market for >50 years but their use as a first-line drug has decreased because of increased incidence of bacterial resistance and the availability of other more effective and less toxic antibiotics. They remain highly effective, however, to treat some infections such as Rocky Mountain spotted fever, cholera, Lyme disease, and pneumonia from *Mycoplasma pneumoniae*. Doxycycline (Vibramycin) is effective for postexposure prophylaxis to anthrax (see also amoxicillin and ciprofloxacin). Tetracyclines are an alternative therapy to treat many infections when the drug of choice is not suitable for the patient (eg, due to allergy or resistance).

The mechanism of action of the tetracyclines is to inhibit protein synthesis. An active transport mechanism is necessary for sufficient drug to reach the site of action inside the bacteria. Tetracyclines bind to specific active sites on the ribosomal *RNA* to inhibit protein synthesis. Mammalian cells do not have the active transport system necessary to attain sufficient concentrations of tetracyclines at the *site of action*, and also the structure of mammalian ribosomal RNA is different than for bacteria. Inhibition of protein synthesis with tetracyclines will diminish the growth of the bacteria (bacteriostatic), but will not kill the microorganism. All of the tetracyclines are broad-spectrum antibiotics, effective for many *gram-positive* and *gram-negative* bacteria.

A major difference among the tetracyclines is the duration of action (Table 5-4), with the two most lipid soluble tetracyclines, doxycycline and minocycline, having the longest duration of action. These two tetracyclines also have the greatest ability to penetrate into the brain and CSF compared with the other tetracyclines. Although all of the tetracyclines are effective orally, they are not completely absorbed and the presence of food will further diminish their absorption. However, the greater lipid solubility of doxycycline and minocycline contributes to their more complete absorption from the gastrointestinal tract and the diminished impact from food on the absorption. The extent of absorption is an important factor because unabsorbed tetracycline can alter the intestinal flora and result in the development of resistant organisms and bacterial and fungal superinfections.

Table 5-4. Selected Characteristics of Tetracyclines

Generic Name	Trade Name	Lipid Solubility	Approximate t½	Extent of Oral Absorption
democlocycline	Declomycin	Intermediate	14 hours	Intermediate
doxycycline	Vibramycin	High	20 hours	High[1]
minocycline	Minocin	High	15 hours	High[1]
oxytetracycline	Terramycin	Low	9 hours	Intermediate
tetracycline	Panmycin	Intermediate	9 hours	Intermediate

[1]Oral absorption not significantly affected by food.

All tetracyclines bind to certain minerals, primarily calcium, magnesium, aluminum, zinc, and iron, although doxycycline and minocycline are affected to a lesser extent. When tetracycline molecules bind to these minerals that are contained in foods, laxatives, and mineral supplements, the drug is not absorbed from the gastrointestinal tract. Consequently, except for doxycycline and minocycline, oral doses of these drugs should only be taken 1 hour before or 2 hours after the consumption of food, particularly dairy products. The binding of tetracyclines to the calcium in bones and teeth causes these drugs to affect bone development and causes permanent discoloration of tooth enamel. Therefore, the tetracyclines should not be administered to children aged <8 years or to pregnant or nursing mothers because these drugs cross the placenta and are found in breast milk.

In addition to the potential to affect teeth and bones in children, the tetracyclines may also cause other adverse effects. Gastrointestinal symptoms such as epigastric burning, nausea, vomiting, and diarrhea can occur, especially when the tetracycline is administered on an empty stomach. These antibiotics can also produce photosensitivity in some patients, which may cause the patient to become sunburned more readily when exposed to direct sunlight or sunlamps. Protective clothing is advised to avoid direct sunlight and sunscreens are of little benefit. Some patients may need to discontinue therapy, and photosensitivity may persist for weeks after the drug is discontinued.

In addition to treatment of some systemic and respiratory infections, tetracyclines have three other specific uses. Oxytetracycline and chlortetracycline, in particular, are used in agriculture as an additive to animal feed to increase the growth rate of livestock. This use continues to be controversial due to its possible impact on contributing to the development of resistant strains of bacteria. Another use particularly of tetracycline, in combination with other drugs, is to treat peptic ulcers caused by *Helicobacter pylori (H. pylori)*, a bacterium that is a major cause of peptic ulcer disease (see Chapter 11). A third use is to treat acne. The mechanism involved in acne therapy is through inhibition of *Propionibacterium acnes*, which produce fatty acids that initiate an inflammatory response. Daily, oral use of tetracycline as low-dose therapy is effective to treat acne with minimal adverse effects (Box 5-4).

Macrolides

This group of antibiotics includes the original macrolide, erythromycin (E-Mycin), and the newer macrolides, clarithromycin (Biaxin), azithromycin (Zithromax), and dirithromycin (Dynabac). These drugs can be administered orally and are generally bacteriostatic although at higher concentrations they become bactericidal to some bacteria. The macrolides inhibit protein

Box 5-4. Facts About Tetracyclines

- Mechanism of action: Inhibit protein synthesis.
- Bacteriostatic.
- Spectrum of activity: Broad.
- Adverse effects: Epigastric burning, nausea, vomiting, and diarrhea, photosensitivity (up to 2% of patients). May affect bones and teeth in patients <8 years old.
- Primary uses: Infections such as Rocky Mountain spotted fever, cholera, Lyme disease, and pneumonia form *Mycoplasma pneumoniae*; alternative therapy to treat many infections when the drug of choice is not suitable for the patient.
- Other uses: Additive to animal feed to increase the growth rate of livestock, treat peptic ulcers caused by *H. pylori*, and treat acne.
- Excretion: Primarily urine but some excreted in bile.
- Other notes: Absorption is affected by the presence of food. Unabsorbed tetracycline can alter the intestinal flora and result in the development of resistant organisms and bacterial and fungal superinfections.

synthesis of sensitive bacteria. The spectrum of activity of these antibiotics is somewhat similar to the penicillins, but like the tetracyclines the macrolides are often the alternate drug recommended in penicillin-allergic patients. They are used as an alternative to penicillins and other antibacterial therapy to treat infections of gastrointestinal, genital, and respiratory tract, as well as skin and soft tissue infections. Resistance can occur by several mechanisms: an altered transport mechanism that decreases the amount of macrolide inside the bacterial cell; a change in the structure of the binding site; or due to an increased production of an enzyme that inactivates the macrolide. Erythromycin is also used topically to treat acne by inhibiting *P acnes*, which contribute to the inflammation.

The most common adverse effects from macrolides are gastrointestinal and include epigastric irritation, nausea, and vomiting. Among the macrolides, erythromycin has the highest incidence of these effects but they can be minimized by administration of the drug with food. However, erythromycin is not stable to stomach acid and food diminishes absorption. Consequently, various dosage formulations, such as acid-resistant coatings (also known as *enteric* coatings), have been developed to facilitate adequate absorption even when given with food. Clarithromycin is not affected by stomach acid or presence of food as much as erythromycin but it does undergo first pass effect, which diminishes its *bioavailability*. This macrolide is also manufactured in an extended release dosage form, which should be administered with food. The food slows the rate at which the drug passes through the small intestine, and thus increases the bioavailability of the extended release clarithromycin. Azithromycin is affected by food and thus should be given either 1 hour before or 2 hours after meals.

The macrolides are good examples of some of the pharmacokinetic principles discussed in Chapter 2. Erythromycin is an ionizable base and also is inactivated by stomach acid, and thus is incompletely absorbed. Administration with food decreases the absorption of the acid-sensitive erythromycin base. Erythromycin is also manufactured as several inactive *prodrug* forms, such as erythromycin estolate, which are more lipid soluble and less affected by stomach acid, thus more completely absorbed from the gastrointestinal tract. The prodrug is converted to the active erythromycin. Erythromycin is also manufactured with acid-resistant coatings, which allow adequate absorption even when given with food (Box 5-5).

Box 5-5. Facts About Macrolides

- Mechanism of action: Inhibit protein synthesis.
- Bacteriostatic.
- Spectrum of activity: Narrow to broad, depending on the specific drug.
- Adverse effects: Epigastric irritation, nausea, and vomiting.
- Primary uses: Treat infections of the gastrointestinal, genital, and respiratory tracts as well as skin and soft tissue infections. Alternative for penicillin-allergic patients.
- Excretion: Bile and urine.
- Other notes: Absorption is not affected by food, except for erythromycin.

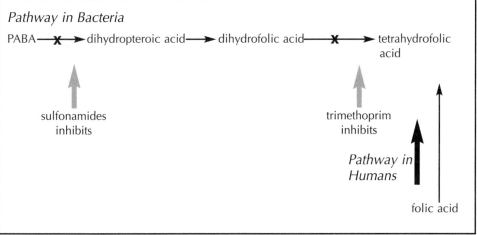

Pathway in Bacteria

PABA —X—▶ dihydropteroic acid —▶ dihydrofolic acid —X—▶ tetrahydrofolic acid

sulfonamides inhibits

trimethoprim inhibits

Pathway in Humans

folic acid

Figure 5-3. Mechanism of action of sulfonamides and trimethoprim. Sulfonamide antibiotics inhibit (X) the enzyme that uses PABA as the substrate in the synthesis of tetrahydrofolic acid in some bacteria. Humans cannot use PABA in this manner but rather ingest the vitamin folic acid, which is more directly converted to tetrahydrofolic acid. Consequently, the sulfonamide antibiotics do not inhibit folic acid metabolism in humans. Trimethoprim is not a sulfonamide but it also inhibits the synthesis of tetrahydrofolic acid at another step along the same pathway. Trimethoprim is often used concurrently with a sulfonamide because the two drugs together produce a synergistic antibacterial effect.

Sulfonamides

Sulfonamides were the first systemic antibacterial agents used therapeutically. They have been referred to as "sulfa drugs" because of the sulfur atom in the chemical structure. The use of these drugs has diminished as additional antibiotics have become available and strains of sulfonamide-resistant bacteria have developed. Sulfonamides are broad-spectrum bacteriostatic antibiotics. Their mechanism of action (Figure 5-3) is to inhibit an enzyme needed for synthesis of tetrahydrofolic acid (THFA) from para-aminobenzoic acid (PABA). THFA is necessary for the synthesis of *DNA, RNA,* and proteins, and therefore sulfonamides are referred to as metabolic inhibitors. A deficiency of THFA will prevent cell growth and division. Tetrahydrofolic acid must be synthesized inside certain bacteria because they cannot transport extracellular folic acid into the cell as an alternative means to make THFA. Mammalian cells cannot synthesize THFA from PABA but must obtain folic acid from the diet; it is a vitamin. Consequently, sulfonamides do not affect folic acid use in mammals.

Box 5-6. Facts About Sulfonamides ("Sulfa Drugs")

- Mechanism of action: Inhibit an enzyme needed for synthesis of THFA from PABA.
- Bacteriostatic.
- Spectrum of activity: Broad.
- Adverse effects: Crystallization of sulfonamides in the urine if not enough water is consumed resulting in renal damage; skin rashes, photosensitivity; hypersensitivity to topical sulfonamides.
- Primary uses: Urinary tract infections, pneumonia, and upper respiratory infections. Topical sulfonamides used to treat eye infections and second- and third-degree burns.
- Excretion: Urine.

Bacterial resistance to sulfonamides can be due to several mechanisms. Sometimes bacteria acquire a different enzyme that uses PABA but to which sulfonamides bind less effectively. Some bacteria develop characteristics that diminish the rate of entry of sulfonamides into the cell. Alternatively, other bacteria develop resistance by synthesizing much more PABA to compete for the active site on the enzyme that uses PABA as substrate.

The sulfonamides such as sulfisoxazole (Gantrisin), sulfamethoxazole (Gantanol), sufacytine (Renoquid), and Sulfamethizole (Thiosulfil Forte) are excreted by the kidney and thus reach a relatively high concentration to be useful in treating urinary tract infections. Other uses for these sulfonamides include treatment of pneumonia and upper respiratory tract infections caused by susceptible bacteria. Topical use of sulfonamides results in a high incidence of hypersensitivity reactions and therefore is confined to treatment of eye infections with sulfactamide (Sulamyd) and to prevent infections following second- and third-degree burns, silver sulfadizine (Silvadene) being the preferred sulfonamide. Mefenide (Sulfamylon) can also be used to prevent topical infections although unlike silver sulfadizine, mefenide causes pain on application to wounds and can cause blood acid-base imbalance.

It is common to use another antibiotic, trimethoprim, together in the same dosage as the sulfonamides to obtain a synergistic effect. As shown in Figure 5-3, trimethoprim also inhibits the synthesis of folic acid but in an enzymatic step in the pathway following the site of action of sulfonamides. Use of trimethoprim with sulfamethoxazole together (Bactrim) has extended the usefulness of this and other sulfonamides. This combination is often the treatment of choice for urinary tract infections.

Several adverse effects are of significant concern when sulfonamides are being used. If sulfonamides crystallize in the urine, they can cause renal damage. This is less of a problem with the currently used sulfonamides, but nonetheless patients should be cautioned to drink enough liquid to produce 1200 to 1500 mL of urine per day. Mild hypersensitivity reactions are relatively common and are usually manifested by skin rash or photosensitivity. Infants should not be given sulfonamides because they can displace bilirubin from the albumin-bound sites to increase the concentration of free bilirubin in the blood, which can reach toxic levels. Near-term pregnant women and nursing mothers should also not be treated with sulfonamides (Box 5-6).

Aminoglycosides

The aminoglycosides are bactericidal antibiotics that are used primarily to treat infections from gram-negative bacteria. These antibiotics inhibit protein synthesis, which typically results in bacteriostatic activity. However, aminoglycosides also disrupt other aspects of the bacterial cell,

Box 5-7. Facts About Aminoglycosides

- Mechanism of action: Inhibit protein synthesis.
- Bactericidal.
- Spectrum of activity: Narrow.
- Adverse effects: Potential for ototoxicity and nephrotoxicity and this must be monitored.
- Uses: Systemically to treat serious gram-negative infections of urinary and respiratory tracts as well as topically to treat infections of eyes, ears, and skin.
- Excretion: Urine.
- Other notes: None are absorbed orally, used parenterally and topically; synergic effect when used with cell wall synthesis inhibitors (eg, penicillins, cephalosporins).

such as cell membrane integrity, which contribute to the bactericidal activity. As with the other antibiotics, resistance can develop to these antibiotics by several mechanisms, including a change in the cell permeability to the drug and inactivation of the drug by the resistant bacteria.

Streptomycin was the first antibiotic developed among this group but is used less frequently since the advent of more active aminoglycosides such as gentamicin (Garamycin), tobramycin (Nebcin), and amikacin (Amikin). None of the aminoglycosides are absorbed orally due to their highly polar nature. Thus, they are used only parenterally for a systemic effect and some are used topically to treat eye infections. Neomycin, another aminoglycoside, is too toxic for systemic use but is used orally to suppress intestinal bacteria prior to surgery and is used in several topical antibiotic preparations, both alone and in combination with other drugs (see page 119). A unique characteristic of aminoglycosides is their synergistic activity when used in combination with cell wall synthesis inhibitors (eg, penicillins, cephalosporins). These combinations enhance the activity of the aminoglycosides against certain gram-negative bacteria that cause urinary tract infections, pneumonia, upper respiratory tract infections, and bacteremia.

The aminoglycosides have a relatively low therapeutic index. A significant adverse effect of the aminoglycosides is their potential to cause ototoxicity and nephrotoxicity. Ototoxicity results in impaired balance and hearing, which may be irreversible if the drug dosage is not decreased. Nephrotoxicity may result in diminished renal function but this is usually reversible upon discontinuation of the drug. Patients on aminoglycoside therapy must be monitored for early signs of ototoxicity (eg, tinnitus, dizziness) and nephrotoxicity (eg, elevated blood creatinine) (Box 5-7).

Fluoroquinolones

The fluoroquinolones (Table 5-5) is a group of antibiotics with several favorable characteristics. These antibiotics:
- Are bactericidal and broad spectrum; thus, one or more of these drugs can be used to treat infections caused by many gram-negative and gram-positive bacteria.
- Penetrate into many tissues and thus are effective in treating infections of the urinary tract, respiratory tract, prostate, gastrointestinal tract, bones, joints, and soft tissues.
- Are effective orally (however, the absorption of fluoroquinolones is reduced by certain minerals; therefore, these antibacterial drugs should not be given with food, drugs, or mineral supplements that contain calcium, magnesium, aluminum, zinc, and iron).
- Have relatively mild adverse effects; the most frequently reported include nausea, vomiting, headache, and dizziness.

Table 5-5. Fluoroquinolone Antibiotics

Generic Name	Trade Name	Administration*
ciprofloxacin	Cipro	PO, IV
gatifloxacin	Tequin	PO, IV
levofloxacin	Levaquin	PO, IV
lemefloxacin	Maxaquin	PO
moxifloxacin	Avelox	PO, IV
norfloxacin	Noroxin	PO
ofloxacin	Floxin	PO, IV
sparfloxacin	Zagam	PO

IV = intravenous; PO = oral

In addition, ciprofloxacin (Cipro) is approved for postexposure prophylaxis to anthrax (see also doxycycline and amoxicillin).

Some adverse effects are of particular note to the athletic trainer. The fluoroquinolones have demonstrated some potential to cause rupture of tendons; thus, the drug should be discontinued if symptoms of tendonitis occur and should be avoided in patients with any symptoms of tendonitis. These drugs may also cause lesions on the cartilage of weight-bearing joints. Consequently, fluoroquinolones are not currently recommended for use in patients aged <18 years or in pregnant women. Additionally, some fluoroquinolones (particularly lomefloxacin) cause phototoxicity to direct or indirect sunlight or to artificial ultraviolet light (eg, sunlamps). Symptoms such as skin burning, redness, rash, or itching are indications the drug should be discontinued.

The mechanism of action for fluoroquinolones is to inhibit DNA synthesis. The corresponding process in mammalian cells is not affected by the fluoroquinolones. As with other antibiotics, resistance can develop to the fluoroquinolones by more than one mechanism (Box 5-8).

Topical Antibacterial Drugs

Several antibacterial drugs are available for topical use as creams, ointments, lotions, and ophthalmic solutions. Some antibiotics are available as prescription products to treat or prevent infections on the skin from wounds or burns and to treat ophthalmic infections. Many of these antibiotics have already been discussed and include sulfonamides, fluoroquinolones, erythromycin, and tobramycin.

Some topical antibiotics are available without a prescription and are used primarily to prevent infection from minor wounds and burns. To treat infections from a wider array of bacteria, several products contain more than one antibiotic. Examples of these products are listed in Table 5-6. They typically include the following antibiotics:

- *Bacitracin.* This is a bactericidal antibiotic that inhibits cell wall synthesis. It is primarily effective against gram-positive bacteria.
- *Neomycin.* As previously discussed, neomycin is a bactericidal aminoglycoside antibiotic. It is primarily effective against gram-negative bacteria and some Staphylococcus species. Potentially any topical antibiotic could cause an allergic skin reaction although neomycin has the highest incidence (approximately 5%) among these OTC antibiotics.

Box 5-8. Facts About Fluoroquinolones

- Mechanism of action: Inhibit DNA synthesis.
- Bactericidal.
- Spectrum of activity: Broad.
- Adverse effects: Nausea, vomiting, headache, and dizziness and have demonstrated some potential to cause rupture of tendons and articular cartilage lesions; phototoxicity.
- Primary uses: Infections of the urinary tract, respiratory tract, prostrate, gastrointestinal tract, bones, joints, and soft tissues.
- Excretion: Varies within the group, some primarily in urine but other through gastrointestinal tract.
- Other notes: Should not be given with foods, drugs, or mineral supplements that contain calcium, magnesium, aluminum, zinc, or iron, as this can affect absorption.

Table 5-6. Topical OTC Antibacterial Products

Trade Name	Generic Contents	Dosage Form
Achromycin	tetracycline HCl	Ointment
Baceguent	bacitracin	Ointment
Myciguent	neomycin	Ointment, cream
Neosporin	neomycin	Cream
	polymyxin B	
Polysporin	polymyxin B	Ointment
	bacitracin	
Triple Antibiotic	bacitracin	Ointment
	neomycin	
	polymyxin B	Ointment

- *Polymyxin B.* This is bactericidal primarily against gram-negative bacteria and is available OTC to treat skin infections and also by prescription as an ophthalmic solution. It alters cell membrane structure and thus changes the permeability characteristics of the membrane.
- *Tetracycline.* As previously discussed, this is a broad-spectrum, bacteriostatic agent used topically to treat wound infections. It stains the skin yellow and some patients experience a stinging sensation when it is applied. Tetracycline is also available for use topically to treat acne but because of these adverse effects, other topical prescription antibiotics are preferred such as erythromycin or clindamycin.

Summary

There are many chemical categories of antibacterial drugs but they can also be grouped by mechanism of action. Antibiotics that inhibit the synthesis of bacterial cell walls are bactericidal and include the penicillins, cephalosporins, and carbapenems. These are also called β-lactam antibiotics because they contain a chemical structural entity called a β-lactam ring. Protein synthesis inhibitors are bacteriostatic and include the tetracyclines and macrolides. Aminoglycosides inhibit protein synthesis but also disrupt other cellular activity and thus are bactericidal. The sulfonamides inhibit the production of tetrahydrofolic acid, a compound synthesized by some bacteria and necessary for their cell growth; inhibition of tetrahydrofolic acid synthesis does not kill the cell. Fluoroquinolones inhibit DNA synthesis and are bactericidal.

Resistance can develop to the β-lactam antibiotics as a result of some bacteria being able to produce enzymes called β-lactamases that break apart the β-lactam ring. Antibiotics that are inactivated by these enzymes are β-lactamase sensitive; those that are not inactivated are β-lactamase resistant. Penicillinases and cephalosporinases are subgroups of these enzymes. Numerous penicillins and cephalosporins are effective in treating infections of many tissues. The primary differences among these drugs are their effectiveness against specific bacteria, their effectiveness when administered orally, and their sensitivity to β-lactamases. The most significant adverse effect is the potential for allergic reactions; cross-reactivity among the β-lactam antibiotics exists in some patients.

The tetracyclines are broad-spectrum agents; doxycycline and minocycline are the tetracyclines most commonly used to treat systemic infections. Tetracyclines bind to calcium, magnesium, aluminum, zinc, and iron although doxycycline and minocycline are affected the least. Therefore, these drugs should not be administered within about 1 to 2 hours of using nutritional supplements or foods that are rich in these minerals. The tetracyclines should also be avoided in children and during pregnancy because they bind to the calcium in teeth and bone. These antibiotics are especially useful as an alternative therapy for many infections. Macrolides are useful to treat many of the same infections as the tetracyclines.

The aminoglycosides are only used parenterally to treat systemic infections. They have the potential to cause ototoxicity and nephrotoxicity and thus blood concentrations and adverse effects are monitored closely.

The fluoroquinolones are broad-spectrum, bactericidal, and effective when administered orally. Because they have the potential to cause tendons to rupture and lesions on cartilage, fluoroquinolones are not recommended for patients aged <18 years, for use during pregnancy, or in patients with tendonitis.

Antifungal Agents

The key biochemical processes that are targets of antibacterial drugs are different for fungi, and thus drugs used to treat bacterial infections are not effective against fungi. The biochemical processes of fungi more closely resemble human cells than bacteria cells, which makes it more difficult to treat fungal infections (called mycoses) without also affecting human cells. Treatment of fungal infections is a serious concern because of the increase in incidence of these infections and the development of resistance to antifungal therapy. Contributing to the increased incidence of fungal infections is the use of broad-spectrum antibiotics that may result in fungal superinfections, more medical procedures that have the potential to introduce fungal infections, and an increased number of immunocompromised patients (eg, cancer, transplant, and AIDS patients).

Compared with superficial fungal infections, systemic fungal infections have a greater potential for morbidity. However, to the athletic trainer, superficial fungal infections are important because they occur much more frequently and they can hinder the performance of the athlete. Yeasts and molds are fungi; yeasts are multicellular and thread-like in appearance, whereas molds are oval-shaped single cell organisms. Yeasts are typically in a parasitic form that infects tissue. Fungi can cause systemic infections through the respiratory, gastrointestinal, or urinary tracts as well as through compromised skin. Fungal infections increase in patients whose immune defenses are diminished through disease or drugs (eg, corticosteroids), or as superinfections through the disruption of normal flora due to use of broad-spectrum antibiotics. *Candida*, for example, is a part of the normal flora of skin and mucous membranes. The number of *Candida* organisms at these sites is usually relatively low because the predominance of the normal flora competes for nutrients with *Candida* and prevents them from proliferating. The use of a broad-spectrum antibiotic, however, can cause the number of normal bacterial flora to be diminished sufficiently to allow the *Candida* to proliferate, thus becoming an infection of the skin, gastrointestinal tract, mouth, or vagina.

Antifungal Agents for Systemic Infections

Except for fungal infections that may be obtained due to invasive medical procedures or use of broad-spectrum antimicrobial agents, most systemic fungal infections are contracted by inhalation of the fungus. Once the lungs are infected, the fungus can spread to other organs and become life threatening. Patients who are immunocompromised, such as those receiving certain cancer therapies or immunosuppressive drugs (eg, corticosteroids) or with HIV/AIDS, are more susceptible.

The mechanism of action of many antifungal agents is to disrupt the normal functioning of the cell membrane causing leakage of cellular contents. For some of these drugs, whether they have fungistatic or fungicidal activity depends on the concentration of the drug at the site of action; higher concentrations being fungicidal. Amphotericin B (Fungizone) is a very effective antifungal agent and remains the treatment of choice for some fungal infections, but it has the significant disadvantages of not being absorbed orally and causing a relatively high incidence of nephrotoxicity. It is also associated with other adverse effects such as fever, chills, nausea, and headache. For many years, amphotericin B was the primary antifungal agent but other drugs have been developed that are less toxic and are effective orally, particularly the azole group. This is a group of broad-spectrum antifungal agents and includes ketoconazole (Mylan), fluconazole (Diflucan), and itraconazole (Sporanox). Nausea and vomiting are the most common adverse effect but can be reduced by administration of the drug with food. Other adverse effects vary among the antifungal agents but include headache and abdominal pain. Systemic use of some antifungal agents (eg, itraconazole, ketoconazole, terbinafine) has the potential to cause hepatotoxicity, and thus monitoring liver function is recommended.

Antifungal Agents for Superficial Infections

Superficial fungal infections affect mucous membranes (eg, vaginal, oral, gastrointestinal), skin, scalp, and nails. Examples of topical antifungal drugs are listed in Table 5-7 and additional antiseptic agents used for ringworm of the scalp are listed in Table 5-8. Some antifungal therapy for superficial infections requires oral administration because of the site or severity of the infection. For example, nystatin (Mycostatin) can be used orally to treat gastrointestinal fungal infections because the drug is not absorbed from the gastrointestinal tract. When topical therapy alone is ineffective, oral dosage forms of griseofulvin (Fulvicin), ketoconazole (Nizoral), itraconazole (Sporanox), fluconazole (Diflucan), and terbinafine (Lamisil) are used to treat fungal infections of the skin, scalp, and/or nails because these drugs penetrate into these sites. Although improvement in symptoms is typically observed after 1 week of treating some fungal infections, weeks to months of treatment are usually necessary to eliminate the infection, depending on the drug used and the site of the infection. Consequently, compliance throughout the duration of therapy is sometimes a challenge to achieve but necessary to attain success.

Table 5-7. Topical Antifungal Agents

Generic Name	Trade Name	OTC/Rx	Dosage Form
amphotericin B[1]	Fungizone	Rx	Cream, lotion
butenafine	Mentax	Rx	Cream
ciclopirox	Loprox	Rx	Cream, lotion
clioquinol	Clioquinol	OTC	Cream
clotrimazole	Lotrimin	OTC, Rx	Cream, lotion, solution
	Gyne-Lotrimin	OTC	Vaginal suppositories, cream
econazole	Spectazole	Rx	Cream
haloprogin	Halotex	Rx	Cream, solution
ketoconazole	Nizoral	Rx	Cream
miconazole	Micatin	OTC	Cream, powder, spray
	Monistat	OTC	Vaginal suppositories, cream
naftifine	Naftin	Rx	Cream, gel
nystatin[1]	Mycostatin	Rx	Cream, ointment, powder
	Nystatin	Rx	Vaginal tablets
oxiconazole	Oxistat	Rx	Cream, lotion
sulconazole	Exelderm	Rx	Cream
terbinafine	Lamisil AT	OTC	Cream
tolnaftate[2]	Tinactin	OTC	Cream, powder, solution, spray
triacetin[2]	Fungoid	Rx	Cream, solution, tincture
undecylenic acid[3]	Desenex	OTC	Cream, foam, ointment, powder, soap, spray

Except where indicated, these products are effective against infections of tinea pedis, tinea cruris, and tinea corporis.

[1]Not for tinea infections.
[2]Also used for onychomycosis although tolnaftate only as adjunct to systemic therapy.
[3]Also used to treat diaper rash as fungal infection can be a contributing component.

Fungal infections of skin, scalp, and nails are most often caused by several species of fungi referred to dermatophytes. These fungal infections are collectively termed tinea, dermatomycoses, or ringworm (which are not worms or rings but produce an itching and painful red-ringed patch). Some characteristics of these and other superficial infections are:

- *Tinea pedis, ringworm of the foot, athlete's foot.* This is the most common dermatomycoses. Infection is facilitated through the moist environment of sweating feet and poorly ventilated shoes. Symptoms vary from cracking and itching between the toes to swelling, severe inflammation, and occurrence of secondary bacterial infection. Treatment with appropriate OTC products is typically sufficient unless there is serious inflammation, the toenails are affected, or the infection prevents normal activity. Treatment may be necessary for 2 to 6 weeks to resolve the infection.
- *Tinea capitis, ringworm of the scalp.* Occurs more frequently in children and is spread by direct contact with animals, humans, or inanimate objects (eg, combs) that are contaminated with the fungus. Symptoms include painful inflammation, which may result in tem-

Table 5-8. OTC Antiseptics

Generic Name	Trade Name	Dosage Forms	Used Against
benzalkonium chloride	Zephiran	Solution, tincture	Bacteria, fungi, viruses
benzalkonium chloride/salicylic acid	Ionil	Shampoo	Tinea capitis
camphor/phenol	Campho-Phenique	Gel, liquid	Bacteria, fungi, viruses
chlorhexidine	Hibiclens	Solution, towelettes	Antibacterial
hydrogen peroxide	hydrogen peroxide	Liquid	Bacteria, viruses
iodine	Iodine Tincture	Tincture	Bacteria, fungi, viruses
isopropyl alcohol	isopropyl alcohol	Liquid	Bacteria
phenol	Unguentine	Cream, ointment	Bacteria, fungi, viruses
povidone-iodine	Betadine	Aerosol, cream, gel, ointment, shampoo	Bacteria, tinea capitis and other fungi, viruses
selenium sulfide	Selsum Blue	Shampoo	Tinea capitis
thimerosal	Mersol	Solution, tincture	Bacteria, fungi
triclosan	Septisol	Soap, solution	Bacteria

porary or permanent hair loss. Treatment requires systemic antifungal therapy (eg, griseofulvin, itraconazole) for 1 to 3 months. Topical agents can also be used but cannot cure the infection and are generally antiseptic (see below) rather than specifically antifungal.

- *Tinea corporis, ringworm of the body.* Occurs on the skin of the trunk and limbs. The infection is spread by direct contact with animals, humans, or inanimate objects infected with this microorganism. Topical agents are usually sufficiently effective (see Table 5-7) although systemic agents such as griseofulvin, ketoconazole, and terbinafine are also available.
- *Tinea cruris, ringworm of the groin, jock itch.* Tight-fitting clothes and moisture facilitate the infection and recurrence is common. Symptoms are typically redness and itching in the groin area and the inside of the thigh. Recurrence of the infection is common. Topical OTC antifungal therapy is usually sufficient although a systemic antifungal drug may be necessary if severe inflammation exists. Treatment should continue for 1 to 2 weeks although symptoms may disappear after a few days. Topical hydrocortisone (see Chapter 6) for 2 to 3 days may also be used to relieve itching.
- *Tinea ungulum, ringworm of the nails (onychomycosis).* Infected nails become discolored with debris accumulating underneath and may eventually be destroyed. Topical antifungal agents are usually not as effective as systemic therapy. Oral itraconazole and terbinafine are effective. Because nails are slow growing, treatment with systemic antifungal agents is necessary for 6 weeks to 12 months, depending on the severity and the drug used.
- *Tinea versicolor, pityriasis versicolor.* Not a ringworm but similar in appearance. A mild, chronic skin infection, usually of the upper trunk, caused by a fungus that is part of the normal skin flora (*Malassezia furfur*). Some patients experience mild pruritus, otherwise it is usually asymptomatic. As the fungus is part of the normal flora, the disease is recurrent, occurring more frequently in hot, humid weather, during excessive sweating, or as a result of corticosteroid therapy (see Chapter 6). Typical lesions are scaly and have discoloration

as patches of white, tan, or pink. Almost all topical or oral antifungal drugs are effective treatment.

- *Vaginal candidiasis. Candida albicans* is a part of the normal vaginal flora and causes most vaginal yeast infections. Use of topical therapy such as intravaginal tablets or creams for a few days to 2 weeks is necessary, depending on the antifungal agent. *Candida* infections are also referred to as monilial infections.

- *Oral candidiasis, thrush. Candida* infection of the mucous membranes of the mouth. Topical therapy is usually effective with treatment continuing for 1 to 2 weeks after symptoms relieved. Asthma patients using corticosteroids by inhalation have a higher incidence of thrush, especially if they do not rinse their mouth with water after using the inhaler or do not use a spacer with it (see Chapter 9).

Summary

Fungal infections can occur from inhalation of airborne fungus, contamination of a wound, as a superinfection during treatment with broad-spectrum antibiotics, or in immunocompromised patients. There are several antifungal agents available to treat systemic fungal infections and although resistance to these drugs can occur, it is less frequent than bacterial resistance to antibiotics. Examples of superficial fungal infections are athlete's foot, jock itch, and ringworm of the scalp and nails. Both topical and systemic antifungal agents are used to treat certain superficial fungal infections. Unlike most bacterial infections, which require days to weeks of treatment, fungal infections typically require weeks to months of antifungal therapy.

ANTIVIRAL AGENTS

As previously mentioned, the development of drug therapy to treat viral infections poses unique challenges because viruses use the enzymes and genetic processes of the host cell to propagate. Consequently, drugs used to treat bacterial and fungal infections are not effective for treatment of viral infections. Nonetheless, millions of prescriptions are written each year for antibiotics to treat infections that are not bacterial. This inappropriate use of antibiotics costs hundreds of millions of dollars, unnecessarily exposes the patient to potential adverse effects, and contributes to the occurrence of antimicrobial resistance.

Viruses contain *DNA* or *RNA* enveloped within a protein coat. Examples of diseases caused by DNA viruses include small pox, chicken pox, shingles, herpes simplex infections, hepatitis B, and warts. German measles, rabies, common cold, influenza, and mumps are caused by RNA virus. Drugs used to treat the RNA virus that causes AIDS will not be discussed because of the complexity of the disease, the medical complications that arise as ramifications of the disease, and the varied drug regimens that have been used to treat the disease.

Many of the antiviral drugs have chemical structures similar to the building blocks of RNA and DNA (Figure 5-4). These drugs, therefore, interfere with the synthesis of viral RNA and DNA. As with antibacterial and antifungal agents, resistance can also develop to the antiviral agents. Adverse effects range from neurotoxicity and nephrotoxicity to nausea and vomiting, depending on the drug. Each drug is effective against only a narrow-spectrum of viruses and most are effective orally but some are also available for parenteral or topical use.

Acyclovir (Zovirax) is the drug of choice to treat the *herpes simplex virus* (eg, genital herpes and encephalitis) or *varicella-zoster virus* (eg, chicken pox and shingles). Gastrointestinal upset and headache are common adverse effects from oral use. Valacyclovir (Valtrex) is a prodrug, metabolized to acyclovir after oral administration and provides better bioavailability than acy-

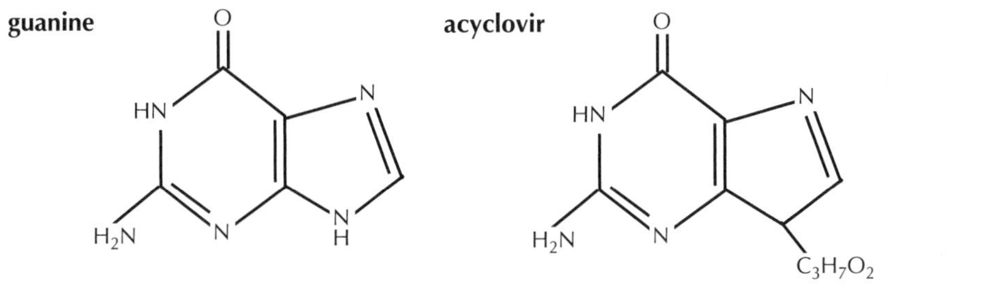

Figure 5-4. Chemical comparison of antiviral drug, acyclovir, with DNA component, guanine. Some antiviral drugs have a chemical structure very similar to components of RNA and DNA. Acyclovir is an antiviral drug that has a structure similar to guanine, a building block for DNA. Thus acyclovir interferes with DNA synthesis in cells infected with certain viruses.

clovir. Famciclovir (Famvir) is also a prodrug but converted to a different metabolite that is not orally absorbed. Idoxuridine (Herplex), vidarabine (Vira-A), and trifluridine (Viroptic) are available as ophthalmic dosage forms for treatment of herpes simplex keratitis. Penciclovir (Denavir) is also topical but used to treat cold sores, a herpes simplex virus.

Amantadine (Symmetrel) and rimantadine (Flumadine) are effective in preventing and treating influenza A, and zanamivir (Relenza) impacts influenza A and B. These drugs can be used to protect high-risk patients (eg, elderly, immunocompromised patients, health care workers) who are not immunized until after an epidemic has started. Adverse effects include anorexia, nausea, nervousness, anxiety, lightheadedness, and insomnia. Amantadine is also used to treat Parkinson's disease but the mechanism is not related to its antiviral activity.

ANTISEPTICS AND DISINFECTANTS

Antiseptics and disinfectants are used only externally to kill (germicide) or inhibit the growth (germistatic) of microorganisms. *Antiseptics* are preparations applied to tissue such as hands or a site of injection or incision. *Disinfectants* are products applied to inanimate objects such as surgical areas or instruments. The mechanism of action of these compounds is generally nonspecific compared to the site-specific action of the antimicrobials previously discussed and consequently they are too toxic for internal use. Some antiseptics and disinfectants are toxic to bacteria, fungi, and viruses. They may facilitate the physical removal of cells from surfaces, denature protein, or physically disrupt membranes due to the harsh chemical nature of the compound. See Table 5-8 for some examples of antiseptics used primarily as skin and wound cleansers. Continuous exposure of wounds to some antiseptic products may delay wound healing through a cytotoxic effect on some cells necessary for the healing processes.

TREATMENT OF SEXUALLY TRANSMITTED DISEASES

Sexually transmitted diseases (STDs) are a significant health problem in the United States. The number of sexual partners is the biggest risk factor for contracting STD; the more partners, the larger the risk. The incidence is also greater for homosexual men than for heterosexuals. For some infections, the treatment regimen differs depending on the age of the patient (child versus adult), location of the infection, and whether the patient is pregnant. Treatment of some STDs

Table 5-9. Examples of Sexually Transmitted Diseases and Treatment[1]

Disease	Infecting Organism	Generic Name	Trade Name	Administration
Chlamydia	Chlamydia trachomatis	azithromycin or doxycycline	Zithroma or Vibramycin	Oral Oral
Gonorrhea	Neisseria gonorrhoeae	cefixime or ciprofloxacin or ceftriaxone or ofloxacin	Suprax or Cipro or Rocephin or Floxin	Oral Oral IM Oral
Syphilis	Treponema pallidum	penicillin G or doxycycline	Bicillin LA or Vibramycin	IM Oral
Trichomoniasis	Trichomonas vaginalis	metronidazole	Flagyl	Oral
Bacterial Vaginosis	Gardnerella vaginalis, Mycoplasma hominis	metronidazole	Flagyl	Oral
Genital Herpes	herpes simplex virus (HSV)	acyclovir or valacyclovir or famciclovir	Zovirax or Valtrex or Famvir	Oral Oral Oral
Genital Warts	human papillomavirus (HPV)	podofilox or imiquimod	Condylox or Aldara	Topical Topical
Pubic lice (crabs)	Phthirus pubis	permethrin	Nix[2]	Topical
Pubic mites (scabies)	Sarcoptes scabiei	permethrin	Elimite	Topical

[1]In adults. Selection of drug may vary depending on the site of the infection.
[2]Available over the counter. All other by prescription.

has changed over the years because of the development of resistant strains of some organisms. Table 5-9 lists the causative organism for common STDs and a drug of choice for treating the disease in adults. Most of the drugs in Table 5-9 have been previously mentioned in this chapter; the others are:

- *Metronidazole* (Flagyl). This drug is effective against certain bacteria and protozoa. Bacterial infections include *H. pylori* in some people with ulcers (see Chapter 11) and bacterial vaginosis; protozoal infections include amebiasis and trichomoniasis. Metronidazole interferes with DNA function in these organisms. It is absorbed orally, metabolized by the liver, and excreted primarily by the kidney. The most common adverse effects include dizziness, headache, nausea, vomiting, diarrhea, metallic taste in the mouth, and loss of appetite. Metronidazole may be taken with food if gastrointestinal upset occurs. The drug discolors the urine dark or reddish-brown. An unpleasant disulfiram-like reaction occurs if the patient ingests alcohol or is exposed to topically applied products with alcohol within 72 hours of taking metronidazole.

- *Podofilox* (Condylox). Podofilox is used topically as a solution or gel to treat genital warts. It is applied twice daily in a cycle of 3 days with application followed by 4 days without applying the drug. It causes erosion of the wart tissue. Adverse effects are pain, inflammation, burning, and itching.
- *Imiquimod* (Aldara). Imiquimod is a topical cream used to treat genital warts. It induces cytokines and other factors that enhance the immune response at the local site. Imiquimod is applied at bedtime three times per week and then removed by washing in the morning. Adverse effects are local itching, burning, erosion, flaking, and edema.

> *Disulfiram (Antabuse) is a drug that is used in the management of chronic alcoholism. It produces an unpleasant response if alcohol is consumed while taking disulfiram. Some other drugs, such as metronidazole, also produce a similar unpleasant disulfiram-like reaction when combined with alcohol. The unpleasant reaction is characterized by headache, nausea, vomiting, flushing, sweating, and tachycardia.*

- *Permethrin* (Elimite, Nix). Permethrin is used topically as a liquid (Nix) to treat lice infestation (also called pediculosis) and as a cream (Nix) to treat mite infestation (also called scabies). It is effective against not only pubic lice (crabs) but also head and body lice. It causes paralysis and death of the parasite. For treatment of scabies or lice, a single application is usually sufficient. Adverse effects are mild and include temporary burning or stinging.

ROLE OF THE ATHLETIC TRAINER

- *Educate regarding infections.* Many patients do not understand that the occurrence of an infection does not mean automatic treatment with an antibiotic. Antibiotics are not effective in the treatment of viral infections, the most common cause of most upper respiratory infections. Unnecessary use of antibiotics can lead to unnecessary adverse effects, including the occurrence of superinfections.
- *Educate regarding compliance.* As with therapy for many diseases, noncompliance with appropriate antimicrobial therapy is a significant cause of treatment failures. Typical antibiotic therapy requires 7 to 14 days of the prescribed dosage regimen for a cure, although the recommended length of therapy varies with the type of infection, site of infection, and treatment regimen. Sometimes patients discontinue use of the drug after a few days because the symptoms disappear; treatment for the entire prescribed time is necessary to most efficiently eradicate the infection. It is particularly difficult to continue with treatment of fungal infections that require weeks to months of therapy. The athletic trainer can encourage the patient to continue treatment for successful recovery.
- *Monitor for allergies.* Patients who develop a rash during systemic or topical treatment with any antimicrobial drug may not realize that the rash could be the result of an allergic response to the drug. The athletic trainer can be observant concerning these connections so that a change in antimicrobial therapy can be initiated if necessary.
- *Monitor for common adverse effects.* The athletic trainer can help avoid adverse effects other than allergic reactions. Tetracyclines, for example, should not be used by children <8 years old. Also, potential problems associated with photosensitivity with these drugs and the fluoroquinolones should be monitored so that the adverse effects can be minimized through use of protective clothing or the therapy can be changed. Also, fluoroquinolones should be avoided in athletes <18 years old and in athletes with tendonitis. The occurrence of any symptom that did not exist before therapy was initiated should be suspected as potential adverse effect.

- *Monitor for effectiveness.* Because infections are caused by so many microorganisms, and because resistance to antimicrobial agents is a significant problem, some patients on antimicrobial therapy may not have improved symptoms as therapy progresses. The athletic trainer can check with the athlete to be sure the infection is being responsive to the drug therapy. For example, are the symptoms ameliorating; if they are not, re-evaluation of the therapy may be necessary.

BIBLIOGRAPHY

APhA Special Report. Combating antibiotic resistance. Washington, DC: American Pharmaceutical Association; 2001.

Pflomm J. Strategies for minimizing antimicrobial resistance. *Am J Health Syst Pharm.* 2002;59(Suppl 3):S12-S15.

Post-exposure anthrax prophylaxis. *The Medical Letter.* 2001;43:91-92.

Rabenberg VS, Ingersoll CS, Sandrey MA, Johnson MT. The bacterial and cytotoxic effects of antimicrobial wound cleansers. *Journal of Athletic Training.* 2002;37:51-54.

Scholar EM. Fluoroquinolones: past, present and future of a novel group of antibacterial agents. *Am J Pharm Educ.* 2002;66:164-172.

The choice of antibacterial drugs. *The Medical Letter.* 2001;43:69-78.

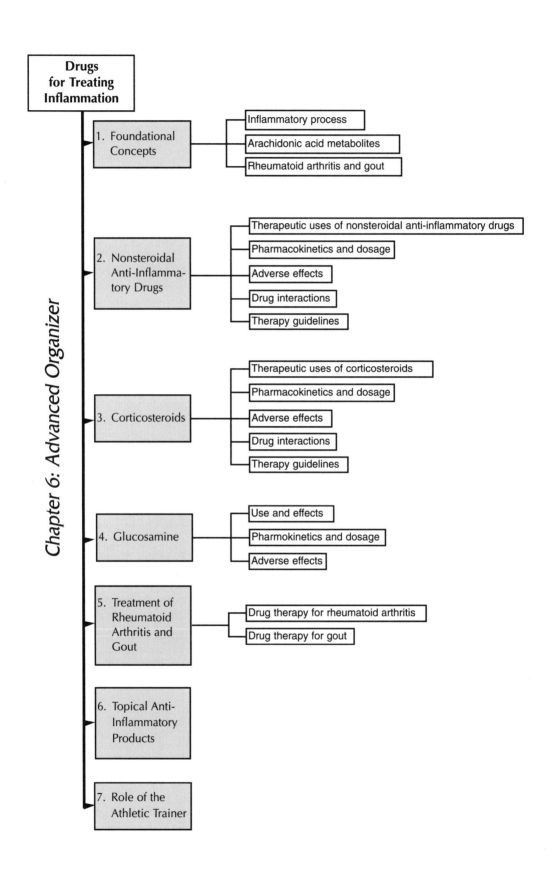

DRUGS FOR TREATING INFLAMMATION

CHAPTER OBJECTIVES

At the end of this chapter, the reader will be able to:

- Describe and explain the inflammatory process.
- List the common chemical mediators, explain how they affect physiological functions, and summarize their role in the inflammatory process.
- Differentiate how the pathophysiology of rheumatoid arthritis and gout differ from other inflammatory reactions.
- Explain the difference between COX-1 and COX-2 enzymes.
- Explain how nonsteroidal anti-inflammatory drugs (NSAIDs) effect blood clotting and how aspirin differs from other NSAIDs in this mechanism.
- Describe the pharmacokinetics of NSAIDs and corticosteroids.
- Recall the general dosing regimen for NSAIDs and corticosteroids.
- List the signs and symptoms and explain the pathophysiology of specific adverse effects and drug interactions with NSAID and corticosteroid therapy.
- Explain the physiological effects of increased dosage and treatment duration for corticosteroids.
- Describe how corticosteroids exert their therapeutic effect on the inflammatory process.
- Recall the most appropriate drug therapy for the treatment of rheumatoid arthritis and gout.
- Recall the three types of drugs that can be components in a topical over-the-counter (OTC) anti-inflammatory medication.
- Describe the potential value of glucosamine to treat osteoarthritis.
- Explain how topical anti-inflammatory medications exert their therapeutic effects.
- Summarize the role of the athletic trainer for patients who are on NSAID or corticosteroid drug therapy.

Inflammation can be caused by a variety of stimuli, including physical injury, infections, heat, and *antigen*-antibody interactions. The inflammatory response is generally a beneficial mechanism that allows the body to combat the injury or infection more effectively. However, sometimes the inflammatory response is excessive in duration or intensity and the use of drug therapy to reduce the response is beneficial. This chapter discusses the key cellular components of the inflammatory response as a basis for an understanding of the *mechanism of action* of anti-inflammatory drugs, the pharmacological characteristics that are common among the agents within the

Table 6-1. Drugs Only Used to Treat Inflammation Caused by a Specific Disease Process

Generic Name	Trade Name	Use	Mechanism
cromolyn	Intal	Asthma	Mast cell-stabilizer
montelukast	Singulair	Asthma	Diminishes effect of leuko-trienes
nedocromil	Tilade	Asthma	Mast cell-stabilizer
zafirlukast	Accolate	Asthma	Diminishes effect of leuko-trienes
zileuton	Zyflo	Asthma	Diminishes effect of leuko-trienes
allopurinol	Zyloprim	Gout	Inhibits uric acid formtion
colchicine	none	Gout	Inhibits leukocyte infiltration
probenecid	Benemid	Gout	Increases urinary excretion of uric acid
sulfinpyrazone	Anturane	Gout	Increases urinary excretion of uric acid
azathioprine	Imuran	Rheumatoid arthritis	Immunosuppression, but mechanism unknown
etanercept	Enbrel	Rheumatoid arthritis	Prevents inflammatory activity of tumor necrosis factor
gold compounds (eg, auranofin)	Several (eg, Ridaura)	Rheumatoid arthritis	Immunosuppression, but unknown mechanism
hydroxychloroquine	Plaquenil	Rheumatoid arthritis	Immunosuppression, but unknown mechanism
leflunomide	Arava	Rheumatoid arthritis	Inhibits T-cell and antibody production
methotrexate	Rheumatrex	Rheumatoid arthritis	Several, including immuno-suppression
penicillamine	Cuprimine	Rheumatoid arthritis	Immunosuppression, but mechanism unknown

nonsteroidal and steroidal categories of anti-inflammatory drugs, and some specific examples of drugs in each of these two categories.

The NSAIDs and *corticosteroids* discussed in this chapter have a direct effect on the inflammatory response mechanism. There are other drugs that also diminish inflammation indirectly by improving the inflammatory-causing disease and thus are used to relieve the inflammation associated with that specific disease. For example, *antimicrobial drugs* (see Chapter 5) reduce the inflammation associated with an infection by affecting the infecting organism, but these drugs do not have direct anti-inflammatory activity. In a similar fashion, inflammation is abated by some drugs that are unique to the treatment of rheumatoid arthritis, gout, or asthma (Table 6-1) because of the impact of these drugs on the disease process. Drugs used to treat asthma will be discussed in Chapter 9; drugs used selectively for rheumatoid arthritis and gout are discussed later in this chapter.

FOUNDATIONAL CONCEPTS

The major purpose for using anti-inflammatory drugs, obviously, is to reduce inflammation. Consequently, a brief discussion of the inflammatory process is provided. The mechanism of action of steroidal and nonsteroidal anti-inflammatory agents center on the biochemical production of *arachidonic acid* metabolites, and therefore those pathways will also be a focus of the Foundational Concepts.

Inflammatory Process

The inflammatory process is normally a beneficial process, initiated immediately after injury and intended to facilitate repair and expedite a return of the tissue to normal function. Often times the inflammatory process is either bothersome or excessive in intensity or duration so that it must be treated to reduce the negative impact of the process, which may merely be acute discomfort or pain, or may be chronic and debilitating. Regardless of the cause of the inflammation, there are many chemical mediators, numerous types of activated cells, and a few *plasma protein systems* that become a part of the inflammatory response (Figure 6-1). *Chemical mediators* are compounds that are released by one cell type, attach to the receptor of a second cell type, and affect the response of that second cell (see histamine example below). There is considerable interaction among these mediators, various cell types, and plasma protein systems, which are intended to regulate the rate and extent of the inflammatory response. In other words, some of these interactions stimulate the progress of the inflammatory response whereas other interactions prevent the process from spreading beyond certain limits.

The inflammatory response is initiated within seconds after cellular injury caused by a wide range of stimuli, including physical trauma, radiation (eg, ultraviolet light, X-rays), chemicals (toxins, caustic substances), heat, infectious microorganisms, or hypersensitivity reactions. These stimuli cause the release of several chemical mediators by mast cells and *basophils*, which are key cells in initiating the inflammatory response. *Mast cells* are located in connective tissue near blood vessels whereas basophils are circulating in the blood. Both of these cell types have storage pockets (granules) for specific chemical mediators. Histamine, for example, dilates local capillaries and increases vascular permeability, which increases blood flow and access to the site by other components of the inflammatory response. Chemotactic factors are also released; these are compounds that cause *chemotaxis*, the attraction of specific types of cells to the area. *Leukotrienes* and *prostaglandins* are also chemical mediators that are released by mast cells and play a role in vascular permeability, chemotaxis, and pain response; these mediators are discussed in more detail below. See Table 6-2 for a list of other chemical mediators.

Besides mast cells and basophils, many other cell types accumulate at the site of inflammation, either through chemotaxis or adhesion mechanisms, which hold the cells in the area of inflammation. Some cells are phagocytic, which remove dead cells, debris, and bacteria from the site by engulfing them (*phagocytosis*). *Neutrophils* are at the scene early to carry out this task, whereas *macrophages* arrive later and persist longer. The regulatory processes that control the activity of these and other phagocytic cells (eg, *eosinophils* and basophils) are complex but are important to prevent an excessive inflammatory response. Platelets and lymphocytes are examples of nonphagocytic cells that also have specific roles during inflammation (see Table 6-2).

The *plasma protein systems* are biochemical sequences that produce several proteins with specific important functions in the inflammatory response. The clotting system, for example, is a sequence of proteins that activates other proteins leading to the formation of a clot. Some of the proteins generated through the clotting process also have other functions such as chemotaxis and enhancing the *kinin system*. The kinin system is another plasma protein system, the most notable

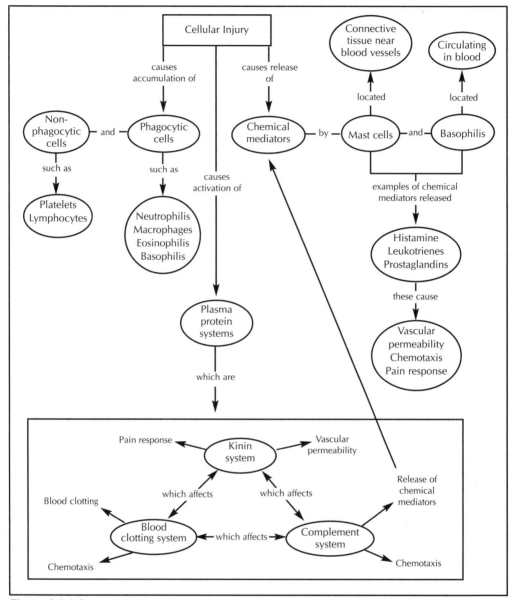

Figure 6-1. Inflammation process.

protein is *bradykinin*, which increases vascular permeability and produces pain. The *complement system* is also a plasma protein system that impacts inflammation. This biochemical sequence of activated proteins can be initiated by the presence of bacterial or fungal cells. Among the many functions of the complement system are to kill microorganisms, cause chemotaxis, and initiate the release of chemical mediators from mast cells.

The inflammatory response is a complex process and therefore it is difficult to completely control. Drug therapy can have an impact on the process; however, the prime focus of their mechanism of action is to alter the effect that chemical mediators have on the inflammatory response.

Table 6-2. Major Components of Inflammatory Process

	Components	*Function*
Chemical mediators	Bradykinin	Causes vasodilation and pain response.
	Cytokines	Cause wide range of effects in inflammation and immune response; subgroups include interleukins (IL) and interferons (INF) of which there are several of each, such as IL-1, IL-2, INF-α, INF-β, etc.
	Eosinophil chemotactic factor	Attracts eosinophils to inflammatory site.
	Histamine	Increases capillary blood flow and vascular permeability.
	Leukotrienes	Increases vascular permeability and chemotaxis.
	Neutrophil chemotactic factor	Attracts neutrophils to inflammatory site.
	Platelet-activating factor	Stimulates activity of platelets.
	Prostaglandins	Increases vascular permeability and hemotaxis; induces pain; suppresses some aspects of inflammation.
	Serotonin	Increases capillary blood flow and vascular permeability.
Cell types	Basophils	Storage/release of several chemical meditors.
	Eosinophils	Phagocytic; inactivates some chemical mediators (eg, histamine, leukotrienes).
	Lymphocytes	Key cells of immune reactions; production/release of antibodies, including during inflammation.
	Macrophages	Key phagocytes; primarily after 24 hours from initial inflammatory response.
	Mast cells	Storage/release of chemical mediators.
	Neutrophils polymorphonuclear Neutrophils [PMNs])	Key phagocytes; within 6 to 12 hours of initial inflammatory response.
	Platelets	Interact with clotting system for clot formation; releases chemical mediators.
Plasma protein systems	Clotting system	Prevents bleeding and traps debris; affects chemotaxis; increases kinin response.
	Complement system	Initiates inflammation; chemotaxis; destroys microorganisms; increases vascular permeability.
	Kinin system	Increases vascular permeability and vasodilation; affects clotting system; causes pain response with prostaglandins.

Figure 6-2. Pathways for the synthesis of arachidonic acid metabolites. Phospholipase A_2 releases arachidonic acid from the stored site as a component of membrane phospholipid. The released arachidonic acid is converted to various metabolites by either lipoxygenase or COX (see text for discussion). COX = cyclooxygenase, PGs = prostaglandins, PGI_2 = prostacyclin, TXs = thromboxanes, LTs = leukotrienes.

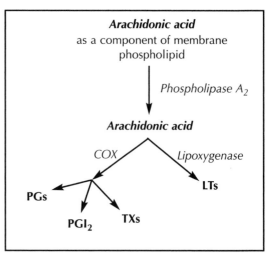

Arachidonic Acid Metabolites

The metabolism of arachidonic acid plays an important role in the inflammatory process and is worthy of separate consideration as much of anti-inflammatory drug therapy affects these pathways. Arachidonic acid is an unsaturated fatty acid that is the starting point (substrate) for the biosynthesis of several groups of compounds. In other words, these compounds are metabolites of arachidonic acid that contribute to the inflammatory response. These metabolites of arachidonic acid are also called *eicosanoids*. The eicosanoids are a part of a larger group of compounds referred to as chemical mediators. As discussed above, the extent of inflammation is largely controlled by the extent of release of chemical mediators from various cell types. Aside from eicosanoids, other chemical mediators that are noneicosanoids include *histamine, cytokines*, and *platelet-activating factor* (see Table 6-2).

As shown in Figure 6-2, arachidonic acid is attached to phospholipids that are components of the membrane structure. An enzyme, *phospholipase A_2*, catalyzes the intracellular release of arachidonic acid from the membrane-bound phospholipid. Arachidonic acid then follows one of two pathways depending on which enzymes are active within that cell type. The two pathways are the cyclooxygenase (COX) pathway and the lipoxygenase (leukotriene) pathway. These pathways lead to four groups of eicosanoid mediators: *prostaglandins* (PGs), *prostacyclin* (PGI_2), *thromboxanes* (TXs), and *leukotrienes* (LTs). The specific eicosanoids produced in these pathways were given letter designations as they were discovered, such as prostaglandins A through I (ie, PGA, PGB, PGC, etc) and leukotrienes A through E. The names for the eicosanoids also have a subscript that designates the number of carbon-carbon double bonds in the molecule. For example, PGE_2 and LTC_4 have two and four such double bonds, respectively. Table 6-3 identifies some physiological functions that have been attributed to individual eicosanoids.

One or more of the eicosanoids are produced by virtually all cells and they play an important role of regulating many physiological functions in addition to inflammation. In some cases, one eicosanoid modulates the response from another eicosanoid to maintain homeostasis. Trauma, disease, or drugs can offset the balance between these and other eicosanoids. One example is regarding the physiological effects of prostaglandin I_2 (PGI_2, also called prostacyclin) and thromboxane A_2 (TXA_2). Prostacyclin is produced in blood vessel walls and inhibits platelet aggregation whereas TXA_2 is produced by platelets and enhances platelet aggregation (Figure 6-3). The

Table 6-3. Physiological Effects of Selected Arachidonic Acid Metabolites (Eicosanoids)

Eicosanoid[1]	Physiological Effect
LTB$_4$	Chemotactic for polymorphonuclear neutrophils (PMNs)
LTC$_4$ LTD$_4$ LTE$_4$	Bronchoconstriction, increases mucus secretion, increases microvascular permeability
PGD$_2$	Bronchoconstriction
PGE$_2$	Protects gastric mucosa by increasing mucus and decreasing acid secretion, increases edema during inflammation, potentiates bradykinin-induced pain, increases renal blood flow by renal vasodilation, bronchodilation, causes fever and increased perception of pain in the brain
PGF$_{2\alpha}$	Bronchoconstriction
PGI$_2$	Inhibits platelet aggregation, increases local vasodilatation, increases edema during inflammation, potentiates bradykinin-induced pain, protects gastric mucosa by increasing mucus production and decreasing acid secretion, increases renal blood flow by renal vasodilation
TXA$_2$	Bronchoconstriction, increases platelet aggregation, increases local vasoconstriction, decreases renal blood flow

[1]*LT = leukotriene; PG = prostaglandin; TX = thromboxane*

normal balance between the effects of PGI$_2$ and TXA$_2$ is disrupted when the blood vessel wall is damaged by a laceration or by atherosclerosis. In this situation, the production of PGI$_2$ is reduced and the effects of TXA$_2$ predominate; hence, platelets aggregate and contribute to blood clot formation. A disruption of this normal balance also occurs as a result of some cardiovascular diseases, resulting in unwanted platelet aggregation and eventual thrombosis.

Related to inflammation, the arachidonic acid metabolites contribute to the symptoms of inflammation, including redness, swelling, and pain. During an allergic reaction or the bronchial hyper-responsiveness of an asthma attack, these same mediators are released as an exaggerated response to stimuli (see Chapter 9).

Because the COX pathway leads to the production of TX, PG, and PGI$_2$, drugs that block this pathway (COX inhibitors) will affect the processes controlled by these eicosanoids. There are two forms of the COX enzyme, *COX-1* and *COX-2*, referred to as *isoforms*. Although these two enzymes catalyze the same reaction, they are produced under different conditions and by different tissues. COX-1 is produced in virtually all tissues at a relatively stable rate so that there is a sufficient amount of the appropriate eicosanoid necessary to regulate certain normal ("housekeeping") functions. Similarly, COX-2 is produced in the brain, female reproductive tract, blood vessel walls, and kidneys. However, the production of COX-2 is also *induced* in response to inflammation and tissue injury, resulting in an increase in the synthesis of mediators that contribute to inflammation. Prostaglandins increase blood flow and *erythema* in the local area of the inflammatory response, initiate chemotaxis, sensitize pain receptors at the local site of inflammation, and cause a central nervous system pain response.

Figure 6-3. Platelet aggregation effects of PGI_2 and TXA_2. As platelets flow through blood vessels, they produce and release thromboxane A_2 (TXA_2) which causes platelets to aggregate. The cells that comprise the blood vessel wall produce and release PGI_2, which inhibits platelet aggregation, thus off-setting the potentially deleterious effects of TXA_2. Under normal conditions there is no need for platelet

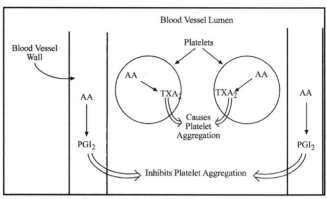

aggregation and the proper balance between the effects of PGI_2 and TXA_2 is important to prevent an unwanted blood clot. If there is trauma to the blood vessel wall (eg, laceration or atherosclerosis), some of the cells are damaged and production of PGI_2 is diminished. Since PGI_2 is not produced to off-set the effect of TXA_2, platelets aggregate at the site of the laceration and facilitate blood clot formation. PGI_2 and TXA_2 are made from arachidonic acid (AA) as shown in Figure 6-2.

Various hormones and physical stimuli activate phospholipase A_2, which increases the release of stored arachidonic acid from the phospholipid structure. After the eicosanoids are produced from arachidonic acid, they are released by the cell. These mediators have a relatively short half-life and thus their primary site of action is at or near the tissue that produces them; they are "local hormones." For example, PGE_2

Recall from Chapter 3 that when an enzyme is induced the number of molecules of enzyme synthesized by the cell is increased due to an effect on the regulatory mechanism at the gene level. The result is an increased level of enzyme activity.

affects gastric acid secretion and is produced by gastric cells (see Chapter 11), the LTs that constrict bronchial smooth muscle are produced in the respiratory tract (see Chapter 9), and kidney function is altered by eicosanoids produced by renal cells. Once in the extracellular space, the eicosanoids can attach to their corresponding receptors to initiate an intracellular sequence through a *second messenger system* similar to the process described in Chapter 3. These intracellular reactions lead to the physiological responses shown in Table 6-3, including swelling, redness, and pain at the site of inflammation.

Rheumatoid Arthritis and Gout

Although the etiology for rheumatoid arthritis and gout is different, inflammation is the principal characteristic of both. In addition to the inflammatory mechanism already discussed, other mechanisms also contribute to these diseases and thus a discussion of additional drugs is necessary.

Rheumatoid arthritis is a common systemic inflammatory disease caused by an autoimmune response, possibly initiated as a result of a bacterial or viral infection. As discussed above, chemical mediators are released and contribute to the inflammatory response. Among these is *tumor necrosis factor* (TNF), a cytokine that has been identified as one of the chemical mediators that contributes to the autoimmune process in rheumatoid arthritis. Symptoms of rheumatoid arthritis often begin with joint stiffness and progress at varying rates among patients but can lead to total destruction of the cartilage, erosion of the bone, and destruction of the joint. Stiffness and swelling in the small joints of the hands, wrists, and feet are the most common, although other joints can also be involved. Chronic inflammation leads to deformity. Other tissues, such as lungs, heart, and eyes, may also be affected and pose serious complications. Some patients experience periods of spontaneous remission. The disease can occur at any age and is more common in women than in men.

Gout is inflammation and joint pain as a result of elevated uric acid blood concentration. Uric acid is a waste product of purine metabolism. The purines are a group of compounds produced in the body for use as part of the building blocks of *DNA* and *RNA* synthesis and they are also one of the breakdown products of DNA and RNA. Patients with gout have an increased production or reduced excretion of uric acid and therefore have an elevated blood level of uric acid (ie, hyperuricemia). When the blood concentration of uric acid becomes too high, some crystallization of sodium urate (the sodium salt of uric acid) occurs in the synovium of joints and surrounding tissue. The deposit of these crystals initiates the inflammatory response at these sites, resulting in pain and swelling. Although symptoms can eventually occur at any joint, the most distal joints are most frequently affected, the first metatarsophalangeal joint often being the first of all. A possible explanation for the distal sites being favored is that the solubility of sodium urate is temperature dependent and the more distal joints are cooler. Although deposit of sodium urate in other tissues (eg, hips, shoulders, Achilles tendon, hands) is an eventual occurrence if untreated, drug therapy has immensely reduced this effect. Crystallization of uric acid and sodium urate in the kidney, however, remains a concern. Problems range from the more common formation of uric acid stones in urine to the less common acute renal failure.

Patients with gout experience acute, extremely painful attacks at varying intervals (initially months), which become shorter as the disease progresses. Initially, the time between acute attacks is pain free but as chronic gout develops, the periods between acute attacks are not completely pain free. Duration of acute attacks also varies from hours to weeks if untreated. The incidence of gout peaks at age 30 to 50 and is higher in men than women during this age group but becomes more evenly distributed in the elderly. Genetic factors related to the synthesis and excretion of uric acid can predispose a patient to develop gout, but other factors that cause increased uric acid blood levels are obesity, alcoholic beverages, hyperlipidemia, renal disease, hypertension, diuretic therapy (see Chapter 12), and low-dose aspirin therapy (aspirin at low doses blocks normal renal excretion mechanism of uric acid whereas doses >5 g/day increase uric acid excretion).

Summary

The inflammatory response involves numerous types of cells, chemical mediators, and plasma protein systems, which, when functioning properly, produce an inflammatory response that aids in the repair of damaged tissue. There are regulatory mechanisms as a part of the inflammatory response that affect the rate and extent of the response. The chemical mediators play a significant role in these regulatory mechanisms. These are compounds that are released by certain cells, or in some cases, produced by a plasma protein system and affect the response from other cells. The major mechanism of most anti-inflammatory drugs is to alter the response from chemical mediators.

Among the chemical mediators is a group called eicosanoids. These are compounds produced from the metabolism of arachidonic acid. There are two pathways that produce the eicosanoids: the COX enzyme initiates the COX pathway, which produces the PG, TX, and PGI eicosanoids; whereas the lipoxygenase enzyme initiates the pathway that produces the LT eicosanoids. There are two forms of the COX enzyme, referred to as COX-1 and COX-2. Although most cells contain COX-1 activity, some cells contain a significant amount of COX-2 (Figure 6-4). These include cells at the site of an inflammatory response and cells of the kidney and blood vessels.

Rheumatoid arthritis and gout are inflammatory diseases but with unique pathophysiology. The basis of rheumatoid arthritis is an autoimmune reaction that may be initiated by an infection whereas gout results from crystallization of sodium urate. In both diseases, the joints are the prime site of pain and inflammation.

Nonsteroidal Anti-Inflammatory Drugs

NSAIDs are among the most frequently prescribed drugs and frequently used OTC drugs; one estimate places the use of aspirin in the United States at >10,000 tons per year. Aspirin, also abbreviated ASA for the chemical name, *acetylsalicylic acid*, has been used since the late 1800s. There are other compounds that also have salicylic acid as part of the chemical structure and thus are referred to as salicylates, but aspirin is the most frequently used.

Aspirin is the prototype NSAID to which the effects of other NSAIDs are often compared. There are now >20 NSAIDs on the market. Table 6-4 lists selected NSAIDs with the typical anti-inflammatory adult daily dosage. The major mechanism of action of these drugs is to decrease PG production (see Figure 6-2) by inhibiting either one or both of the cyclooxygenase isoforms (COX-1, COX-2). The NSAIDs have little or no clinically significant effect on the lipoxygenase pathway, which produces LT. Because LTs and several noneicosanoid mediators contribute to the inflammatory response, the extent to which noneicosanoids are involved may impact the effectiveness of NSAIDs in relieving the symptoms of inflammation.

As previously discussed, COX-2 activity is enhanced in response to pain and inflammation and thus for anti-inflammatory effectiveness it is advantageous for NSAIDs to primarily inhibit this isoform rather than inhibiting both COX-1 and COX-2 (see Table 6-4). Inhibition of COX-1 will diminish the beneficial effects of prostaglandins, ie, cause some of the adverse effects, especially in the gastric and kidney cells. Selective COX-2 NSAIDs have been developed in recent years. These are highly specific for COX-2, have no clinically significant effect on COX-1 at therapeutic doses, and as discussed below, may have a lower incidence of some adverse effects. The other NSAIDs are nonselective inhibitors because they also affect COX-1 although the relative selectivity for COX-1 and COX-2 varies among this group. For example, aspirin has a greater selectivity for COX-1 whereas etodolac (Lodine) has greater selectivity for COX-2 than for COX-1.

Therapeutic Uses of Nonsteroidal Anti-Inflammatory Drugs

NSAIDs are used to treat both acute and chronic inflammation. All of the NSAIDs are equally effective although response varies from one patient to another; one particular NSAID may not be effective in a patient whereas another may be. A week or 2 of therapy is typically long enough to determine whether the anti-inflammatory effect of the drug is sufficiently effective. There are no clinical guidelines to determine which NSAID will be most effective in a particular patient. Selection of an NSAID should be made based on experiences of the physician, preference of the patient, cost, and adverse effects. The principle use of NSAIDs is to treat the inflammation associated with musculoskeletal disorders such as osteoarthritis, rheumatoid arthritis, gout, tendonitis, sprains, and strains. Treatment with an NSAID reduces pain, swelling, stiffness, and increases mobility. Because eicosanoid-induced inflammatory responses are a COX-2 response, either selective or nonselective COX inhibitors are effective treatment.

Although it is clear that NSAIDs reduce pain and inflammation, it is not as clear whether they decrease the healing time to allow the athlete to more quickly return to activity. Several factors may impact whether healing is expedited. As mentioned previously, mediators other than

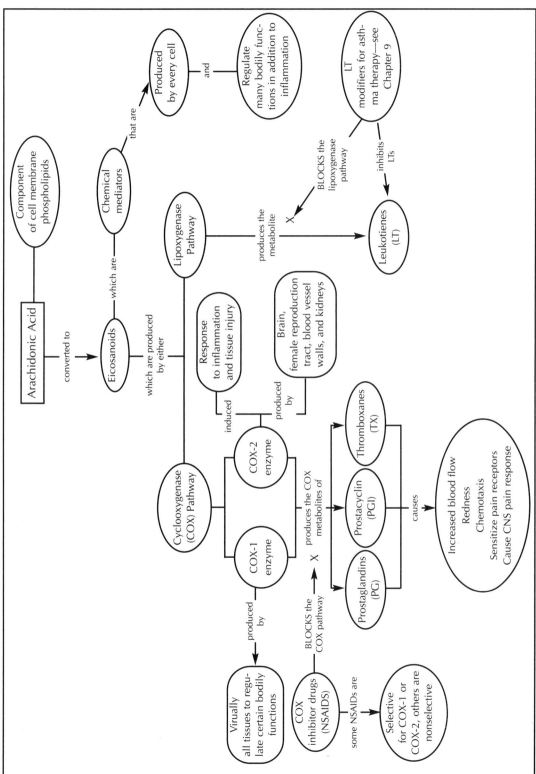

Figure 6–4. Effects of arachidonic acid metabolites and sites of drug action.

Table 6-4. Selected Nonsteroidal Anti-Inflammatory Drugs

Generic Name	Trade Name	Anti-Inflammatory Typical Dose (mg)	Doses/Day	OTC
aspirin	Many	650 to 975	4	Yes
celecoxib[1]	Celebrex	200	1	No
diclofenac	Voltaren	50	3 to 4	No
etodolac	Lodine	300	2 to 3	No
fenoprofen	Nalfon	300 to 600	3 to 4	No
flurbiprofen	Ansaid	50 to 75	2 to 4	No
ibuprofen	Advil	400 to 800	3 to 4	Yes
indomethacin	Indocin	50	2 to 4	No
ketoprofen	Orudis	50 to 75	3 to 4	Yes
meloxicam	Mobic	7.5	1	No
nabumetone	Relafen	1000	1	No
naproxen Na	Aleve	275 to 550	2	Yes
oxaprozin	Daypro	600 to 1200	1	No
piroxicam	Feldene	20	1	No
sulindac	Clinoril	150	2	No
tolmetin	Tolectin	200 to 600	3	No
valdecoxib[1]	Bextra	10	1	No

[1]Indicates selective COX-2 inhibitor.

eicosanoids are involved to various extents during the inflammatory response and therefore the type and extent of injury may influence the effectiveness of the NSAID. Timing between injury and drug therapy may also be important as the NSAIDs inhibit the synthesis of eicosanoids but do not affect the response of the eicosanoids once they are produced. Obviously, there are pharmacokinetic and/or pharmacodynamic factors that are significantly different from patient to patient as there is a wide range of intrapatient responses with any particular NSAID. Consequently, selection of the NSAID, dosing, and duration of therapy can also impact the potential for improved healing rate. Use of other treatment modalities (eg, ice, compression, ultrasound, etc) along with NSAID therapy may be of particular benefit when excessive inflammation is involved.

All of the NSAIDs also have analgesic and antipyretic (fever reducing) activity; however, not all of them are approved for these uses. Use of NSAIDs as analgesics are covered in the next chapter. Fever production is a COX-2 response that occurs in the brain. Aspirin and ibuprofen are the two NSAIDs most frequently used to reduce fever. Acetaminophen (Tylenol), which is not an NSAID, is also frequently used to reduce fever and is discussed in the next chapter with the other analgesics. NSAIDs and acetaminophen do not lower body temperature below normal or lower body temperature when it has been elevated by exercise.

NSAIDs are effective in inhibiting uterine synthesis of eicosanoids that contribute to cramps and excessive bleeding during menstruation. Therefore, these drugs are effective treatment of dysmenorrhea.

NSAIDs that inhibit COX-1 have antiplatelet activity and thus have an anticoagulant effect. The importance of the balance between TXA_2 and PGI_2 regarding platelet aggregation has been discussed (see Figure 6-3). COX-1 produces TXA_2, which stimulates platelet aggregation; COX-2 produces PGI_2, which inhibits platelet aggregation. Platelet aggregation stimulates activation of blood coagulation factors that can lead to a thromboembolism and subsequent myocardial infarction (MI), transient ischemic attack (TIA), or stroke. Therefore, inhibition of TXA_2 production in platelets is useful therapy to prevent the development of thromboemboli in susceptible patients. Aspirin differs from other NSAIDs in this respect because it is an irreversible inhibitor of the COX enzymes (ie, when aspirin binds to a molecule of COX, the enzyme remains inactive). All other NSAIDs are reversible inhibitors (they bind and release, back and forth) and thus are less effective for antiplatelet therapy. Unlike most other cells, platelets do not have significant protein synthesis capacity so platelets cannot regenerate more molecules of COX. Because aspirin binds irreversibly to COX, it prevents the production of TXA_2 for the lifespan of the platelet (about 8 days). Once TXA_2 production is inhibited, the PGI_2 effect of inhibiting platelet aggregation will predominate. Low-dose aspirin (40 to 325 mg/day) is effective for antiplatelet therapy and is used to reduce the risk of TIAs and stroke, to decrease the risk of MI in patients with previous MI or unstable angina, and to decrease the incidence of emboli formation in patients with various cardiovascular disease. The other NSAIDs are less effective because they are not irreversible inhibitors of COX. Because the production of PGI_2 is catalyzed by COX-2, selective COX-2 inhibitors may be counterproductive for these patients. In fact, some evidence indicates an increased incidence of thrombotic cardiovascular events (eg, MI, unstable angina, ischemic stroke, TIA) with COX-2 inhibitors compared with COX-1 inhibitors or placebo. In other words, a deleterious effect associated with cardiovascular events.

Another use for aspirin is to prevent the intense upper body flushing associated with high-dose niacin, which is used for treatment of elevated blood cholesterol. This flushing is caused by release of PGD_2, which can be inhibited by low-dose aspirin.

Pharmacokinetics and Dosage

All NSAIDs are absorbed rapidly from the gastrointestinal tract, and thus almost all NSAIDs are available only as oral preparations. Administration with food or milk is generally advised to reduce gastric upset. Use of enteric-coated aspirin will also reduce gastric upset but will delay absorption. This delay is not of clinical significance for chronic anti-inflammatory use, but may be important if quick pain relief is desired.

Recall from Chapter 2 that there is an acid secretion transporter in the kidney that actively transports acids from the blood into the renal tubule.

NSAIDs distribute into the central nervous system (CNS). They also distribute into breast milk and cross the placenta; thus, they are generally not recommended for use by pregnant or lactating women. NSAIDs, including selective COX-2 inhibitors, are extensively bound to plasma protein. Ibuprofen, fenoprofen, naproxen, and tolmetin are 99% bound to plasma protein.

Clearance of NSAIDs generally involves liver metabolism to form various metabolites followed by excretion in the urine. Aspirin, for example, is rapidly converted by the liver to several metabolites, which are excreted in the urine, including the active metabolite salicylic acid. Both glomerular filtration and/or renal tubular excretion are used in the kidney to get NSAIDs and their metabolites into the renal tubule.

The antipyretic dose for aspirin and ibuprofen is similar to the dose for relief of mild to moderate pain. However, there is a risk of potentially fatal Reye's syndrome associated with the use of aspirin in children with fever, and therefore aspirin and other NSAIDs should be avoided as antipyretic therapy in children <19 years of age; acet-aminophen (Tylenol) is preferred. The mechanism for the development of Reye's syndrome as a result of aspirin therapy is unknown.

The anti-inflammatory and analgesic dosage for NSAIDs will vary among patients depending on the extent of inflammation and pain, but generally the maximum anti-inflammatory dosage is greater than the maximum analgesic dosage. A typical analgesic dose for ibuprofen (Advil) in treating mild to moderate pain is 400 mg four times a day, whereas a typical anti-inflammatory dose is 600 mg four times a day. Similarly, for aspirin, the maximum daily analgesic and anti-inflammatory doses are 4 g and 6 g per day, respectively.

Reye's syndrome is a potentially fatal condition that causes liver and brain damage. It occurs in some children who have chickenpox or influenza and are treated with aspirin. Because these two diseases are viral infections, and because it is often difficult to distinguish between influenza symptoms and other viral upper respiratory infections, use of aspirin and aspirin-containing products should be avoided in children and teenagers with any cold or flu-type symptoms.

A typical adult "aspirin tablet" is 325 mg whereas a "baby aspirin" and "adult low strength" aspirin is 81 mg. These amounts of aspirin per tablet seem to be an odd strength considering that all dosage forms for virtually all other NSAIDs are round numbers such as 10 mg, 100 mg, or 150 mg per tablet. The reason for the difference is that aspirin and some other drugs that have been available for >100 years (eg, morphine and codeine) were originally marketed in tablet strengths based on the system of weight called grains. Adult-strength aspirin tablets have historically been marketed as 5-grain tablets, which is approximately 325 mg; baby-strength aspirin as 1.25 grain, which is 81 mg. Consequently, these strengths are still used today. The extra strength or maximum strength products were marketed later and contain 500 mg per tablet although some extended release products continue to use multiples of 325 mg (ie, 650, 975). Some naproxen products are also marketed in an unusual strength because they exist in the product as the sodium salt of naproxen. Consequently, as stated on the OTC packaging, 220 mg naproxen sodium (Aleve) contains 200 mg of naproxen. Similarly, one drug company markets 500 mg/tablet of naproxen under one trade name and 550 mg/tablet of naproxen sodium under another trade name; both products contain the same amount of active drug (500 mg naproxen/tablet).

Aspirin overdose is a significant concern, especially regarding accidental poisoning in children. The initial symptom of toxicity often is tinnitus, but other symptoms may include nausea, vomiting, hyperthermia, sweating, disorientation, lethargy, and hyperventilation followed by respiratory depression, coma, and death. Toxicity from other NSAIDs rarely causes death. Outdated bottles of aspirin will have an odor of vinegar (acetic acid) because the acetylsalicylic acid has decomposed to acetic acid and salicylic acid. These should be discarded because the salicylic acid will have greater gastric irritation effects.

Adverse Effects

The morbidity and mortality of the adverse effects associated with NSAID use are significant, especially with daily use and in certain at-risk patients (see page 145). Over 16,000 patients die each year and >100,000 are hospitalized as a result of NSAID-related adverse effects. The toxicity from NSAIDs may be underestimated by patients because of the ready accessibility of NSAIDs as OTC products.

The most common adverse effects of NSAIDs are gastrointestinal irritation, heartburn, nausea, upper gastrointestinal bleeding, and gastric and duodenal ulcers. Patients may experience gastric upset without ulceration, and on the other hand, patients with a developing ulcer may be asymptomatic until ulceration has occurred. Two mechanisms are involved in the development of these gastrointestinal adverse effects. A direct local irritation effect occurs when the drug is in direct contact with gastric mucosa. Almost all NSAIDs are acids and thus exist primarily in the unionized state in the acid environment of the stomach. Thus, the drug readily diffuses across the cell membrane but becomes trapped inside as it converts to the ionized form in the higher intracellular pH.

> *Recall from Chapter 2 that acids are more highly unionized in acidic pH and in this form are more lipophilic and will cross membranes more readily.*

The high intracellular concentration of NSAID causes cell damage. The other mechanism for gastrointestinal damage is by the systemic action of inhibiting COX. Gastric upset and some blood loss are a result of local irritation and can occur with the first dose, whereas the incidence of serious gastrointestinal bleeding (potentially to the point of anemia) or ulceration increases significantly with higher doses of NSAID and with longer duration of therapy. Risk of these serious adverse effects is also greater in patients >60 years old, patients who have a history of peptic ulcer disease, and patients who are also using oral corticosteroids, anticoagulants, alcoholic beverages, or cigarettes. Among the OTC NSAIDs, gastrointestinal adverse effects occur most frequently with aspirin and least with ibuprofen. Contrary to initial reports, there is some uncertainty as to whether all COX-2 selective inhibitors have a lower incidence of these adverse effects compared with nonselective NSAIDs. Also, because the incidence of gastrointestinal effects is most significant with long-term use, there may be no advantage of COX-2 inhibitors for short-term use (<2 weeks) in patients with no other risk factors for gastrointestinal ulceration. Symptoms of gastrointestinal toxicity include dark, tarry stools; indigestion; nausea; vomiting; and abdominal pain.

Gastric irritation can be minimized by administration of NSAIDs with milk, food, or antacids (except for enteric-coated products, as milk and antacids may cause the coating to dissolve prematurely). A disadvantage of antacid use with chronic aspirin therapy is that antacids can alkalinize the urine, which increases the excretion rate of aspirin. Enteric-coated aspirin also reduces gastric mucosal damage by preventing dissolution of the aspirin until it reaches the small intestine and may be particularly useful, compared to buffered or plain aspirin, for patients on chronic aspirin therapy. Another means of protecting the gastric mucosa during NSAID therapy is the administration of the prostaglandin substitute, misoprostol (Cytotec), or a *proton pump inhibitor*. Misoprostol is a chemical modification of PGE_1 and acts by the same mechanism as PGE_2 and thus is a PGE_2-substitute during NSAID therapy, but is contraindicated in women of child-bearing age because it has *abortifacient* properties. Proton pump inhibitors such as omeprazole (Prilosec) reduce the amount of acid pumped into the stomach lumen by the stomach cells (see Chapter 11). The incidence of peptic ulcers associated with long-term NSAID therapy can be reduced when misoprostol or proton pump inhibitors (eg, omeprazole) are used in conjunction with NSAID therapy.

> *Recall from Chapter 2 that alkalinization of the urine keeps drugs that are acids in the ionized form and thus prevents reabsorption back into the blood.*

Hypersensitivity to NSAIDs is another adverse effect of significant concern. Symptoms typically occur within 3 hours of ingestion of the drug and range from rhinitis, urticaria, and flushing to bronchospasm and asthmatic attack. Hypersensitivity reactions to NSAIDs are more frequent in patients with chronic urticaria, asthma, or nasal polyps. Fatal reactions of anaphylaxis or asthma are rare but have occurred. There is a *cross-sensitivity* among the NSAIDs and therefore these drugs should be avoided in patients who have experienced any allergic symptoms from use of any of the NSAIDs. Currently, this recommendation also applies to the COX-2 inhibitors although there is some evidence that COX-2 inhibitors may not cause the pulmonary effects in patients with aspirin-induced asthma.

One theory for the hypersensitivity mechanism is that as the NSAIDs inhibit COX-1, additional arachidonic acid is available as a substrate for the lipoxygenase pathway (see Figure 6-2), resulting in increased levels of LTs, which are the cause of asthmatic bronchospasms and anaphylaxis in susceptible patients. Patients with known intolerance to NSAIDs must be careful when selecting OTC medication because NSAIDs are components of many analgesic and anti-inflammatory products as well as combination products such as for cold and sinus relief. Examples of OTC products containing NSAIDs are shown in Table 6-5. Patients who are allergic to aspirin also have a greater likelihood of being allergic to tartrazine (FDA yellow #5), which is a coloring agent added to some foods and drugs. Finally, patients who are allergic to sulfonamides (sulfur-containing drugs), such as sulfa antibiotics, certain diuretics, and oral antidiabetic drugs are likely to also be allergic to celecoxib (Celebrex), which also contains a sulfur. Therefore, this selective COX-2 inhibitor should not be used in these patients.

All NSAIDs have the potential to cause renal toxicity. Prostaglandins play a role in maintaining appropriate salt and water balance and also cause renal vasodilation as a counter measure to maintain renal blood flow when it is diminished by other factors such as age, heart failure, hypertension, or kidney disease. Consequently, all NSAIDs should be used with caution in patients with these or any other condition associated with fluid retention and edema because the NSAID may reduce kidney function and thus accentuate the problem. These patients should also be aware that reduced urine output and edema are symptoms of diminished kidney function.

The incidence of liver toxicity is less than the risk of renal toxicity. Nonetheless, caution is necessary when using NSAIDs in patients with reduced liver function or history of liver disease. If NSAIDs are used in these patients, reduced dosage may be necessary as most NSAIDs have a significant liver metabolism component to the clearance. If symptoms of nausea, fatigue, jaundice, *pruritus*, right-upper-quadrant abdominal pain, and flu-like symptoms occur, hepatotoxicity should be considered.

Because of the antiplatelet action of aspirin, it should be avoided in patients with blood clotting disorders. Similarly, other nonselective NSAIDs should be used with caution in these patients. Selective COX-2 inhibitors do not diminish platelet aggregation. As mentioned earlier, inhibition of PGI_2 (and not TXA_2) by COX-2 selective inhibitors may be deleterious for patients with cardiovascular risk factors.

Of additional interest for the athletic trainer are animal studies that have shown delayed new bone growth with use of NSAIDs, including selective COX-2 inhibitors, which may have a larger impact than nonselective COX inhibitors on delaying bone healing. Use of non-NSAID analgesics (see Chapter 7) rather than NSAIDs for pain relief is advisable for patients with fractures.

> *As discussed later in this chapter, methotrexate is used to treat rheumatoid arthritis, but it is also used as an anticancer drug. Doses are higher for cancer treatment than typically used for rheumatoid arthritis. Methotrexate inhibits folic acid use and therefore folic acid or a derivative of folic acid is used to reduce adverse effects associated with methotrexate.*

Drug Interactions

Because aspirin prolongs clotting time through its antiplatelet activity, it will enhance the effect of other anticoagulants such as warfarin (Coumadin), a frequently used oral anticoagulant.

Aspirin must be used with caution with warfarin, especially considering that aspirin can cause gastric bleeding, which may be enhanced significantly in conjunction with the anticoagulant effects of warfarin. Although the antiplatelet activity is less pronounced with the other NSAIDs, caution is also warranted when these drugs are used with warfarin. Even selective COX-2

Table 6-5. Examples of OTC Products Containing Aspirin or Other Nonsteroidal Anti-Inflammatory Drugs

Trade Name Product	*NSAID Component[1]*
Actron	ketoprofen
Advil Cold & Sinus	ibuprofen
Aleve	naproxen
Anacin	aspirin
Arthritis Pain Formula	aspirin
Ascriptin Regular Strength	aspirin
Bayer Low Adult Strength	aspirin
Buffex	aspirin
Cope	aspirin
Dristan Sinus Pain	ibuprofen
Ecotrin Adult Low Strength	aspirin
Empirin	aspirin
Excedrin Migraine	aspirin
Excedrin Extra Strength	aspirin
Genpril	ibuprofen
Genprin	aspirin
Haltran	ibuprofen
Heartline	aspirin
Midol Maximum Strength	ibuprofen
Motrin IB	ibuprofen
Nuprin	ibuprofen
Orudis KT	ketoprofen
Saleto Tablets	aspirin
Vanquish	aspirin

[1] *The product may contain other active components in addition to the NSAID.*

inhibitors may affect warfarin response, possibly by releasing warfarin from plasma protein binding sites or by inhibiting CYP450 enzyme metabolism (see Chapter 2) of warfarin. For mild to moderate analgesia, acetaminophen is preferred for patients on warfarin therapy because acetaminophen does not have anticoagulant effects.

Because aspirin and other NSAIDs are extensively bound to plasma protein, they may displace other drugs besides warfarin from their plasma protein binding site and thus increase the response from the displaced drug. For example, adding aspirin (or other NSAIDs) to the therapy of patients taking oral antidiabetic drugs may increase the hypoglycemic effect from some antidiabetic drugs. Similarly, NSAIDs can cause potentially toxic effects of methotrexate when it is used at anticancer dosages because the NSAID can release some of the methotrexate that is bound to plasma protein.

NSAIDs also diminish the effects of some drugs. The effectiveness of antihypertensive drugs (see Chapter 12) such as diuretics, *angiotensin-converting enzyme inhibitors*, and β-*blockers* are diminished by the use of NSAIDs.

Use of systemic corticosteroid or alcoholic beverages has the potential to cause peptic ulcers. Consequently, patients on NSAID therapy, particularly aspirin, should be warned about the additional risk of using alcoholic beverages concurrently with NSAIDs. The enhanced risk of ulcer formation from the concurrent use of corticosteroids and long-term NSAID therapy warrants that consideration be given to using misoprostol (Cytotec) or a proton pump inhibitor as a preventative measure.

There are other such potential interactions, but the point is that because NSAIDs affect pathways that have an impact on so many physiological functions, NSAIDs have the potential for several adverse effects as well as a significant potential for drug interactions. Therefore, the patient's response to multiple drug therapy should be monitored by a physician and/or pharmacist. As a general rule, if a patient experiences a change in symptoms or response after the addition of another drug, it is reasonable to suspect a drug interaction; an adjustment in therapy may be necessary.

Therapy Guidelines

Because NSAIDs have the potential for several significant adverse effects and because the goal of therapy with these drugs is generally to attain specific symptomatic relief, the lowest dose for the shortest duration of therapy that accomplishes the therapeutic goal should be used. Because response varies significantly among patients, it may be necessary to switch from one NSAID to another before an acceptably effective one is identified for a specific patient. A suitable therapeutic response is generally evident within 2 weeks after beginning therapy.

There is no clinically effective means of determining which NSAID may be effective for a patient. However, the patient's medical history, the anticipated duration of therapy, cost, and prior experiences can be a guide to the selection. For example, an OTC NSAID of the patient's choice may be suitable for short-term therapy to treat pain and inflammation of an acute sprain in a young and otherwise healthy athlete. On the other hand, long-term therapy to treat arthritis in an active older adult may require consideration of a COX-2 selective agent, the cost, and other medications the patient is taking.

Treatment with NSAIDs should be limited to one of these drugs at a time. There is no significant therapeutic advantage to combining NSAIDs. In fact, because some NSAIDs have a greater tendency for one adverse effect or drug interaction, using a combination of two NSAIDs at the same time adds the potential for adverse effects from both drugs.

Studies regarding the use of NSAIDs in children are limited; therefore, dosing recommendations for use in children and children's dosage forms are not available for most NSAIDs. The exception is for ibuprofen. Studies have demonstrated that ibuprofen is safe and effective for use in children, and appropriate pediatric dosage forms are available. Approved dosages for children >2 years of age are also reported for naproxen and tolmetin.

Summary

Arachidonic acid is a fatty acid that is a component of membrane phospholipids in virtually all cells. The arachidonic acid is converted to a series of metabolites, also known as eicosanoids, by either the COX or lipoxygenase pathways. The metabolites of the COX pathway include prostaglandins, prostacyclin, and thromboxanes. These metabolites affect many physiological functions, including decreasing the production of stomach acid, increasing the production of protective mucus in the stomach, producing renal vasodilation, contracting uterine smooth muscle, promoting and inhibiting platelet aggregation, sensitizing pain receptors at peripheral and CNS sites, causing fever, and contributing significantly to the inflammatory response by increasing blood flow, edema, and release of other inflammatory mediators. There are two isoforms of COX and each tissue produces a predominance of one or the other. COX-1 is produced by gastric mucosal and renal cells, and inhibition of COX-1 by NSAIDs is the cause of the most frequent significant adverse effects. Production of COX-2 occurs at sites that cause pain, inflammation, menstrual cramps, and fever. Inhibition of COX-2 is usually the intent of therapy (the exception is to prevent platelet aggregation). Therefore, NSAIDs that selectively inhibit COX-2 have a therapeutic advantage when treating pain and inflammation (see Figure 6-4).

Aspirin is a nonselective NSAID and is the prototype to which both selective and nonselective NSAIDs are often compared. Therapy with NSAIDs should be tailored to the needs of each patient and involve the lowest dose used for the shortest time necessary to achieve the desired therapeutic outcome. The patient should be aware of potential adverse effects, particularly gastric upset and ulceration. Use of NSAIDs with food or milk helps diminish gastric adverse effects. NSAIDs should be used with caution in patients with kidney or liver disease. Selective COX-2 inhibitors may be deleterious to patients with risk factors associated with cardiovascular disease. NSAIDs also inhibit healing of bone fractures. The primary potential for drug interactions exists with patients who are also using corticosteroids, alcoholic beverages, or warfarin.

CORTICOSTEROIDS

The adrenal cortex produces two types of *corticosteroids*: the glucocorticoids and the mineralocorticoids. The primary endogenous glucocorticoid is cortisol (hydrocortisone) and the primary mineralocorticoid is aldosterone. As the name suggests, the mineralocorticoid response has a significant impact on mineral balance; aldosterone increases urinary reabsorption of sodium and excretion of potassium. The glucocorticoid response has a significant impact on glucose metabolism, but also affects several other physiological processes. The extent to which corticosteroids exhibit these glucocorticoid physiological effects generally increases as dose and duration of therapy increase. Box 6-1 lists the most significant physiological effects.

Because there is some chemical structure similarity between cortisol and aldosterone, it is not surprising that cortisol has some degree of mineralocorticoid effect (eg, sodium retention). Development of corticosteroids for therapeutic use has focused on increasing the relative potency of the anti-inflammatory, compared with mineralocorticoid, effect. Hydrocortisone, for example, has equal potency of anti-inflammatory and sodium retention activity. Dexamethasone, on the hand, is 25 times more potent than hydrocortisone regarding anti-inflammatory activity and has no sodium retention effects. Prednisone is four times more potent than hydrocortisone but has almost the same degree of mineralocorticoid effect as hydrocortisone. Table 6-6 lists some corticosteroids and their anti-inflammatory dosages.

Therapeutic Uses of Corticosteroids

The major use of corticosteroids is to suppress the immune and inflammatory responses. These two processes are interconnected such that immune responses often have an inflammatory component. The anti-inflammatory mechanism of action for the corticosteroids encompasses a broader effect than that of the NSAIDs. The corticosteroids inhibit the activity of phospholipase A_2 (see Figure 6-2) to decrease both prostaglandin and leukotriene production. Inhibition of these eicosanoid chemical mediators reduces the swelling and pain associated with inflammation. However, they also inhibit the infiltration of phagocytes and lymphocytes at the site of inflammation and inhibit the release of additional chemical mediators that affect the inflammatory and immune responses, such as histamine and some cytokines.

Box 6-1. Physiological Effects of Increased Dosage and Treatment Duration of Corticosteriods

- Glucose production by the liver is increased using glycerol and amino acids (gluconeogenesis), and the glucose is released into the blood (hyperglycemia).
- The rate of protein breakdown is increased to supply amino acids to the liver for glucose synthesis.
- Skeletal muscle wasting occurs with high-dose, long-term use.
- Triglyceride hydrolysis (lipolysis) is increased to supply glycerol for glucose synthesis. Fatty acids become more available as the other product of lipolysis and thus there is an increased use of fatty acids as an energy source in peripheral tissues.
- Fat is redistributed away from extremities with high-dose, long-term use.
- Calcium absorption from the gastrointestinal tract is diminished and excretion of calcium by the kidney is increased.
- The aldosterone-like effects (ie, sodium and water retention, potassium excretion) from corticosteroids is generally low but varies depending on which corticosteroid is used.
- Several components of the immune and inflammatory responses are diminished.

Table 6-6. Dosage Range of Selected Corticosteroids

Generic Name	Trade Name	Dosage Range[1] (mg/day)
betamethasone	Celestone	0.6 to 0.75
cortisone	Cortisone	25 to 300
dexamethasone	Decadron	0.75 to 9
hydrocortisone	Cortef	20 to 240
methylprednisolone	Medrol	4 to 48
prednisolone	Delta-Cortef	5 to 60
prednisone	Deltasone	5 to 60
triamcinolone	Aristocort	4 to 60

[1]*Represents initial oral adult dosage range but dosage must be individualized based on patient's response and the specific disease being treated.*

Corticosteroids are used to treat rheumatoid and gouty arthritis (see below), systemic lupus erythematosus (SLE), bronchial asthma (see Chapter 9), inflammatory bowel disease (see Chapter 11), tendonitis, bursitis, inflammatory ocular disorders, allergic reactions, and dermatologic diseases. Table 6-6 lists examples of corticosteroids used to treat these conditions. Aside from these conditions, which have an inflammatory component, corticosteroids are also used to treat certain cancers, suppress organ transplant rejection, and as replacement therapy for adrenocortical insufficiency.

Pharmacokinetics and Dosage

Doses and duration of therapy with corticosteroids varies considerably depending on the specific inflammatory or immune disorder being treated. For example, long-term, low-dose therapy with prednisone for a patient with SLE may be 15 mg/day given as a single dose in the morning. On the other hand, short-term therapy at 60 mg/day in divided doses may be used to treat ulcerative colitis until remission occurs. Except for life-threatening situations, such as immuno-suppressive therapy in organ transplantation or as cancer chemotherapy, corticosteroid therapy should be initiated at the lowest dose and for the shortest time possible to achieve the therapeutic outcomes. Determining the dosage regimen for each patient for systemic treatment is somewhat trial and error and necessitates monitoring the extent of therapeutic, as well as adverse, effects. As therapy extends beyond 1 week, the incidence of adverse effects generally increases in a dose-related fashion.

Corticosteroids are available for use by several routes of administration. Inhalation products used to treat asthma are discussed in Chapter 9. Topical application of corticosteroids is used only for local, not systemic, effects and should be used whenever possible in place of systemic therapy to treat dermatological inflammatory conditions. Local injections are also useful to minimize systemic adverse effects in situations where inflammation is limited (eg, in a specific joint or soft tissue such as tendons). For a systemic effect, the oral route is preferred as corticosteroids are almost completely absorbed from the gastrointestinal tract. Intramuscular injections are available in which the corticosteroid exists as an ester form, which has lower aqueous solubility and thus slowly dissipates from the site of injection. These forms of the corticosteroid have a longer duration of action of several days to weeks depending on the specific product. Examples are betamethasone acetate (Celestone Soluspan), dexamethasone acetate (Decadron-LA), methylprednisolone acetate (Depo-Medrol), and triamcinolone diacetate (Aristocort Forte).

> *An ester form means that another molecule (eg, acetate) is chemically bonded to the corticosteroid. The addition of the acetate makes the corticosteroid less polar and thus it will not be dissolved in the extracellular fluid as rapidly. These are sometimes referred to as "depot" injections.*

The primary mechanism of clearance for corticosteroids is liver metabolism to form inactive metabolites that are excreted in the urine.

Adverse Effects

An alteration of the normal physiological regulation of corticosteroid production is the cause of significant adverse effects associated with corticosteroid therapy. The amount of corticosteroid produced by the adrenal gland is regulated through a feedback regulation process by the amount of corticosteroid in the blood. The corticosteroid level in the blood fluctuates; when it starts decreasing, the hypothalamus releases corticotropin-releasing hormone (CRH), which signals the anterior pituitary to release adrenocorticotropic hormone (ACTH), which signals the adrenal gland to produce more corticosteroid (ie, cortisol). When the cortisol level in the blood is sufficient, it signals the hypothalamus and pituitary to stop releasing hormone.

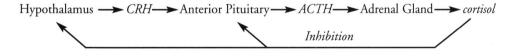

This control system is referred to as the *hypothalamic-pituitary-adrenal (HPA)* axis. If a corticosteroid is given as drug therapy, it mimics the action of cortisol on the HPA axis and thus suppresses the synthesis of cortisol by the adrenal gland. The amount of HPA suppression, and subsequent adrenal suppression, is dependent on the dose and duration of corticosteroid therapy. There is also variation among patients as to the time it takes to recover from adrenal suppression.

It could take weeks to months for normal HPA axis function to return. If adrenal suppression occurs and the dose of corticosteroid is removed too quickly, the patient can experience various symptoms including nausea, vomiting, anorexia, headache, lethargy, fever, and pain in the muscles and joints. Abrupt discontinuation after long-term therapy can be fatal.

Treatment with corticosteroids for only a few days usually does not elicit the significant adrenal suppression or the other adverse effects listed in Box 6-2. However, even when short-term treatment is warranted for acute inflammation, it may be worth considering whether the metabolic effects on glucose, protein, and lipid metabolism may have an impact on the athlete's performance. The incidence and extent of adverse effects increases with duration of therapy and increased dose. The impact on athletic performance will depend on the extent of the adverse effect, level of athletic participation, and the specific athletic event of concern. Muscle weakness from long-term corticosteroid therapy, for example, would likely impact the performance of all athletes on this therapy, whereas a fungal infection, with treatment, would not.

Drug Interactions

The major drug interactions are related to the adverse effects discussed above. Patients on NSAIDs have an increased risk of peptic ulcers when corticosteroids are added to therapy. Also, because corticosteroids can cause hyperglycemia, they are working against the desired effect of insulin or oral hypoglycemic drugs used to treat diabetic patients; adjustment of diabetic therapy may be necessary. The effect on potassium excretion can accentuate the potassium loss associated with certain diuretics that can cause hypokalemia.

Therapy Guidelines

Although dosages of corticosteroids vary considerably depending on the disease and the individual responses, there are some general therapy guidelines. Among the major concerns with corticosteroid therapy is the existence of adrenal suppression. It is difficult to determine exactly what dose, duration of therapy, and dosing schedule will result in adrenal suppression. In general, however, short-term therapy is considered to be <1week. In general, as doses of prednisone increase above 5 mg/day, the dose is considered supraphysiologic and therefore capable of causing adrenal suppression. When corticosteroid therapy is to be discontinued in patients who are likely to have adrenal suppression, the dose of corticosteroid is tapered to provide time for HPA axis to recover. There are many protocols that have been reported for tapering corticosteroid dosages, but the process can take weeks to months depending on the duration and dosage of corticosteroid that the patient received. Alternate-day dosing is sometimes used in patients receiving long-term therapy after initial management of the disease has been accomplished. This dosing schedule provides a means of diminishing some of the adverse effects associated with corticosteroid therapy as well as reducing the effect on the HPA axis.

Summary

Use of corticosteroids is an effective means of treating inflammation associated with rheumatoid arthritis, bronchial asthma, tendonitis, bursitis, osteoarthritis, allergic reactions, SLE, and dermatologic diseases. However, systemic use poses the potential for several significant adverse effects. Consequently, except for life-threatening conditions, use of systemic corticosteroids should be at the lowest dose for the shortest time necessary. The mechanism of action of corticosteroids is multifaceted and includes inhibition of the synthesis of arachidonic acid metabolites, diminished action of phagocytic cells, and reduced release of other mediators. Besides adre-

Box 6-2. Potential Adverse Effects of Corticosteroid Therapy

- Adrenal suppression is a significant concern, especially as dose and duration of therapy increase. Consequently, withdrawal of long-term corticosteroid therapy must be tapered over a period of time determined by the extent of adrenal suppression. Using alternate-day dosing of systemic corticosteroids, rather than dosing every day, helps minimize the adrenal suppression.

- Flare-up of the disease being treated is a problem associated with the withdrawal of corticosteroid therapy because the symptoms of the disease are no longer being suppressed.

- Hypertension and hypokalemia can occur in part as a result of sodium and water retention (edema) and potassium depletion. This is minimized by use of corticosteroids with predominantly glucocorticoid rather than mineralocorticoid activity (see Table 6-6). Consequently, corticosteroids should be used with caution in patients on diuretics that deplete potassium (see Chapter 12) or patients with reduced kidney function.

- Osteoporosis is a frequent result of long-term corticosteroid therapy. Steps to minimize this effect include use of calcium supplements, vitamin D supplements, and any one of a group of drugs called bisphosphonates (brand name examples are Fosamax, Didronel, Aredia), which inhibit bone resorption. However, caution is needed with the use of corticosteroids in patients with existing osteoporosis.

- Increased susceptibility to infection as a result of suppression of the immune response, or activation of an infection that had been held under control by the immune system. Because inflammation often contributes to the infection symptoms, corticosteroids may also mask the existence of an infection. It is reasonable advice for patients on oral corticosteroid therapy to take extra precautions to avoid contact with people who have a communicable disease. Also, because of the immune suppression effects of corticosteroids and because fungal infections are often difficult to treat, patients with fungal infections should avoid corticosteroid therapy if possible.

- Increased risk of peptic ulcers, especially when combined with other ulcer-causing agents such as NSAIDs.

- Suppression of growth in children can occur with relatively small doses of systemic corticosteroids. This effect can be reduced by alternate-day dosing.

- Myopathy can occur but is more frequently associated with prolonged, high-dose use of corticosteroids. The muscle weakness is primarily of the arms and legs but may include generalized weakness. Discontinuation of therapy is warranted and reversal of the effect occurs after several months.

- Cataracts are a relatively common adverse effect from long-term corticosteroid use. Consequently, periodic eye exams are recommended for early detection. Glaucoma can also occur, especially in patients with diabetes or a family history of glaucoma.

- A variety of effects on the central nervous system results in an array of possible responses, including elevated mood, euphoria, insomnia, irritability, nervousness, insomnia, and depression. These effects occur within days of initiating therapy and are more likely to occur with higher daily doses.

- In addition to the central nervous system effects, there are various other adverse effects that can occur with short-term therapy (eg, appetite stimulation, gastrointestinal irritation, headache, and exacerbation of acne).

- Many of the corticosteroids cross the placenta and also enter breast milk and can affect the infant.

- Increased blood glucose may diminish control of hyperglycemia in diabetic patients and therefore should be used with caution in these patients.

- Fat redistribution can occur with long-term, high-dose therapy. The fat moves from the extremities to the face and trunk, causing a moon face, buffalo hump, and enlarged abdomen.

nal suppression, examples of other adverse effects are hypertension, osteoporosis, cataracts, behavioral disturbances, infection, peptic ulcer, glucose intolerance, increased appetite, and muscle weakness. Adverse effects are minimized when corticosteroids are used topically, by inhalation, or by local injection at the site of inflammation. Alternate-day dosing is another means of decreasing adverse effects and HPA axis effects in patients who require long-term therapy. Drug interactions are primarily associated with concurrent use of NSAIDs and drugs used to treat diabetes.

GLUCOSAMINE

Glucosamine is classified as a dietary supplement and thus does not fall under the same scrutiny by the Food and Drug Administration (FDA) as drugs. Although the product labeling includes a statement that the product is not intended to treat or prevent disease, glucosamine is becoming more widely accepted as a means of treating osteoarthritis and thus is included in this chapter.

Use and Effects

Glucosamine is not an analgesic and is not considered an anti-inflammatory agent; it does not affect the COX pathway. Glucosamine is an aminomonosaccharide that is used to make glycosaminoglycans, which are components of proteoglycans used to make cartilage. Use of glucosamine is based on the belief that it stimulates the production of cartilage to replace damaged cartilage. Unlike the anti-inflammatory drugs, glucosamine reportedly may stop or reverse the progression of osteoarthritis, a disease characterized by continued breakdown of articular cartilage. Effects of glucosamine therapy have included reduced restriction of active and passive movement, articular pain, and joint tenderness and swelling.

Many clinical studies have demonstrated some effectiveness of glucosamine in reducing the symptoms of osteoarthritis compared with placebo. Some of these studies have been interpreted with caution due to poor study design and/or small sample size. These, as well as most of the other studies have been short-term (4 to 8 weeks), although a 3-year study demonstrated a significant benefit in the treatment of osteoarthritis with glucosamine therapy. A few additional studies have compared the effectiveness of ibuprofen (400 mg 3 times/day) with glucosamine therapy (500 mg 3 times/day) and generally found that it took about 2 weeks of glucosamine therapy to equal the effectiveness achieved within 1 week of ibuprofen therapy. However, after 2 weeks of therapy, the relief of symptoms was as effective or more effective with glucosamine compared with ibuprofen. The accumulating body of evidence seems convincing that glucosamine is effective for the short-term treatment of osteoarthritis; limited data for long-term studies are promising.

Pharmacokinetics and Dosage

Glucosamine is absorbed by the oral route, although the first pass effect (see Chapter 2) reduces bioavailability to about one-fourth the oral dose. The majority of the unaltered glucosamine is excreted by the kidney. The most common oral dosage used in clinical trials is 500 mg three times a day given as glucosamine sulfate. Glucosamine is available in most pharmacies and food supplement stores. Because dietary supplements are not subject to the same standards of potency and purity (nor efficacy and safety) as drug products, the characteristics of each glucosamine product are unknown.

Glucosamine is sometimes marketed in the same dosage form with chondroitin sulfate, which is a glycosaminoglycan. The proposed action of this compound is similar to glucosamine. Compared with glucosamine, less research has been reported regarding the effect of chondroitin sulfate on osteoarthritis. The molecular size of chondoitin is quite large, making it unlikely that a significant amount of the compound can be absorbed intact from the gastrointestinal tract. Compared with glucosamine, chondroitin is more expensive and its relative therapeutic effectiveness is unclear.

Adverse Effects

The adverse effects reported for glucosamine have been quite minimal although the focus has been regarding short-term use. When adverse effects have been reported, the major complaint has been gastrointestinal discomfort, but other complaints include headache, skin rash, and itching. Although no systematic study has been conducted regarding drug interactions with glucosamine, some of the clinical trials of therapeutic effectiveness of glucosamine included patients taking medications for various diseases; no significant drug interactions were reported.

Summary

The use of glucosamine to treat osteoarthritis is gaining acceptance. An increasing number of clinical trials, particularly regarding short-term therapy, have demonstrated significant improvement in symptoms of osteoarthritis compared to placebo. In addition, therapeutic benefit approximately equal to ibuprofen therapy after 2 weeks of treatment with glucosamine has been reported. Adverse effects are minimal, the most predominant being gastrointestinal discomfort.

TREATMENT OF RHEUMATOID ARTHRITIS AND GOUT

NSAIDs and corticosteroids are used to treat rheumatoid arthritis and gout, but unique features of these diseases also necessitate the use of other drugs.

Drug Therapy for Rheumatoid Arthritis

For treatment of rheumatoid arthritis, the NSAIDs are usually part of initial therapy and are useful to provide anti-inflammatory activity and as an analgesic to quickly reduce the pain. All of the NSAIDs are effective in reducing these symptoms, although some patients respond better to one drug compared to another. The likelihood of toxicity from the long-term use of anti-inflammatory doses of NSAIDs limits their use. Additionally, NSAIDs only reduce the symptoms; they do not affect the progression of the disease. More aggressive therapy is recommended as a part of initial therapy and includes *disease-modifying antirheumatic drugs* (DMARDs) along with NSAIDs. Long-term use of DMARDs may be able to delay or stop the progression of the disease, but it takes weeks to months for the effects of DMARDs to develop. In the meantime, NSAIDs are useful to alleviate the symptoms but then can be discontinued when the effect of the DMARD is sufficient. Table 6-7 lists DMARDs and summarizes their characteristics. Among the DMARDs, methotrexate (Rheumatrex) is often the first choice. Hydroxychloroquine (Plaquenil) and sulfasalazine are also used to treat mild to moderate rheumatoid arthritis. These drugs are also used in combination with methotrexate or with other DMARDs to treat patients who do not respond sufficiently to a single agent. The mechanism of action of some DMARDs is unknown whereas some specific immunosuppressive and/or anti-inflammatory activity has been identified for others.

Table 6-7. Drugs to Treat Rheumatoid Arthritis

Generic Name	Trade Name	Selected Characteristics	Onset of Effectiveness
adalimumab	Humira	Made from human IgG. Given by subcutaneous injection every other week. May cause flu-like symptoms and increase risk of infections, including serious respiratory infections. Use if other DMARDs not effective.	1 week
auranofin	Ridaura	Orally effective gold compound. May cause rash, renal toxicity, oral lesions, metallic taste, and GI effects.	3 to 6 months
azathioprine	Imuran	Monitor liver function and signs of bone marrow suppression. Contraindicated during pregnancy.	3 to 12 weeks
cyclosporine	Neoral	Monitor kidney function. May cause hypertension, hyperglycemia, increased incidence of infection, and GI effects. Use if other DMARDs not effective.	4 to 12 weeks
etanercept	Enbrel	Made from human IgG. Given by subcutaneous injection twice/week. May cause headache and increase risk of infections, including serious respiratory infections. Use if other DMARDs not effective.	2 to 3 weeks
hydroxychloroquine	Plaquenil	Relatively safe but monitor for retinal toxicity. Give with food to minimize GI effects.	1 to 6 months
infliximab	Remicade	Made from portions of mouse and human IgG. Must be given with methotrexate to prevent antibody production against infliximab. May increase the risk of infections, including serious respiratory infections. Dose given by IV infusion at certain week intervals.	2 weeks
leflunomide	Arava	Monitor liver function. Contraindicated during pregnancy. May cause reversible hair loss, respiratory infections, GI effects. Long $t\frac{1}{2}$ so loading dose given.	4 weeks
methotrexate	Rheumatrex	Monitor liver and kidney function and blood cell counts. GI effects. Contraindicated during pregnancy. Dosage is once/week.	3 to 6 weeks
penicillamine	Cuprimine	May cause autoimmune diseases, GI effects, metallic taste, skin rash, oral mucosal lesions. Use when other DMARDs not effective. Caution if penicillin allergy.	4 to 12 weeks
sulfasalazine[1]	Azulfidine	Prodrug converted to active sulfapyridine by GI bacteria and then absorbed. GI effects common but decreased by using enteric-coated dosage forms, take with food, or using divided daily dosage. May cause rash and harmlessly turn skin and urine yellow-orange.	4 to 8 weeks

[1]Sulfasalazine also used to treat inflammatory bowel disease; see Chapter 11.

IgG=Immunoglobulin G; DMARDs=disease-modifying antirheumatic drugs; GI=gastrointestinal; IV=intravenous; $t\frac{1}{2}$=half-life

Three relatively new drugs available for treatment of rheumatoid arthritis are etanercept (Enbrel), adalimumab (Humira), and infliximab (Remicade). These are proteins and thus must be administered by injection. They are TNF antagonists; they bind to TNF and block its effects as a chemical mediator of inflammation. Tumor necrosis factor antagonists are used alone or in combination with other DMARDs to treat moderate to severe rheumatoid arthritis that is not responding to other DMARDs. A significant concern is the occurrence of serious infections, including tuberculosis and fungal infections. Patients should be screened with tuberculin skin test.

Similar to NSAIDs, corticosteroids alleviate symptoms of rheumatoid arthritis but do not delay the progression of the disease. Several days of high-dose corticosteroid therapy are useful in controlling flare-ups of rheumatoid arthritis. Corticosteroid therapy is also used to control symptoms while DMARD therapy is being initiated if NSAIDs are not effective. Intra-articular and intramuscular injections are an alternative to oral therapy and slow release forms of the corticosteroid provides weeks to months of relief. Long-term therapy, even at low doses, is not preferred but is useful in patients who do not respond sufficiently to any other therapy. As always, long-term use poses the problems of potentially serious adverse effects such as osteoporosis, glaucoma, cataracts, hyperglycemia, hypertension, and increased susceptibility to infections. Consequently, some precautions that should be taken are to monitor blood pressure and blood glucose, watch for symptoms of osteoporosis (eg, bone pain), and use calcium and vitamin D supplements to prevent osteoporosis.

Drug Therapy for Gout

Drug therapy of gout centers on two approaches: alleviate the pain associated with acute attacks and prevent recurrent attacks by decreasing the blood uric acid level. The most frequently used drugs to treat acute gout (Table 6-8) are colchicine and indomethacin (Indocin). The exact mechanism for colchicine is not clear but it does not have generalized anti-inflammatory or analgesic activity; its effectiveness is relatively specific for gout. Colchicine is most effective if given within 48 hours after onset of symptoms. Pain is diminished within hours of the first dose and inflammation is usually gone within 3 days. This drug has a low therapeutic index and therefore the dosage regimen is quite specific (0.5 to 1.2 mg orally, then 0.5 to 0.6 mg every 1 to 2 hours or 1 to 1.2 mg every 2 hours until relief or nausea, vomiting, or diarrhea occur, or a maximum of 8 mg is taken. Wait 3 days before initiating another course of therapy). Gastrointestinal adverse symptoms are an indication of toxicity and these symptoms often occur prior to 8 mg, necessitating dosage termination. Death has occurred with <10 mg. Although colchicine is very effective, patients must be well advised regarding the use of this drug.

Indomethacin is considered the drug of choice to treat acute gout attacks. It has a quick onset of action, is comparable to colchicine in effectiveness, and is much less toxic than colchicine. After an initial higher oral dose, the dose of indomethacin is reduced until symptoms are gone and then the dose is tapered off over several days. Many other NSAIDs are also effective (eg, naproxen, fenoprofen, ibuprofen) and can be used to treat acute attacks. Aspirin, however, should not be used as it can block the excretion of uric acid, depending on the dose. Although there are some advantages of indomethacin and NSAIDs compared with colchicine, patients with a history of gastrointestinal bleeding or renal disease should avoid indomethacin and other NSAIDs.

If colchicine or NSAIDs are not effective or inappropriate for a patient, corticosteroid therapy can be used to treat acute attacks. Oral, parenteral, or intra-articular administration are effective. The oral dose must be tapered gradually after the acute attack subsides.

Table 6-8. Drugs Used to Treat Gout

Generic Name	Trade Name	Selected Characteristics	Use
colchicine	generic	Low therapeutic index. GI effects are sign of toxicity. Also effective intravenously. Avoid in pregnancy. Must be taken within 48 hours of onset of symptoms. Pain subsides within hours; swelling subsides within few days. Not effective for other inflammatory conditions.	Treat acute episodes
indomethacin	Indocin	Pain subsides within hours; swelling subsides within few days. May cause severe frontal headache, GI effects, and gastric ulcers. Avoid use if history of ulcers or kidney disease.	Treat acute episodes
allopurinol	Zyloprim	May cause hypersensitivity reaction; discontinue if skin rash. May increase likelihood of acute attack within first several months but use with colchicine or NSAID decreases incidence. Use with large volume of fluid/day to prevent uric acid damage to kidney. No anti-inflammatory/analgesic effect.	Long-term preventative; blocks uric acid synthesis
probenecid	Benemid	GI effects; use with food. May increase likelihood of acute attack within first several months but use with colchicine or NSAID decreases incidence. Use with large volume of fluid/day to prevent uric acid damage to kidney. No anti-inflammatory or analgesic effect. Avoid in patients with impaired kidney function.	Long-term preventative; increases uric acid excretion
sulfinpyrazone	Anturane	GI effects; use with food. May increase likelihood of acute attack within first several months but use with colchicine or NSAID decreases incidence. Use with large volume of fluid/day to prevent uric acid damage to kidney. No anti-inflammatory or analgesic effect. Avoid in patients with impaired kidney function.	Long-term preventative; increases uric acid excretion

GI = gastrointestinal

There are three drugs used to lower uric acid blood levels (antihyperuricemic therapy). Two of them, probenecid (Benemid) and sufinpyrazone (Anturane), increase the excretion rate of uric acid by blocking the reabsorption of uric acid from the renal tubule. A third antihyperuricemic drug, allopurinol (Zyloprim), inhibits the synthesis of uric acid from purines. Allopurinol is preferred over the other two if the patient has a history of diminished renal function or urinary stones. The *antihyperuricemic* drugs are of no benefit to treat acute gout attacks but long-term therapy reduces the incidence of acute attacks. However, the incidence of an acute attack is increased during the initial several months of therapy with antihyperuricemic drugs and, therefore, colchicine (0.5 to 0.6 mg/day or every other day) or an NSAID can be added during these months to decrease the incidence of acute attacks. A large daily intake of water is recommended during therapy to avoid the development of uric acid stones. Also, antihyperuricemic therapy should not be started during an acute attack since these drugs may exacerbate the symptoms.

Summary

Drug therapy for rheumatoid arthritis and gout has two major aspects: treat acute pain and inflammation and use long-term therapy to decrease the incidence of acute episodes. NSAIDs play a role to treat acute pain and inflammation for both diseases and corticosteroid therapy can be used if NSAIDs are not effective. Colchicine and indomethacin are particularly useful to treat acute gout. The use of DMARDs is part of the more aggressive therapy to reduce the progression of rheumatoid arthritis. Drugs such as methotrexate, gold salts, and hydroxychloroquine are DMARDs but the response from therapy must be monitored as they can cause serious adverse effects. Sulfinpyrazone, probenecid, and allopurinol are antihyperuricemic drugs, which may be life-long therapy to reduce the incidence of acute gout attacks.

> *Recall from Chapter 2 that there is an active transport mechanism that transports endogenous compounds (eg, amino acids, glucose) back into the blood from the renal tubule. Uric acid is reabsorbed by this active transport mechanism.*

TOPICAL ANTI-INFLAMMATORY PRODUCTS

Topical anti-inflammatory products are available by prescription to treat various topical inflammatory conditions, but there are numerous gels, creams, and ointments available OTC that contain an NSAID (ie, a salicylate), a counterirritant (see page 160), and/or a corticosteroid (eg, hydrocortisone). As discussed below, there may also be an analgesic component added to some of these compounds. Table 6-9 lists examples of these OTC anti-inflammatory/analgesic products.

Salicylate is the only NSAID used topically in the United States. The form of salicylate is usually methyl salicylate or trolamine salicylate (see Table 6-9). Topically applied salicylate may be effective when applied at the site of strains, sprains, and muscle soreness from strenuous exercise, although most of the reports are regarding analgesic rather than anti-inflammatory effectiveness for the treatment of these conditions. Topical application has not been shown to be more effective than oral use of NSAIDs.

Salicylates act primarily by penetrating directly to the tissue rather than by absorption into the systemic circulation and distribution to the tissue site. The rate and extent of absorption into the systemic circulation varies depending on the site of application (eg, greater on abdomen or forearm and less on the foot) and increases with multiple applications at the same site. Regardless of the site of application, the amount absorbed is too low for systemic therapeutic purposes (ie,

Table 6-9. Selected Topical Nonprescription Anti-Inflammatory/Analgesic Products

Trade Name	Dosage Form	Primary Ingredients
Absorbine Jr Arthritis Strength	Liquid	4% menthol, 0.025% capsaicin, Echinacea, wormwood
Aspercreme	Cream	10% trolamine salicylate
Ben-Gay Arthritis Formula	Cream	30% methyl salicylate, 8% menthol
Ben-Gay Original	Ointment	18.3% methyl salicylate, 16% menthol
Ben-Gay Ultra Strength	Cream	30% methyl salicylate, 10% menthol, 4% camphor
Eucalyptamint	Gel	8% menthol, eucalyptus oil
Exocaine Medicated Rub	Ointment	25% methyl salicylate
Exocaine Plus Rub	Cream	30% methyl salicylate
Heet	Liniment	15% methyl salicylate, 3.6% camphor, 0.025% capsaicin
Cortizone-10	Ointment	1% hydrocortisone
Icy Hot Balm	Ointment	29% methyl salicylate, 7.6% menthol
Icy Hot Cream	Cream	30% methyl salicylate, 10% menthol
Icy Hot Stick	Gel	30% methyl salicylate, 10% menthol
Sportscreme	Cream	10% trolamine salicylate
Vicks VapoRub	Ointment	4.8% camphor, 2.6% menthol, 1.2% eucalyptus oil

it is not a transdermal route) and is used for a local response only. Nonetheless, *topically applied salicylates must be used with the same caution as oral NSAIDs in patients with known risk factors such as NSAID-hypersensitivity, renal disease, liver disease, alcohol beverage use, and history of gastrointestinal bleeding.*

Counterirritants are often times a component of OTC anti-inflammatory/analgesic products. These are compounds that are applied topically to relieve pain; they act by producing less severe pain (via skin irritation) to essentially distract the patient from a more severe pain. Although the exact mechanism is unclear, counterirritants appear to indirectly stimulate sensations such as cold, hot, or itching, which directs the attention away from the more severe pain in the muscles, joints, or tendons. This mechanism contributes to the analgesic action of methyl salicylate, allyl isothiocyanate (mustard oil), turpentine oil, camphor, menthol, and capsicum (from hot chili peppers). In addition to the counterirritant effect, methyl salicylate, allyl isothiocyanate, and turpentine oil are also *rubefacients* (ie, they cause redness due to cutaneous vasodilation). Menthol and camphor, on the other hand, cause a cooling effect whereas capsicum causes a feeling of warmth without vasodilation. Although these compounds are considered safe and effective counterirritants, they may also have a placebo component. The feeling of warmth or coolness, and the sensations of irritation, as well as some odors associated with topical application, may give the patient the confidence that the drug is working thus producing a beneficial psychological effect. Methyl salicylate and menthol are also used in smaller amounts as components of wintergreen oil and peppermint oil, respectively, as flavoring agents.

Box 6-3. Considerations for the Topical Use of Corticosteriods

- Because corticosteroids inhibit the immune response, do not use topical corticosteroids to treat inflammation associated with skin infection.
- Prescription topical corticosteroids can cause local skin reactions such as skin atrophy, acneiform eruptions, and perioral dermatitis.
- Topical use of corticosteroids for long periods, particularly the more potent prescription products, can cause systemic adverse effects.
- Systemic absorption of topically applied corticosteroids will increase if applied to inflamed skin.
- In addition to the anti-inflammatory effect, topical corticosteroids also relieve the itching associated with insect bites and contact dermatitis from poison ivy, harsh chemicals, cosmetics, and other minor irritants.

Increased irritation and possible tissue damage (eg, blistering) can occur if methyl salicylate is applied to tissue and then occlusive bandaging or heating pads are used. Use of counterirritants during hot and humid weather or application after strenuous exercise can pose similar problems. Counterirritants should only be applied to intact skin, not to wounds or damaged skin.

Capsicum has been used two to four times daily to reduce the pain associated with osteoarthritis and rheumatoid arthritis by rubbing the product around the affected joints. Capsicum appears to inhibit *substance P*, a neurotransmitter that is thought to be involved in pain sensation at peripheral sites. It may also have some anti-inflammatory properties. For treatment of arthritis, pain relief may not occur until after 1 to 2 weeks of treatment with maximum relief after several weeks. A local burning sensation occurs with initial therapy but subsides with continued use.

Camphor and menthol are also used topically to relieve itching (antipruritic) caused from contact with numerous irritants such as poison ivy, chemicals, and cosmetics. These local analgesics are typically used in combination with other compounds, such as topical anesthetics, which also contribute to the antipruritic response.

Hydrocortisone is the only topical corticosteroid available without a prescription but several more potent corticosteroids are available in topical dosage forms by prescription. The mechanism and therapeutic use of these products has already been discussed but some additional noteworthy points are listed in Box 6-3.

There are other substances that reportedly have anti-inflammatory and/or counterirritant properties and are added to some OTC products, although evidence is less convincing regarding their effectiveness. These substances include eucalyptus oil, wormwood, and Echinacea.

Summary

The advantage of topical application of anti-inflammatory agents is the reduced incidence of systemic effects as well as the potential of some placebo effect. Trolamine salicylate and methyl salicylate are the two NSAIDs most frequently used for topical application, although methyl salicylate exerts its action primarily as a counterirritant. Other counterirritants include camphor, menthol, and capsicum. Pain and itching may be associated with inflammation, and counterirritants are used for their topical analgesic and antipruritic activity rather than for any specific anti-inflammatory action. Hydrocortisone is the only topical corticosteroid available OTC although other topical corticosteroids are available by prescription for their anti-inflammatory effectiveness.

Table 6-10. Characteristics of NSAIDs and Corticosteroids

Characteristic	NSAIDs	Corticosteroids
Availability	OTC and Rx	OTC topical and Rx
Primary route	Oral	Oral, injection, topical
Therapeutic uses	Anti-inflammatory Analgesic Antipyretic Anticoagulant	Anti-inflammatory Immunosuppressant Adrenal replacement therapy Anticancer
Primary clearance route	Liver metabolism Urinary excretion	Liver metabolism Urinary excretion
Primary adverse effects	Gastric irritation Peptic ulcers Diminished kidney function Allergic reaction Increased clotting time	Adrenal suppression Increased blood glucose Peptic ulcers Osteoporosis Susceptibility to infection Muscle weakness

Primary drug interactions	Increased warfarin response
	Increased oral antidiabetic
	  drug effect
	Decreased effect of some
	  antihypertensives
	Increased ulcer risk with
	  corticosteroids
		Decreased effect of insulin and
		  oral antidiabetic drugs
		Increased ulcer risk with
		  NSAIDs

Examples	Apirin, ibuprofen, naproxen	Cortisone, dexamethasone, prednisone
Mechanism	Inhibits COX	Inhibits phospholipase

ROLE OF THE ATHLETIC TRAINER

A comparison of the characteristics of NSAIDs and corticosteroids is summarized in Table 6-10. Regarding the use of NSAIDs by athletes, the athletic trainer can have a positive impact on ensuring therapeutic outcomes and reducing adverse effects. The dose and duration of therapy will depend on the therapeutic goal; low-dose, long-term therapy with aspirin is typical to prevent heart attack or stroke in certain predisposed patients, whereas short-term, higher-dose therapy with any one of many NSAIDs is expected for treatment of an acute inflammatory conditions. The athletic trainer should understand these differences and encourage the athlete to be compliant with the prescribed therapeutic regimen. Regardless of dose and therapeutic intent for use of NSAIDs, the following are important to consider:

- The benefits and risks must be weighed to determine whether anti-inflammatory drugs should be used for any specific athlete. There is significant potential for adverse effects with the use of NSAIDs and corticosteroids and a benefit of faster healing or shorter time before a return to full activity is not assured.
- NSAIDs should be taken with food or milk, or at least with a full glass of water, to reduce gastric discomfort.

- Only one NSAID should be used at a time by an athlete.
- The use of NSAIDs should be avoided in athletes who have had a hypersensitivity response to any NSAID.
- The likelihood of gastric ulceration increases with longer-term, higher-dose use of NSAIDs and in athletes who are elderly, have a history of peptic ulcer disease, are concurrently taking corticosteroids, or are consuming alcoholic beverages. Athletes with severe or persistent gastric pain should be referred to their physician.
- NSAIDs should be avoided in athletes who are pregnant or breast feeding. Aspirin should be avoided in children and teens with viral infections.
- NSAIDs can cause diminished renal function, although athletes at risk for this are primarily those with existing heart, liver, or kidney impairment. NSAIDs should be discontinued and the athlete referred to his or her physician when signs of edema or reduced urine output are present.

Corticosteroids are often used in bursts of short-term therapy to treat acute inflammation; the frequency of adverse effects is greatly reduced when these drugs are used for only a few days. Nonetheless the athletic trainer should be aware of the potential for adverse effects and drug interactions, particularly in athletes who are being treated with corticosteroids for longer time periods. Use of corticosteroids is associated with these key points:

- Diabetic athletes should be keenly aware that they may require an adjustment in anti-diabetic drug therapy.
- Athletes who are also on NSAIDs should know that black, tarry stools may indicate gastrointestinal bleeding.
- Athletes should be alerted that fever and sore throat are often signs of infection.
- Signs of swelling and weight gain may indicate sodium and water retention and may warrant a change in therapy.

BIBLIOGRAPHY

APhA Special Report. Emerging therapies for inflammation and pain: the role of cyclooxygenase selectivity. Washington, DC: American Pharmaceutical Association; 1999.

Barclay TS, Tsourounis C, McCart GM. Glucosamine. *Ann Pharmacother.* 1998;32:574-579.

Cardiovascular safety of COX-2 inhibitors. *The Medical Letter.* 2001;43:99-100.

daCamara CC, Dowless GV. Glucosamine sulfate for osteoarthritis. *Ann Pharmacother.* 1998;32:580-587.

Garnett WR. Clinical implications of drug interactions with coxibs. *Pharmacotherapy.* 2001;21:1223-1232.

Leadbetter WB. Anti-inflammatory therapy in sports injury. *Clin Sports Med.* 1995;14:353-410.

Mukherjee D, Nissen SE, Topol EJ. Risk of cardiovascular events associated with selective COX-2 inhibitors. *JAMA.* 2001;286:954-959.

Postgraduate Medicine Online. A practical approach to gout. Available at http://www.postgradmed.com/issues/1999/10_01_99/davis.htm. Accessed August 29, 2003.

Reginster JY, Deroisy R, Rovati LC, et al. Long-term effects of glucosamine sulphate on osteoarthritis progression: a randomized, placebo-controlled clinical trial. *Lancet.* 2001;357:251-256.

Schuna AA, Megeff C. New drugs for the treatment of rheumatoid arthritis. *Am J Health Syst Pharm.* 2000; 57:225-234.

Simon AM, Manigrasso MB, O'Connor JP. Cyclo-oxygenase 2 function is essential for bone fracture healing. *J Bone Miner Res.* 2002;17:963-976.

Standing JA, Skrabal MZ, Faulkner MA. Seven cases of interaction between warfarin and cyclooxygenase-2 inhibitors. *Am J Health Syst Pharm.* 2001;58:2076-2080.

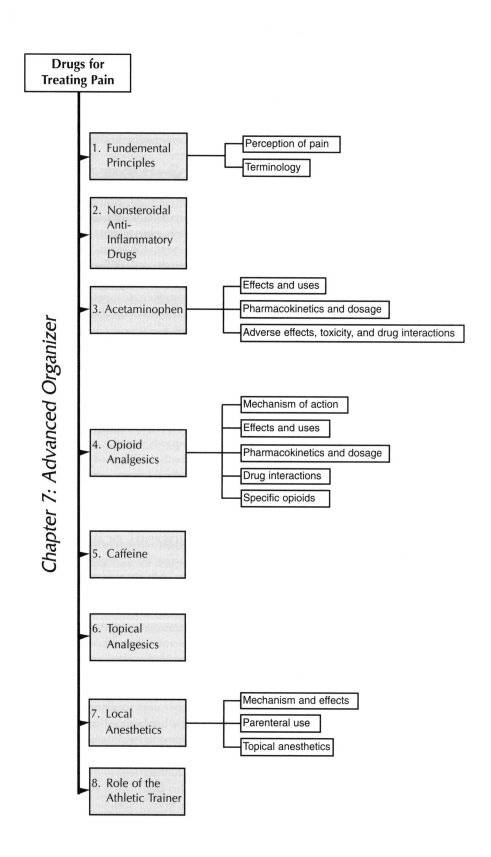

Chapter 7: Advanced Organizer

Drugs for Treating Pain

1. Fundemental Principles
   - Perception of pain
   - Terminology

2. Nonsteroidal Anti-Inflammatory Drugs

3. Acetaminophen
   - Effects and uses
   - Pharmacokinetics and dosage
   - Adverse effects, toxicity, and drug interactions

4. Opioid Analgesics
   - Mechanism of action
   - Effects and uses
   - Pharmacokinetics and dosage
   - Drug interactions
   - Specific opioids

5. Caffeine

6. Topical Analgesics

7. Local Anesthetics
   - Mechanism and effects
   - Parenteral use
   - Topical anesthetics

8. Role of the Athletic Trainer

7

DRUGS FOR TREATING PAIN

CHAPTER OBJECTIVES

At the end of this chapter, the reader will be able to:

- Explain how nonsteroidal anti-inflammatory drugs (NSAIDs) also have an analgesic effect.
- Explain the pharmacokinetics, effects, uses, and dosage regimen for acetaminophen and opioid drugs.
- Recall and recognize the signs and symptoms of possible adverse effects and toxicity for acetaminophen and opioid drugs.
- Identify common drug interactions for acetaminophen and opioid drugs.
- Compare and contrast the therapeutic advantages and disadvantages between aspirin and acetaminophen.
- Describe the mechanism of action for opioid drugs.
- Explain the difference between drug addiction and physical dependence.
- Explain the concept of agonist-antagonist opioids.
- Differentiate between several types of opioid drugs.
- Identify specific drugs that belong to the opioid drug category.
- Explain how caffeine can affect analgesia of other drugs.
- Recall the physiological effects that caffeine has on the body.
- Recall the two main compounds that are used as topical analgesics and how they achieve their topical analgesic effects.
- Explain the mechanism of action, uses, and therapeutic effects of local anesthetics.
- Recall the therapeutic uses of topical anesthetics.
- Summarize the role of the athletic trainer for patients who are taking analgesic medications.

Pain can be a symptom of underlying disease or chronic injury or it may result from obvious acute trauma to musculoskeletal tissue from an athletic injury. The need for pain relief may require a single dose of pain reliever or long-term use of daily medication. Pain is the most common complaint among patients. Not surprising, therefore, is the abundance of analgesic products available by prescription and over-the-counter (OTC) to treat pain. The availability of OTC name brand and generic brand analgesics as single-drug entities and combination products facilitates, even encourages, self-medication by patients, including athletes. In addition, athletic injuries often necessitate the use of prescription pain relievers as part of short-term or long-term rehabilitation therapy. Obtaining optimal therapeutic outcomes of analgesic drug therapy requires not only use of the appropriate drug and dosage for the patient but also appropriate adjustments of therapy if adverse effects or drug interactions occur. Because of the ready availability of OTC analgesic products, achieving optimal outcomes can be a bigger challenge for the athletic trainer than it may seem.

This chapter discusses OTC and prescription analgesics, which include NSAIDs, acetaminophen, opioid analgesics, and caffeine. The uses, adverse effects, and potential drug interactions are discussed. Some of the information regarding the NSAIDs may be repeated from the previous chapter regarding anti-inflammatory drugs whereas other information regarding these drugs will focus on their specific use for analgesia.

FUNDAMENTAL CONCEPTS

Except for a few items of terminology discussed below, the major fundamental principle required to understand this chapter is the mechanism for pain perception as analgesics function by impacting this mechanism.

Perception of Pain

Pain is not a disease but rather a symptom of disease or a result of actual or potential damage to tissue. Alleviating the pain does not cure the underlying disease or repair the damaged tissue, but is an important part of the treatment regimen. Relief from pain may also allow other treatment modalities, such as electrotherapy and heat and cold, to be performed more effectively. There is both a physical and an emotional component to pain and thus it continually interferes with the patient's ability to focus on other tasks (eg, athletic performance). For example, even the anticipation of pain as a result of a previous injury can affect the patient's concentration and performance during athletic competition.

Pain is often described as an unpleasant sensory or emotional experience. It involves both the peripheral and central nervous systems (CNS) and it may be acute (eg, sprained ankle) or chronic (eg, arthritis). Sometimes pain is described as peripheral or visceral; peripheral pain is located in muscles, bones, and joints, whereas visceral is originating from internal organs. Stimuli that damage tissue through chemical, mechanical, or thermal means will cause the activation of pain receptors called *nociceptors*, which exist on nerve endings in nearly all tissue. These stimuli may directly activate or sensitize nociceptors, or may do so indirectly by causing the release of various chemical mediators, which subsequently activate or sensitize the nociceptors. Examples of these mediators are *prostaglandins, leukotrienes, substance P, bradykinin, histamine,* and *cytokines*. These and other chemical mediators may also be involved in the transmission of the nerve impulse (then called neurotransmitters) to the spinal cord and to the brain, which results in pain perception. Other neurotransmitters called *endorphins* (from "endogenous morphine") are released in the CNS as a means to control the pain. These endogenous opioid analgesics combine with specific receptors to inhibit the pain impulse. Other neurotransmitters in the CNS, such as *serotonin* and *gamma amino butyric acid* (GABA), may also be involved in inhibiting pain impulses.

There is no accurate means of quantifying pain because pain is a patient-specific perception of discomfort; pain exists if the patient says it exists. Use of various pain scales, however, is a common means of estimating the extent of pain as perceived by the patient and to determine the relative change in the pain for a given patient. For example, ask the patient to identify the level of pain on a scale of 0 to 10, where 0 is no pain and 10 is the worst pain possible. The visual analog scale (VAS) is another means of obtaining the patient's perception of pain level (Figure 7-1). The VAS uses a 10-cm line that represents a continuum of no pain at one end and the worst possible pain at the other end. The patient visualizes the level of pain on this line and marks the

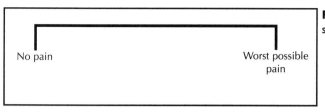

Figure 7-1. Visual analog pain scale (VAS).

place on the line to represent the level of pain. The distance is measured in millimeters from the "no pain" end and can be used to quantify the level of pain. Not only do pain scales give the athletic trainer an idea of the patient's pain level, but they also provide a baseline to determine whether the pain is lesser or greater at another time. Some patients may not give an accurate report of the pain. Athletes, for example, may underreport pain because of a desire to return to activity. Additionally, it is possible to decrease pain perception through relaxation, distraction, or elevated mood. On the other hand, pain perception may be increased by fatigue, anxiety, and depression.

Terminology

An understanding of the following terms will be useful with this chapter:

- An *analgesic* is a drug that is used to alleviate pain without causing the loss of consciousness. Drugs that induce sleep will alleviate the perception of pain while the patient is asleep but they do not selectively inhibit the transmission of pain impulses. Some drugs will alleviate the pain associated with a disease by treating the disease but these drugs are not effective in treating pain associated with other causes. For example, pain from a urinary tract infection is alleviated as a result of treatment with an antibiotic; pain from gout is alleviated by the treatment with a drug that increases uric acid excretion.

- *Opiates* are drugs that are obtained from the opium poppy, opium being the extract from the plant. Morphine and codeine are two of the components of opium and thus are opiates.

- *Opioids* is a term broader than "opiates" and refers to drugs that have effects similar to the opiates. Oxycodone (OxyContin) and meperidine (Demerol) are two examples.

- *Narcotic analgesic* is another term used to refer to opioids. They can produce a state of narcosis (drowsiness or sleep) and relieve pain.

- *Narcotic* is also used in a legal context to refer to any controlled substance. Therefore, morphine is classified pharmacologically as a narcotic analgesic but also as a narcotic in the legal sense because it is a controlled substance. On the other hand, cocaine and amphetamine are classified pharmacologically as CNS stimulants, but because they have an abuse potential, they are also classified from a legal perspective as controlled substances and thus also referred to as narcotics. For clarification and differentiation, narcotic analgesic is the term used to refer to pain relievers that have an abuse potential, whereas the term narcotic can be used to refer to any controlled substance (including the narcotic analgesics).

NONSTEROIDAL ANTI-INFLAMMATORY DRUGS

The previous chapter discussed the mechanism of action of NSAIDs along with their therapeutic uses, pharmacokinetics, dosages, adverse effects, potential drug interactions, and therapy guidelines. As a review, the following points should be kept in mind:

170   *Chapter 7*

Table 7-1. Selected Nonsteroidal Anti-Inflammatory Drug Analgesics

Generic Name	Trade Name	Typical Adult Analgesic Dose	OTC
aspirin	many	500 to 1000 mg every 4 to 6 hours	yes
celecoxib[1]	Celebrex	100 to 200 mg every 12 hours	no
diclofenac	Voltaren	50 mg every 8 hours	no
etodolac	Lodine	200 to 400 mg every 6 to 8 hours	no
fenoprofen	Nalfon	200 mg every 4 to 6 hours	no
ibuprofen	Advil	200 to 400 mg every 4 to 6 hours	yes
ketoprofen	Orudis	12.5 to 25 mg every 6 to 8 hours	yes
naproxen Na	Aleve	275 mg every 6 to 8 hours	yes
valdecoxib[1]	Bextra	20 mg twice/day[2]	no

[1]Indicates selective COX-2 inhibitor.
[2]For dysmenorrhea.

- NSAIDs inhibit cyclooxygenase (COX), an enzyme that catalyzes the production of prostaglandins (PGs).
- There are two isoforms of cyclooxygenase, COX-1 and COX-2. Production of PGs has different function in various tissues. In general, COX-1 is the predominant isoform that produces PGs in most tissues but is particularly significant in the stomach, kidneys, and platelets. COX-2 is the predominant isoform that produces PGs as a result of tissue injury and contributes to pain, inflammation, and fever.
- The most common adverse effects of NSAIDs are gastric irritation and ulceration, reduced renal function, and allergy.
- COX-2 selective NSAIDs may have a diminished incidence of adverse effects in the stomach and kidney.
- NSAIDs should be given with food or milk to reduce the gastric irritation.
- PGs contribute to pain by sensitizing peripheral nerves and relaying the pain impulse in the CNS.
- All NSAIDs have equally effective analgesic and anti-inflammatory activity but the effectiveness of NSAIDs varies among patients, and there is no way to predict which NSAID will be more effective than another in any given patient.

NSAIDs are effective for relief of mild to moderate pain. Generally, the maximum analgesic dose is less than the maximum anti-inflammatory dose although there is overlap for the dosage range for the analgesic and anti-inflammatory effects. NSAIDs are used to treat pain associated with osteoarthritis, rheumatoid arthritis, dental pain, postsurgical pain, menstrual pain, headache, and trauma to tissue such as with musculoskeletal injury. Table 7-1 lists selected NSAIDs with their usual adult analgesic dosage.

ACETAMINOPHEN

A chemical name for acetaminophen is N-acetyl-p-aminophenol and thus it is also referred to as APAP. Another, less common name for acetaminophen is paracetamol. Tylenol is the most common of many brand name OTC analgesics. In addition, there are many generic label combination analgesic products and cold/allergy/sinus products that contain acetaminophen (see Chapter 10).

Effects and Uses

Use of acetaminophen is widespread because it has analgesic and *antipyretic* efficacy comparable to aspirin, but does not have some of the adverse effects associated with aspirin and other NSAIDs. In fact, some names of acetaminophen products incorporate the terms "nonaspirin" or "aspirin free" to emphasize that it is an aspirin-like product but is without aspirin. The following are points of comparison of acetaminophen with aspirin:

- Acetaminophen inhibits COX in the brain but not in the peripheral sites. Consequently, acetaminophen is an effective antipyretic but does not have significant anti-inflammatory activity and hence it is not an NSAID.
- Acetaminophen does not have the risk of causing *Reye's syndrome* as does aspirin (see Chapter 6). Therefore, acetaminophen is safe to use in children and teenagers to treat muscle aches and fever associated with viral infections.
- Except for inhibition of COX in the brain, the mechanism of action of the analgesic activity for acetaminophen is unclear.
- Acetaminophen does not cause gastric irritation or ulceration.
- Platelet aggregation is not affected by acetaminophen and thus it does not affect blood clotting time and can be used in patients with clotting disorders. Occasional use of acetaminophen does not interfere with the effectiveness of *warfarin (Coumadin)* therapy (see Chapter 6), but daily use can inhibit warfarin metabolism and increase bleeding time.
- Acetaminophen does not have adverse effects on the kidney.

As discussed later in this chapter, aspirin and acetaminophen are used in combination with opioid analgesics (see Table 7-2).

Pharmacokinetics and Dosage

Acetaminophen is readily and completely absorbed from the gastrointestinal tract, reaching peak blood concentration within 1 hour after oral administration. The half-life (t½) is about 2 hours. Most of the drug is metabolized by the liver to form metabolites that are more water soluble than the parent drug and thus increase the rate of urinary excretion.

Acetaminophen has similar potency as aspirin. The most effective adult dose is 325 to 1000 mg for acute pain every 4 to 6 hours but daily dosage should not exceed 4000 mg. Like the NSAIDs, but in contrast to the opioids, acetaminophen has a ceiling effect for the analgesic activity such that increasing the dose beyond this ceiling will not achieve additional analgesia. For aspirin and acetaminophen, the ceiling effect for a single dose is usually between 650 and 1300 mg. Acetaminophen is available in many dosage forms, including tablets, capsules, suppositories, chewable tablets, drops for infants, elixirs, and suspensions.

Adverse Effects, Toxicity, and Drug Interactions

There are fewer frequent adverse effects for acetaminophen compared with aspirin. Various allergic reactions, including skin rashes, occur occasionally. Rarely is there cross hypersensitivity with aspirin or the other NSAIDs. Acetaminophen doses of <650 mg also pose little risk of bronchospasm in patients with aspirin-induced asthma.

The most serious adverse effect is due to overdose of acetaminophen. More calls are made to poison control centers for acetaminophen overdose than for overdose with any other drug.

Table 7-2. Selected Opioids and Analgesic Combinations

Opioid (generic)	Trade Name	DEA Schedule	Typical Oral Dose[1]	Other Analgesics
codeine	(generic)	II	15 to 60 mg	
codeine	Fiorinal w/Codeine	III	30 mg	325 mg aspirin 40 mg caffeine
codeine	Tylenol w/Codeine No.3	III	30 mg	300 mg acetaminophen
hydrocodone	Vicodin	III	5 mg	500 mg acetaminophen
hydrocodone	Vicoprofen	III	7.5 mg	200 mg ibuprofen
hydromorphone	Dilaudid	II	2 to 4 mg	
levorphanol	Levo-Dromoran	II	2 to 3 mg	
meperidine	Demerol	II	50 to 150 mg	
methadone	Dolophine	II	2.5 to 10 mg	
morphine	(generic)	II	5 to 30 mg	
oxycodone	OxyContin	II	10 to 20 mg[2]	
oxycodone	Percocet	II	5 mg	325 mg acetaminophen
propoxyphene	Darvocet-N 100	IV	100 mg	650 mg acetaminophen
propoxyphene	Darvon-N	IV	65 mg	

[1]Represents adult dose of the opioid.
[2]Represents 12-hour, controlled-release dose.

Contributing to the incidence of acetaminophen toxicity is the fact that there are so many OTC as well as prescription products that contain this drug. Because of the many combination products, patients often do not know that acetaminophen is one of the components of one or more products they are taking. Toxicity occurs when the amount of acetaminophen exceeds the capacity of the liver to metabolize it (Figure 7-2). Over 90% of an acetaminophen dose is metabolized by the liver by conversion

Recall from Chapter 3 that the blood level of the liver enzymes aspartate and alanine aminotransferase increase in the blood as a result of liver toxicity.

to several products. With therapeutic doses of acetaminophen, a small portion of these products is toxic to the liver cell, but is quickly detoxified within the liver cell. When an overdose occurs, the amount of toxic product produced exceeds the liver's ability to detoxify it and consequently some of the toxic product reacts with other components of the liver cell, which can cause fatal hepatic necrosis. Any dose of acetaminophen >7.5 g is considered potentially toxic in adults and 150 mg/kg in children. Initial symptoms of toxicity may not occur for hours after overdose but include nausea, vomiting, drowsiness, and abdominal pain. Clinical evidence of hepatotoxicity becomes evident 2 to 4 days after overdose as determined by elevated liver enzymes and bilirubin in the blood.

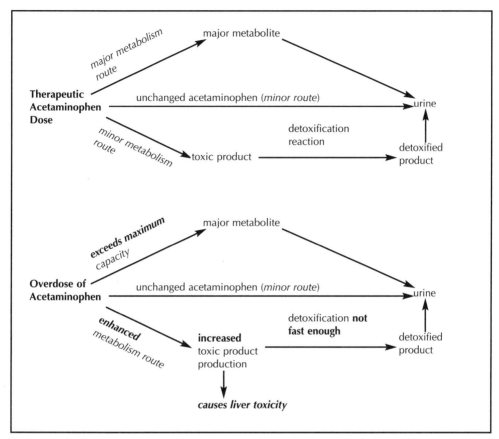

Figure 7-2. Mechanism of acetaminophen toxicity. Two pathways in the liver metabolize most of the acetaminophen. At therapeutic doses, the major pathway metabolizes most of the acetaminophen to form the major metabolite that is excreted in the urine. Because most of the therapeutic dose of acetaminophen is metabolized by this pathway, only a small amount is normally metabolized by another, typically minor pathway. The product of the minor pathway is a toxic product, which is quickly converted to a detoxified product and is then excreted in the urine. When too much acetaminophen is ingested, the capacity of the major pathway is exceeded and more acetaminophen is shunted to the minor pathway. The increased production of the toxic product in the minor pathway exceeds the amount that can be handled by the detoxification reaction. Consequently, some toxic product remains in the liver cell, reacts with other components of the cell, and becomes lethal to the cell.

Treatment of overdose varies depending on the dose of acetaminophen and time since ingestion, but mainstays of treatment are activated charcoal and acetylcysteine (Mucomyst). These are most effective if administered within 1 hour and 10 hours of the acetaminophen, respectively. Acetylcysteine provides a substitute for the natural substance used in the detoxification reaction, thereby increasing the rate of detoxification. Activated charcoal is a nonspecific absorbent that can decrease the absorption of some of the acetaminophen from the gastrointestinal tract. Because of the potential for liver toxicity, patients with existing liver disease should be cautious regarding the use of acetaminophen.

Alcohol consumption provides the most significant potential for drug interaction with acetaminophen. Alcohol increases the amount of toxic product produced from acetaminophen metabolism.

Box 7-1. Facts About Opioid Analgesics

- Used to relieve moderate to severe pain.
- Reduce anxiety and distress.
- Cause drowsiness
- Have an abuse potential for addiction and physical dependence
- All opioids are controlled substances except for tramadol.
- Cause constipation.
- Cough suppression activity.
- Adverse effects: Respiratory depression, miosis, urinary retention, orthostatic hypotension, nausea, and vomiting.
- Tolerance occurs to most of the opioid effects.
- Drug interactions: Significant CNS depressant effects if combined with other CNS depressants, including alcohol.

In addition, liver function may be compromised as a result of chronic alcohol consumption. The Food and Drug Administration (FDA) recommendation is that patients who consume more than three alcoholic drinks per day should consult their physician before using acetaminophen. Another potential drug interaction is with warfarin (Coumadin). Although occasional use of acetaminophen is generally considered acceptable for patients on warfarin therapy, daily use may inhibit warfarin metabolism and increase bleeding time.

Summary

Acetaminophen is a drug that is equipotent with aspirin in relieving mild to moderate pain and reducing fever. Like aspirin, acetaminophen is used in combination with opioid analgesics for relief of moderate to severe pain. In contrast to aspirin, however, acetaminophen does not have an effect on blood clotting; does not cause gastrointestinal adverse reactions; does not elicit the same hypersensitivity reactions; and when used as an antipyretic in children, it is not associated with Reye's syndrome. The major concern regarding the use of acetaminophen is the potential for high doses to cause liver toxicity. Concurrent use of alcohol can cause toxicity at lower doses of acetaminophen. Also, the use of multiple products that each contain acetaminophen can inadvertently cause a toxic dose of acetaminophen.

OPIOID ANALGESICS

Opioid analgesics are drugs that have pharmacological activity similar to morphine, which is the prototype for this drug category. The major characteristics of these drugs are that they relieve moderate to severe pain, produce drowsiness, and have an abuse potential (Box 7-1).

Mechanism of Action

The effects of opioids are the result of them combining with the opioid receptors located primarily in the CNS but also in the peripheral nervous system. There are three main opioid receptor classes, designated mu (μ, MOP), kappa (κ, KOP), and delta (δ, DOP). Evidence indicates that subtypes of these receptors also exist. The brain produces natural analgesics that combine with these receptors to provide natural pain relief. The three main families of endogenous opioids are *peptides* called *β-endorphins, enkephalins,* and *dynorphins*; collectively these are referred to as endorphins. These compounds have various functions as neurotransmitters and neurohormones, but a primary role is to act as natural opioid analgesics to alter the perception of pain and stress. Not surprisingly, the endogenous opioids act through a *second messenger* after combining with the receptor.

Effects and Uses

The effects of most clinically effective opioids, including analgesic and euphoric effects, are a result of their interaction with the mu receptor. Some opioids also combine with the kappa receptor, which contributes to analgesia but has the potential to cause *dysphoria*. Because morphine is the prototype opioid, a look at the effects of this drug is a good picture of the effects of the other opioids. There is, however, some variation in the degree to which each of these effects occurs with each opioid; particularly significant variations will be specified.

> *Recall that second messengers are compounds that are produced within the cell in response to the initial signal received by a receptor outside the cell. The second messenger carries the signal within the cell by initiating a cascade of reactions, a transduction mechanism, that ultimately result in the biochemical response. See also Chapter 3.*

The major therapeutic use of morphine is to relieve moderate to severe pain, such as pain associated with surgery, cancer, and myocardial infarction. Constant, dull pain is more effectively relieved at lower doses than sharp, intermittent pain. Besides analgesia, morphine also causes diminished anxiety and distress, which may contribute to pain relief by affecting the emotional aspect of pain perception. Drowsiness is also common although sleep is not necessary for pain relief. The other senses, such as smell and touch, are not affected.

A specific aspect of opioid analgesics that separates them from acetaminophen and NSAIDs is their abuse potential (ie, their ability to cause addiction/psychological dependence). *Addiction* is a behavioral disorder that is characterized by obsessive drug use typically accompanied by extreme measures to obtain the drug. The driving force that causes addiction is the desire for the euphoria from the drug. However, addiction rarely occurs when opioids are used to treat pain except in patients who have a prior predisposition to drug addiction. Pain seems to antagonize the euphoric effects such that most patients do not experience euphoric effects. Because of the abuse potential, all of the pure opioid *agonists* except tramadol (see below) are controlled substances. They are schedule II drugs with the exception of propoxyphene (Darvon, Class-IV) and the opioid products that are marketed in combination with aspirin or acetaminophen (eg, hydrocodone with acetaminophen [Vicodin, Class-III]).

Physical dependence also exists among all opioid analgesics but is a characteristic separate from addiction. *Dependence* occurs as a result of cellular changes within the body in response to continual exposure to the drug. The nature of these changes is not known, but in essence the many functions of the body that are affected reach a new state of balance. When the drug is removed, the body must readjust to a different state of balance and this abrupt adjustment causes a withdrawal syndrome. The existence of a withdrawal syndrome when the use of a drug is terminated is the only criteria to define the existence of physical dependence.

Opioid withdrawal syndrome is unpleasant, but rarely fatal. The duration and severity of the withdrawal symptoms depend on the duration of action of the specific drug that was used and degree of physical dependence. Drugs with a longer *duration of action* produce a longer but

Box 7-2. Opioid Withdrawal Symptoms

• Sweating	• Nausea
• Runny nose	• Vomiting
• Irritability	• Diarrhea
• Tremor	• Cramps
• Anorexia	• Muscle spasms

milder syndrome. Those with a shorter duration of action produce a shorter but more intense syndrome. The longer the dependence period and the higher the dose that was used, the longer and more intense the syndrome. Symptoms begin several hours after the last dose and are alleviated if any opioid analgesic is used, otherwise the duration of the symptoms is about 7 to 10 days (Box 7-2). Patients on chronic opioid therapy for >1 week are likely to have a degree of physical dependence. For these patients, a gradual reduction of the dosage for a few days will minimize withdrawal symptoms. Consequently, neither addiction nor physical dependence should be a clinical concern when opioids are necessary for pain management.

Morphine combines with opioid receptors in the gastrointestinal tract to reduce intestinal motility and secretion of fluids into the intestine. Consequently, constipation is of significant concern and is one of the most common adverse effects. Constipation develops within days of initiating treatment although it can be minimized by appropriate treatment with laxatives such as stool softeners or milk of magnesia, increased fiber, and adequate hydration. Because of the constipating effect, some opioids are used therapeutically to treat diarrhea. Paregoric (Class-III) and opium tincture (Class-II), which contain opium, and thus contain morphine, are commercially available but are not used very frequently because of the availability of other opioids with less abuse potential. For example, diphenoxylate (Lomotil, Class-V) and difenoxin (Motofen, Class-IV) are effective antidiarrheal agents. Loperamide (Imodium) is also an opioid but has a very low abuse potential and consequently is not a controlled substance. It is available OTC to treat diarrhea.

Morphine also has sedative properties. There are more effective sedatives available than opioids and thus these drugs are not used therapeutically for their sedative properties. However, sedation is sometimes advantageous when treating a patient for pain and may contribute to the reduced perception of acute pain. For other patients, however, drowsiness is an adverse effect as it is not conducive to some activities such as driving a car. Tolerance quickly develops (see below) to the sedative properties.

Opioid analgesics affect the cough center in the medulla to cause cough suppression. Two opioids, codeine and hydrocodone, are each available in combination with various compounds to treat upper respiratory conditions. The antitussive dose is lower than the analgesic dose; codeine dosage, for example, is every 4 to 6 hours at 10 to 20 mg for cough compared with 15 to 60 mg for pain.

Other effects of opioid analgesics include respiratory depression, *miosis* (pupil constriction), urinary retention, orthostatic hypotension (feeling faint when standing up), nausea, and vomiting.

These effects do not offer any therapeutic advantage and hence are adverse. At therapeutic doses, respiratory depression is not of significant concern unless the patient already has compromised respiration such as with chronic obstructive pulmonary disease. However, respiratory depression is the cause of death in most overdose cases. A competitive opioid antagonist can be administered to reverse respiratory depression; an example is naloxone (Narcan). An antagonist combines with the same opioid receptor as the opioid agonists without initiating the effects of the agonist. Consequently, the antagonists reverse the respiratory depression, analgesia, sedation, and euphoria, and will initiate withdrawal syndrome in a physically dependent patient.

Miosis is of relatively little concern although additional lighting may be necessary in some settings. Urinary retention is also a relatively minor problem although the physician should be contacted if the patient is unable to urinate adequately. Because opioids cause some hypotensive effects, patients should be cautioned about the potential for orthostatic

> *Orthostatic hypotension is also called postural hypotension. The patient feels faint or dizzy when standing too quickly from a sitting or lying position. Normally, autonomic reflexes such as increased heart rate and constriction of blood vessels increase blood pressure and prevent orthostatic hypotension. However, drugs like opioid analgesics, which cause dilation of peripheral blood vessels, or antihypertensive drugs (see Chapter 12), which inhibit the autonomic reflexes, will cause orthostatic hypotension.*

hypotension. They should be instructed regarding the potential for experiencing dizziness when standing up, and thus patients may need to stand slowly, especially from a supine position. Nausea and vomiting are CNS responses, occur more frequently in ambulatory patients, and are most pronounced as a result of the first dose.

Tolerance occurs to most of the effects of the opioids. Most importantly, tolerance occurs to the respiratory depression, sedative, and euphoric effects. Tolerance also develops to the analgesic effect but the rate of tolerance varies among patients. Fortunately, however, there is no ceiling effect for the analgesia so the dose of the opioid can be increased as tolerance develops. This is helpful for patients with terminal diseases (eg, some cancer patients) who need long-term pain relief with opioids. Tolerance does not develop significantly to the constipating and pupil constricting effects. Because the opioid analgesics all combine with the mu receptor, it is not surprising that *cross-tolerance* exists among the opioid analgesics (ie, tolerance to one results in tolerance to the others). When tolerance occurs, the duration of the pain relief becomes shorter followed by reduced analgesic effectiveness of each dose.

> *Recall from Chapter 2 that tolerance is a diminished response to a drug as a result of continued use. In other words, the dose of the drug must be increased to achieve the same response that was previously obtained.*

Pharmacokinetics and Dosage

Morphine, as well as most other opioids, is available in dosage forms for use by oral, rectal, and parenteral routes. Morphine undergoes first pass effect in the liver to a larger extent than other opioids; only about 25% of morphine is bioavailable after oral administration. Consequently, the oral dose is considerably higher than parenteral doses. Peak effectiveness occurs about 1.5 hours after oral administration. Most of the morphine is metabolized by the liver and excreted by the kidney. Patients with compromised liver or kidney function will have a higher blood concentration of morphine after repeated doses because of delayed drug clearance; these patients may require a reduced dosage. The typical adult parenteral dose of morphine is 10 mg and the duration of action is about 4 hours. A typical oral starting dosage is 20 to 60 mg every 4 hours although

> *Recall that synergism refers to an effect that occurs when two drugs used in the same therapy provide an effect greater than would be expected from the addition of their individual effects.*

sustained-release tablets and capsules are available that have a duration of action of 8 to 12 hours. Table 7-2 provides a selected list of opioid analgesics and the typical adult oral dosage regimen for comparison, although the dosage regimen for each patient should be individualized to attain adequate pain relief.

Opioid analgesics are often combined with acetaminophen, or sometimes with aspirin or ibuprofen, because the combination of an opioid and nonopioid analgesic provides a synergistic effect, which enhances the analgesia without adding to the adverse effects of either drug.

There are many of these brand name and generic name combination products; some examples are included in Table 7-2.

Drug Interactions

The most notable drug interaction of potentially significant consequence is the combination of opioids with other CNS depressants, including alcohol. The cause of death from an overdose of CNS depressant drugs is respiratory depression. The same result can occur when an opioid is combined with another CNS depressant drug. Examples of CNS depressants (see also Table 8-2) are the barbiturates that are used as sedatives and anticonvulsants (eg, phenobarbital) and the benzodiazepines that are used as sedatives, hypnotics, skeletal muscle relaxants, and antianxiety agents (eg, Valium, Restoril, Xanax, Ativan).

Specific Opioids

Table 7-2 lists examples of opioid analgesics and typical oral doses. Although the pharmacological effects of these drugs are much like morphine, there are some differences in effects and uses among the group. Hydromorphone and levorphenol are more potent than morphine but this is of little clinical significance as the therapeutic dose is adjusted accordingly. Levorphanol has a longer half-life and can be given fewer times per day.

> *Monoamine oxidase inhibitors (MAOIs) are a group of drugs that are categorized therapeutically as antidepressants. They are notorious for adverse effects and drug interactions.*

Codeine is less potent than morphine and is used to treat mild to moderate pain. It is often used in combination with either aspirin or acetaminophen; caffeine is also incorporated in some products. To designate an amount of codeine per dosage unit (ie, per tablet or capsule), the numbers 2, 3, or 4 are sometimes included in the product name to indicate the content of codeine equal to 15, 30, or 60 mg, respectively. For example, aspirin w/codeine No. 3 contains 30 mg of codeine. Much of the analgesic effect is attained as a result of a portion of codeine being metabolized to morphine. Hydrocodone is a chemical derivative of codeine with an analgesic effectiveness between codeine and morphine. It is only available in combination with aspirin or acetaminophen; caffeine is also incorporated in some products. Codeine and hydrocodone are also effective antitussive agents and are available in combination with antihistamines or decongestants for the treatment of colds.

Meperidine has a pharmacological profile similar to morphine but has a shorter duration and can cause additional adverse effects such as tremor, muscle twitching, and seizures. Meperidine should not be used with monoamine oxidase inhibitors (see also Chapter 12) because this combination can cause significant adverse effects (eg, severe respiratory depression, convulsions, and death).

Oxycodone has similar pharmacological effects, potency, and duration as morphine; is available in a controlled-release form; and is frequently combined with aspirin or acetaminophen. Of special note for oxycodone is the abuse associated with the controlled-release product

(OxyContin). This product contains a larger quantity of oxycodone because the drug is meant to be taken every 12 hours rather than every 4 to 6 hours. If the controlled-release tablets are chewed, crushed, or dissolved in water, the controlled-release aspect is eliminated and the entire dose is available quickly by ingesting, snorting, or injecting the drug. Consequently, abuse of the controlled-release product (also known as "oxy") has become a major problem.

Methadone has a longer duration than morphine and has good oral absorption. These are beneficial characteristics for treatment of chronic pain such as is needed for cancer patients. Oral methadone is also used to treat heroin addicts as a means of preventing withdrawal syndrome while gradually diminishing the dependence. Propoxyphene is chemically related to methadone but is much less potent and is used to treat mild to moderate pain. As is the case with some other opioids, a combination of propoxyphene with aspirin or acetaminophen is more effective than propoxyphene alone.

Tramadol (Ultram) is somewhat different than the other opioids in that it is not a controlled substance. It binds to the mu receptor with less effectiveness than codeine but also decreases pain perception through other mechanisms. As a result, tramadol has a significantly reduced risk of respiratory depression in overdose and lower potential for physical dependence and addiction than other opioids. The low abuse potential has warranted nonscheduled status. Like several other opioids, tramadol is available in combination with acetaminophen (Ultracet), which enhances the overall analgesic effectiveness. Tramadol alone or in combination with acetaminophen is recommended for treatment of moderate to moderately severe pain with efficacy similar to codeine and codeine with acetaminophen.

Additional mu-agonist opioids that are not used orally are fentanyl (Sublimaze), alfentanil (Alfenta), sufentanil (Sufenta), and remifentanil (Ultiva). These are analgesic adjuncts to general anesthesia. They are much more potent than morphine (100-fold for fentanyl), thus the dose is much smaller. Fentanyl is also available as a transdermal patch (Duragesic) for treatment of chronic severe pain. Onset is slow and thus is not for acute pain but duration is about 72 hours.

Heroin is not used therapeutically (schedule I) but is available through illicit markets. Heroin is more lipid soluble than morphine and therefore has better access to the brain than morphine, resulting in a high abuse potential but with no advantage as an analgesic. In the heroin-dependent person, withdrawal begins about 6 to 12 hours after the last dose.

Summary

The opioid analgesics mimic the naturally occurring analgesics, endorphins, enkephalins, and dynorphins by combining primarily with the mu, and to some extent the kappa, opioid receptors in the CNS. Morphine is the prototype opioid analgesic to which the effectiveness of others is compared. Besides effectively relieving moderate to severe pain, initial doses of morphine also cause drowsiness, diminished anxiety, orthostatic hypotension, and constipation. Tolerance develops quickly to these effects; however, constipation remains. Although euphoria is also a potential effect from opioids, it usually does not occur in patients being treated for pain. Because euphoria is the driving force for addiction, rarely does addiction occur in these patients. Physical dependence occurs with chronic use of opioids and thus, when the drug is to be discontinued, the dosage of the opioid should be gradually decreased in patients who have been receiving therapy for 5 to 7 days. Several opioids are used in combination with an NSAID or acetaminophen to enhance the analgesic effectiveness. Besides analgesia, other common uses for selected opioids are to treat diarrhea and cough.

Table 7-3. Examples of Over-the-Counter Analgesics That Contain Caffeine

Trade Name	Analgesic (mg)		Caffeine (mg)
	aspirin	acetaminophen	
Anacin Maximum Strength	500		32
APAP-Plus Tablets		500	65
Excedrin Aspirin Free		500	65
Excedrin Extra Strength	250	250	65
P-A-C Analgesic Tablets	400		32
Summit Extra Strength	250	250	65
Vanquish	227	194	33

Box 7-3. Caffeine Withdrawal Symptoms

- Fatigue
- Headache
- Irritability
- Restlessness
- Anxiety
- Yawning
- Runny nose

CAFFEINE

Caffeine is not often thought of as an analgesic but it does enhance the analgesic properties of acetaminophen, aspirin, and ibuprofen when used in combination with them. Used alone, caffeine has little value as an analgesic. Table 7-3 provides examples of some aspirin and acetaminophen-containing OTC products that also contain caffeine. The mechanism by which caffeine enhances the effectiveness of analgesic products is unclear, but studies have demonstrated a shorter onset of action and a longer duration of action for relief of mild to moderate pain with use of OTC analgesics that also contain caffeine.

Although caffeine is frequently used in analgesic products, by far the most common use by the general public is as a CNS stimulant. Approximately 80% of adults in the United States consume caffeine daily; most commonly in the form of coffee, tea, soft drinks, and chocolate containing foods (see Table 13-4). As a stimulant, caffeine will decrease drowsiness and fatigue and increase alertness at doses of 50 to 200 mg. At higher doses, caffeine causes restlessness, insomnia, nervousness, headache, diarrhea, and irritability. Caffeine-containing stimulant products such as NoDoz (available in 100 mg and 200 mg tablets) and Vivarin (available in 200 mg tablets) are marketed to help people stay awake.

Daily use of caffeine can result in physical dependence. Therefore, as with opioid dependency, abrupt discontinuation of caffeine use will cause withdrawal symptoms, which begin within the first day after discontinuing the drug. Peak withdrawal symptoms occur within 48 hours and then taper off, but may last for a week with the primary symptoms being fatigue and headache (Box 7-3). To again highlight the difference between physical dependence and addiction, note that although caffeine can cause physical dependence, caffeine is not listed as an addictive sub-

Table 7-4. Selected Local Anesthetics

Generic Name	Trade Name	Topical	Parenteral	Available OTC[1]
articaine	Septocaine		✓	
benzocaine	Lanacane	✓		✓
bupivacaine	Marcaine		✓	
butamben	Butesin	✓		✓
chloroprocaine	Nesacaine		✓	
cocaine[1]	(generic)	✓		
dibucaine	Nupercainal	✓		✓
lidocaine	Xylocaine	✓	✓	✓
mepivacaine	Polocaine		✓	
pramoxine	Tronothane	✓		✓
procaine	Novocain		✓	
tetracaine	Pontocaine	✓	✓	✓

[1]Only topical dosage forms available.

stance because very few people lose control over the amount of caffeine they ingest or are unable to decrease or eliminate intake if they so choose. Nonetheless, caffeine is a restricted substance in athletic competition (see Chapters 13 and 14).

TOPICAL ANALGESICS

Topical analgesics were discussed in the previous chapter with the topical anti-inflammatory products because some of them are specifically used to relieve the pain associated with inflammation. There are two main groups of compounds used as analgesics, the salicylates and the counterirritants. These compounds are used to relieve pain in muscles, joints, and tendons, but like topical anesthetics (see page 182), are also indicated for the relief of cutaneous pain such as from insect bites, minor burns, and sunburn. Methyl salicylate and trolamine salicylate are components of many products; methyl salicylate is also a counterirritant. Other counterirritants include *menthol, camphor, allyl isothiocyanate,* and *capsicum.* The counterirritants stimulate sensations of cold, warmth, or itching to distract the patient from the greater pain being experienced. These products also have a *rubefacient* effect, in that they cause localized vasodilation, which results in redness and a feeling of warmth. Menthol initially causes a cooling sensation followed by warmth. See Table 6-9 for examples of topical OTC analgesic products.

LOCAL ANESTHETICS

Local anesthetics are used as topical preparations to alleviate pain but are covered separately from the other topically applied analgesics because the mechanism is distinctly different and because some are also injected for a local or regional anesthetic effect. Examples of local anesthetics are shown in Table 7-4.

Mechanism and Effects

Local anesthetics act by inhibiting the nerve impulse transmission in the area where they are applied. Although sensation to pain is readily blocked, transmission of all nerve impulses is also blocked, resulting in diminished perception of hot, cold, and touch. The advantage of these agents is that they act quickly, affect only the localized area, and, even with parenteral administration, do not cause loss of consciousness.

Some absorption occurs into the bloodstream from topical application, especially from mucous membranes. Adverse effects from therapeutic doses of local anesthetics are few, even following parenteral administration. Allergic reactions occur only rarely. At higher concentrations in the blood, local anesthetics can affect cardiac conduction, leading to heart block and cardiac arrest. Elevated blood levels can also stimulate the CNS, resulting in restlessness, tremor, and convulsions, followed by CNS depression. This can progress to coma and respiratory depression.

Parenteral Use

Local anesthetics are often used parenterally by infiltration or nerve block anesthesia in preparation for dental procedures, minor surgery, and diagnostic procedures. Infiltration anesthesia involves the injection of the local anesthetics at or near areas where anesthesia is desired. Nerve block anesthesia involves injection into or near nerves that supply a specific area. The area is usually larger than that which would be covered by infiltration and is also more distant from the injection site. With both of these methods, the duration of anesthesia is dependent on the lipid solubility of the anesthetic and the amount of blood flow at the site of injection; more blood flow carries the drug away from the site more quickly. Sometimes a low concentration of a vasoconstrictor (eg, epinephrine) is added to the local anesthetic to diminish the local blood flow and thus extend the duration of action. For example, procaine (Novocain), has a duration of 15 minutes to 1 hour without epinephrine, and 30 minutes to 1.5 hours with epinephrine.

Topical Anesthetic

Local anesthetics are applied topically to obtain pain relief at that site on the surface of the skin or mucous membranes. Products are available as solutions, sprays, gels, ointments, creams, lozenges, and suppositories. Topically applied local anesthetics are used to treat pain and/or itching due to many causes, including sunburn, minor burns, insect bites, poison ivy, hemorrhoids, sore throat, temporary relief of minor sports injuries, and to prevent pain at the site of parenteral injections.

Ethyl chloride is a topical anesthetic but differs from those listed in Table 7-4 in that its effectiveness is a result of a cooling effect (skin refrigerant). The usefulness of ethyl chloride is similar to the use of ice, but the effectiveness is much quicker. Ethyl chloride is applied as a spray and it cools the skin as it rapidly evaporates. For the temporary relief of sports injuries, ethyl chloride is sprayed on the injured area until the skin just turns white (about 5 seconds). Duration of response is a few seconds to a minute but provides some relief from the initial trauma of the injury. Some caution is necessary in handling and storage of ethyl chloride because it is flammable and the spray containers are pressurized. Inhalation of ethyl chloride should be avoided as general anesthetic and cardiac effects may occur.

Cocaine is a topical anesthetic worthy of specific note. It causes CNS stimulation and euphoria by a mechanism unrelated to the local anesthetic action. Consequently, cocaine has a high abuse potential and is the only local anesthetic that is a controlled substance (C-II). It is, however, an effective local anesthetic that is used topically for anesthesia of the ear, nose, and throat.

Cocaine is also unique from the other local anesthetics in that it causes constriction of the local vasculature and thus eliminates the need for adding epinephrine. Absorption occurs from the mucous membranes and, as indicated, the effects on the CNS are more pronounced than with the other local anesthetics. Stimulatory effects occur first and are followed by depressant effects. Small doses of cocaine cause bradycardia, but moderate doses cause more significant cardiovascular effects such as tachycardia and hypertension.

ROLE OF THE ATHLETIC TRAINER

Use of analgesics by athletes is a frequent occurrence and thus offers many opportunities for the athletic trainer to help ensure proper use of these medications. Unlike the use of antibiotics or long-term asthma medications in which poor compliance does not always initiate symptoms, poor compliance of analgesics initiates a definite undesirable symptom—pain. The desire to relieve pain, coupled with the ready accessibility of OTC pain relievers, contributes to the overuse of analgesic drugs and the potential for significant adverse or toxic effects. The athletic trainer, therefore, can assist the athlete in preventing these effects by being aware of the content of OTC and prescription analgesics and by being alert to the conditions that would cause an athlete to be more susceptible to adverse effects. In this regard, the following are some key points and general statements that should be useful to the athletic trainer:

- Do not doubt the existence of pain reported by an athlete. Everyone's pain threshold is different; pain is in the "eye of the beholder."
- Realize that to treat systemic pain there are two main groups of analgesics: NSAIDs/acetaminophen and opioids. NSAIDs and acetaminophen are effective for mild to moderate pain; opioids are effective for moderate to severe pain.
- Encourage athletes who are using NSAIDs to take them with food or milk to reduce gastric irritation.
- Realize that acetaminophen is often used as an alternative to aspirin and other NSAIDs for relief of mild to moderate pain for athletes who have a history of ulcers, are also taking warfarin, have diminished kidney function, have aspirin-induced asthma, or are allergic to any NSAID.
- Recognize that acetaminophen may be a better choice than NSAIDs as an analgesic for relief of mild to moderate pain while participating in strenuous exercise of long duration as acetaminophen does not impact kidney function as significantly and the termination of its activity is not dependent on kidney function.
- Understand that although certain athletes should not be taking either NSAIDs or acetaminophen, athletes may not realize that they are ingesting an NSAID or acetaminophen as a component of an OTC product(s).
- Advise athletes to be cautious regarding the use of multiple prescription and/or OTC products as they may each contain acetaminophen or aspirin, which can result in toxicity. Initial signs of toxicity for aspirin include tinnitus, dizziness, and headache; for acetaminophen they include nausea, vomiting, and anorexia.
- Alert athletes who require opioid analgesics to the likelihood of constipation as an adverse effect. Recommend use of laxatives (see Chapter 11) for relief of constipation.
- Ensure that all use of opioid analgesics are under the direction of a physician.
- Do not use counterirritants on open wounds or abraded skin. Do not wrap the treated area with occlusive bandages or expose the area to heat because excessive irritation or skin damage can occur (see Chapter 6).

BIBLIOGRAPHY

Drugs for pain. *The Medical Letter.* 2000;42:73-78.

Houglum JE. Pharmacologic considerations in the treatment of injured athletes with nonsteroidal anti-inflammatory drugs. *Journal of Athletic Training.* 1998;33:259-263.

National Drug Intelligence Center. OxyContin diversion and abuse. Available at: http://www.usdoj.gov/ndic/pubs/651/overview.htm. Accessed July 9, 2003.

Schiff PL Jr. Opium and its alkaloids. *Am J Pharm Educ.* 2002;66:186-194.

Zed PJ, Krenzelok EP. Treatment of acetaminophen overdose. *Am J Health Syst Pharm.* 1999;56:1081-1093.

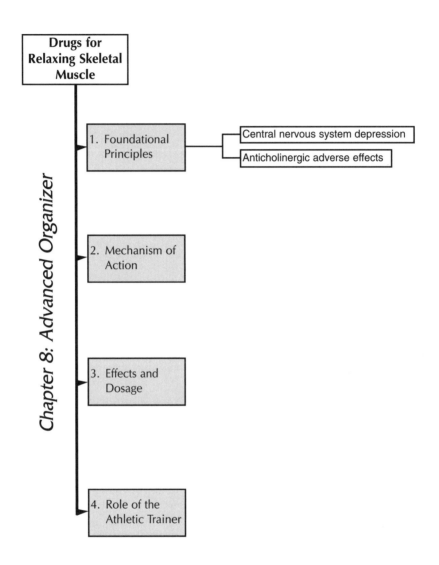

DRUGS FOR RELAXING SKELETAL MUSCLE

CHAPTER OBJECTIVES

At the end of this chapter, the reader will be able to:
- Explain the uses of skeletal muscle relaxant drugs.
- Explain the adverse effects of drugs used to relax skeletal muscles.
- Recognize the signs and symptoms of an anticholinergic adverse effect.
- Identify drug categories that have anticholinergic adverse effects.
- Explain the mechanism of action, therapeutic effects, and dosage regimen for drugs used to relax skeletal muscle.
- Summarize the role of the athletic trainer for patients who are taking skeletal muscle relaxants.

This chapter discusses the use and effects of skeletal muscle relaxants that function through the central nervous system (CNS) (ie, centrally acting) to alleviate muscle spasms. Peripherally acting skeletal muscle relaxants are generally used to block neuromuscular function during surgery or other medical procedures. Examples are tubocurarine, succinylcholine (Anectine), and doxacurium (Nuromax). Another group of muscle relaxants, which include baclofen (Lioresal) and dantrolene (Dantrium), are used to treat spasticity caused by diseases such as multiple sclerosis and cerebral palsy. Neither the peripherally acting muscle relaxants nor those used specifically for treatment of spasticity will be discussed.

Centrally acting skeletal muscle relaxants are a relatively small group of drugs used to prevent or relieve muscle spasms (Table 8-1). Muscle spasms are involuntary localized muscle contractions that are caused by pain, trauma, or muscle inflammation. Pain is often associated with muscle spasms and consequently analgesics may be a part of drug therapy. Some muscle relaxants are available in combination with codeine, acetaminophen, aspirin, or aspirin with caffeine (see Table 8-1). Some physical agents, such as cryotherapy, moist heat, massage, and stretching, are also effective for relieving muscle spasms and associated pain. Muscle relaxants alone, and in combination with analgesics, are also used to treat back and neck pain, although the extent to which they are effective for this use is somewhat unclear.

FOUNDATIONAL CONCEPTS

There are some adverse effects that are predominant among the skeletal muscle relaxants and are also prevalent among other categories of drugs. Therefore, an understanding of the concepts related to these adverse effects is important.

Table 8-1. Skeletal Muscle Relaxants

Generic Name	Analgesic Added (mg)	Trade Name	Typical Adult Oral Maintenance Dose
carisoprodol		Soma	350 mg 3 to 4 times/day
carisoprodol	aspirin (325)	Soma Compound	1 to 2 tablets 4 times/day
carisoprodol	aspirin (325) + codeine (16)	Soma Compound w/codeine	1 to 2 tablets 4 times/day
chlorphenesin		Maolate	400 mg 4 times/day
chlorzoxazone		Paraflex	250 to 750 mg 3 to 4 times/day
chlorzoxazone	acetaminophen (300)	Flexaphen	2 capsules 4 times/day
cyclobenzaprine		Flexeril	10 mg 3 times/day
diazepam		Valium	2 to 10 mg 3 to 4 times/day
metaxalone		Skelaxin	800 mg 3 to 4 times/day
methocarbamol		Robaxin	1 gram 4 times/day
methocarbamol	aspirin (325)	Robaxisal	2 tablets 4 times/day
orphenadrine		Norflex	100 mg 2 times/day
orphenadrine	aspirin (385) + caffeine (30)	Norgesic	1 to 2 tablets 3 to 4 times/day

Central Nervous System Depression

Depression of the CNS can result in drowsiness and dizziness; higher doses result in more significant sedation and respiratory depression. Overdose of CNS depressants results in coma and death from respiratory depression. As shown in Table 8-2, several categories of drugs cause CNS depression. When two or more of these drugs are used concurrently, or used in combination with alcohol, the sedative effects are enhanced. For example, coma and death have resulted from the combination of alcohol and benzodiazepines. Even when therapeutic doses of these drugs are combined, a significantly enhanced drowsiness response can adversely affect the patient's activity, including athletic performance. Drowsiness is a safety concern if the patient is operating a motor vehicle, but this concern is even greater when CNS depressant drugs are combined.

Anticholinergic Adverse Effects

Several of the skeletal muscle relaxants are particularly noted for causing anticholinergic adverse effects. *Anticholinergic effects* is a term that refers to a group of adverse effects that are similar to the effects from drugs in the pharmacological category called anticholinergic drugs, such as atropine and scopolamine. Anticholinergic drugs, and other drugs with anticholinergic effects, block the *cholinergic receptors* at the site where the parasympathetic nervous system innervates smooth muscle and organ tissue. This receptor is also called the *muscarinic receptor* and thus these drugs are also called antimuscarinic drugs or muscarinic blockers. Inhibition of the parasympathetic system by drugs with anticholinergic effects has the potential to cause responses that are opposite of stimulating the parasympathetic system (ie, cause anticholinergic effects as listed in Table 8-3). There are several categories of drugs that cause anticholinergic adverse effects (Box 8-

Table 8-2. Selected Drugs That Have Central Nervous System Depressant Effects[1]

Drug Category	Generic Name	Trade Name
Antianxiety	**benzodiazepines:**	
	alprazolam	Xanax
	clorazepate	Tranxene
	chlordiazepoxide	Librium
	diazepam	Valium
	halazepam	Paxipam
	oxazepam	Serax
Anticonvulsants	**benzodiazepines:**	
	clonazepam	Klonopin
	clorazepate	Tranxene
	diazepam	Valium
	others:	
	carbamazepine	Tegretol
	ethosuximide	Zarontin
	phenobarbital	Luminal
	primidone	Mysoline
Antihistamines	diphenhydramine	Benadryl
	diphenhydramine with acetaminophen	Tylenol Severe Allergy
	promethazine	Phenergan
	hydroxyzine	Vistaril
Opioid analgesics	codeine	(generic)
	hydromorphone	Dilaudid
	meperidine	Demerol
	morphine	(generic)
Sedatives	**benzodiazepines:**	
	estazolam	ProSom
	flurazepam	Dalmane
	temazepam	Restoril
	triazolam	Halcion
	barbiturates:	
	amobarbital	Amytal
	pentobarbital	Nembutal
	phenobarbital	Luminal
	others:	
	chloral hydrate	(generic)
	zaleplon	Sonata
	zolpidem	Ambien

[1]*CNS depressant effects may be enhanced when any of these drugs are used concurrently or with skeletal muscle relaxants in Table 8-1. Alcohol is also a CNS depressant but is not shown.*

Table 8-3. Anticholinergic Adverse Effects

Response	Comments
Blurred vision	Affects near vision
Constipation	Increase fluid/fiber; may require stool softener or laxative
Decreased sweating	Potential for hyperthermia, especially on hot day
Dry mouth	Increase fluids; stimulate saliva with hard candy or gum
Increased heart rate	Potential problem for patients with cardiac problems
Pupil dilation	May cause sensitivity to light; prefer dim light/sunglasses
Increased IOP[1]	Avoid anticholinergic drugs in patients with glaucoma
Urinary hesitancy	If significant, should consider change in therapy
Urinary retention	If significant, should consider change in therapy

[1]IOP = intraocular pressure

Box 8-1. Examples of Drug Categories That Have Anticholinergic Adverse Effects

- Antihistamines such as diphenhydramine (Benadryl) that are used to treat colds and allergies (see Chapter 10), but also are used to treat motion sickness and contained in OTC sleep-aid products to treat insomnia. These antihistamines are not the H_2 antihistamines (H_2-receptor antagonists) that are used to treat peptic ulcers (see Chapter 11).

- Opioid analgesics (see Chapter 7).

- Tricyclic antidepressants such as amitriptyline (Elavil) and imipramine (Tofranil). The term "tricyclic" identifies a specific chemically related group of drugs that share a common therapeutic role as drug therapy for depression.

- Phenothiazines such as trifluoperazine (Stelazine) and chlorpromazine (Compazine). The term "phenothiazine" identifies a specific chemically related group of drugs that are used to treat psychoses; some phenothiazines are used at lower doses as antiemetics.

- Anticholinergic drugs such as atropine and scopolamine. Atropine has varied uses such as treatment of bradycardia and to prepare the eye for certain eye examinations; scopolamine is available OTC and is effective in the treatment of motion sickness.

- Selected skeletal muscle relaxants, particularly cyclobenzaprine (Flexeril) and orphenadrine (Norflex).

1) but at therapeutic doses not all of the drugs in these categories cause all of the responses listed in Table 8-3; the type of response and extent of response varies among these drugs and is dependent on the dosage being used.

MECHANISM OF ACTION

The skeletal muscle relaxants exert their activity on skeletal muscle through the CNS although the exact mechanism is unknown. All of these drugs have some CNS sedative properties and it is possible that these properties contribute to muscle relaxation. Diazepam (Valium) is a drug from the chemical category of drugs called benzodiazepines. Besides having sedative

Box 8-2. Summary of Adverse Effects Related to Skeletal Muscle Relaxants

- Drowsiness.
- Dizziness.
- Diminished liver and kidney function.
- Hypersensitivity reaction.
- Centrally-acting skeletal muscle relaxants can cause physical dependence.
- Anticholinergic effects.

properties, diazepam combines with the *gamma aminobutyric acid* (GABA) receptor. Stimulation of this receptor causes an inhibitory effect on nerve impulse transmission in the CNS, which may also contribute to muscle relaxation.

EFFECTS AND DOSAGE

Skeletal muscle relaxants relieve muscle spasms and, as a result, they also relieve the accompanying pain and increase the patient's range of motion. No single muscle relaxant is recognized as superior to the others in muscle relaxant properties and thus the selection of muscle relaxant depends largely on its adverse effect profile and the preference of the physician and/or the patient. For example, drugs with pronounced anticholinergic effects should not be used in patients with glaucoma. Several skeletal muscle relaxants along with their typical adult oral maintenance dosage for treating muscle spasms are listed in Table 8-1.

Glaucoma is a condition in which the intraocular pressure is elevated. As pressure increases, optic nerve damage occurs, vision is impaired, and blindness can result. Drugs with anticholinergic effects can increase intraocular pressure in patients with glaucoma.

Several adverse effects and related cautions are common among the skeletal muscle relaxants (Box 8-2). For example, because all of these drugs function through CNS depressant effects, they all cause drowsiness and dizziness. Consequently, patients being treated with these drugs must be cautious when driving a motor vehicle. Alcohol and other CNS depressants (see Table 8-2) must also be avoided because the depressant effects from other drugs are enhanced when used concurrently with muscle relaxants. Liver and kidney function may also be diminished by skeletal muscle relaxants, with the risk increasing as the duration of therapy and dosage increases. Consequently, these organs are sometimes monitored to detect early signs of compromised function. The potential for hypersensitivity reaction is also a caution regarding treatment with most of these drugs. Hypersensitivity reactions can range from a dermatological rash to anaphylaxis.

The centrally acting skeletal muscle relaxants have the potential to cause physical dependence, although Diazepam (Valium) and carisoprodol (Soma) are particularly noteworthy in this respect. The incidence of dependence increases as higher doses are used for a longer time. These drugs should be slowly discontinued to avoid withdrawal syndrome.

Some adverse effects are more unique to one or two drugs listed in Table 8-1. For example, chlorzoxasone (Paraflex) and methocarbamol (Skelex) have the unusual characteristic of discoloring the urine. There

Recall from Chapter 7 that physical dependence is a function of the drug's effect on cellular function and is not the same as addiction.

is no symptom associated with this effect but patients should be informed so they are not alarmed at the change. As already mentioned, a response unique to cyclobenzaprine (Flexeril) and orphenadrine (Norflex) are the anticholinergic adverse effects.

Diazepam (Valium) is a member of the chemical category of drugs called benzodiazepines. The term *benzodiazepine* refers to a portion of the chemical structure that these drugs have in common. There are over a dozen benzodiazepines. As a group, these compounds have many uses, such as to treat insomnia, anxiety, alcohol withdrawal syndrome, various seizures, as well as muscle spasms. Although each of the benzodiazepines may be effective to some degree for these uses, some drugs in this group are significantly more effective for one or more of these therapeutic uses than others. Consequently, not all benzodiazepines are approved by the Food and Drug Administration for each of these uses. All benzodiazepines have an abuse potential and thus are controlled substances (schedule IV) and all cause CNS depression and thus produce drowsiness. Examples of benzodiazepines and the therapeutic category for selected drugs are listed in Table 8-2.

Summary

Skeletal muscle relaxants have CNS depressant effects that may contribute to their mechanism of action. Use of these drugs relieves symptoms associated with muscle spasm and improves use of the affected muscles but may also cause adverse effects such as drowsiness, dizziness, diminished liver function, hypersensitivity, and anticholinergic effects. The potential for enhanced adverse effects exists if other drugs are used concurrently that also cause CNS depression or anticholinergic effects. Examples of such drugs include alcohol, antihistamines in cold remedies, anticonvulsants, antianxiety drugs, opioid analgesics, and benzodiazepines.

ROLE OF THE ATHLETIC TRAINER

As always, the athletic trainer can play a role in ensuring that the athlete adheres to the proper dosage regimen and is aware of common adverse effects. Among the skeletal muscle relaxants, the most common adverse effects are drowsiness and dizziness. The potential for enhanced drowsiness exists if the skeletal muscle relaxant is combined with any of the other CNS depressants. Drug-induced drowsiness and dizziness are especially significant problems in athletes competing in sports that require exceptional balance, such as gymnastics or cycling. Drowsiness is also a safety concern (eg, while driving a motor vehicle). Anticholinergic adverse effects are also problematic and the potential exists for enhanced responses of this type due to the concurrent use of more than one drug that causes anticholinergic effects. The athletic trainer, therefore, can be sure that the athlete is aware of the drugs that may exacerbate these problems (see Table 8-2), including over-the-counter drugs that contain antihistamines or alcohol. Consequently, by understanding these drug interactions, the athletic trainer may help prevent undesirable effects and should refer the athlete to a physician when such drug combinations exert an excessive adverse response.

BIBLIOGRAPHY

Browning R, Jackson JL, O'Malley PG. Cyclobenzaprine and back pain: a meta-analysis. *Arch Intern Med.* 2001;161:1613-1620.

Henderson JM. Therapeutic drugs: what to avoid with athletes. *Clin Sports Med.* 1998;17:229-243.

Waldman HJ. Centrally acting skeletal muscle relaxants and associated drugs. *J Pain Symptom Manage.* 1994; 9:434-441.

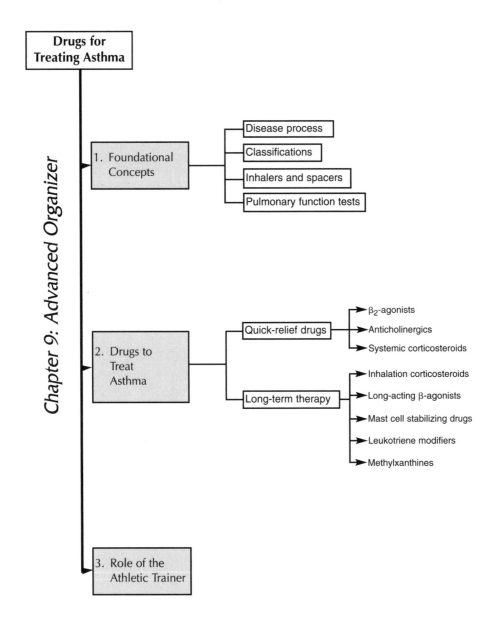

Chapter 9: Advanced Organizer

Drugs for Treating Asthma

1. Foundational Concepts
   - Disease process
   - Classifications
   - Inhalers and spacers
   - Pulmonary function tests

2. Drugs to Treat Asthma
   - Quick-relief drugs
     - β₂-agonists
     - Anticholinergics
     - Systemic corticosteroids
   - Long-term therapy
     - Inhalation corticosteroids
     - Long-acting β-agonists
     - Mast cell stabilizing drugs
     - Leukotriene modifiers
     - Methylxanthines

3. Role of the Athletic Trainer

DRUGS FOR TREATING ASTHMA

CHAPTER OBJECTIVES

At the end of this chapter, the reader will be able to:

- Recall the goals of asthma therapy and the interventions that aid in achieving therapy goals.
- Explain why asthma therapy compliance is problematic and the interventions that can be implemented to improve therapy compliance.
- Describe the disease process that results in the chronic inflammation of the airway and how acute exacerbations of asthma occur.
- Explain a categorical classification system for asthma based on severity and summarize a therapeutic management approach for each category of severity.
- Recall the advantages and disadvantages of metered dose inhalers (MDIs).
- Explain how the use of a spacer with a MDI can improve the likelihood of better drug delivery to the lungs.
- Compare and contrast the three types of inhalers available for asthma treatment.
- Explain the procedure for correct MDI technique.
- Recall the problems associated with inhaler and spacer use and how to overcome them.
- Explain the use of nebulizers, forced expiratory spirometer tests, and peak flow meters in the management of asthma.
- Make recommendations regarding asthma therapy based on peak flow meter readings.
- Identify drug categories used for quick-relief and long-term therapy for asthma.
- Describe the mechanism of action for quick-relief and long-term therapy drug categories for treating asthma.
- Recognize the adverse effects for quick-relief and long-term asthma medications.
- Summarize the role of the athletic trainer for patients who are on an asthma drug therapy regimen.

There is an arsenal of over 20 drugs in six different pharmacological categories that are available to combat asthma. These drugs are used to treat the approximately 15 million people in the United States who have asthma. As will be discussed in this chapter, although there are many drugs available to treat asthma, the approach to drug therapy management can be simplified by dividing asthma drugs into two major therapeutic groups: drugs used to obtain quick relief of acute asthma attacks (rescue therapy), and drugs to obtain long-term control so as to reduce the occurrence of acute attacks. Athletic trainers can have a significant impact on the therapeutic

Box 9-1. Asthma Therapy Goals and Keys to a Successful Therapy Regimen

Goals of Asthma Therapy

- Prevent chronic and troublesome symptoms (eg, coughing or breathlessness in the night, in the early morning, or after exertion).
- Maintain (near) "normal" pulmonary function.
- Maintain normal activity levels (including exercise and other physical activity).
- Prevent recurrent exacerbations of asthma and minimize the need for emergency department visits or hospitalizations.
- Provide optimal pharmacotherapy with minimal or no adverse effects.
- Meet patients' and families' expectations of and satisfaction with asthma care.

Keys to Achieving Therapy Goals

- Using the appropriate medications at the appropriate dosage.
- Avoiding factors that exacerbate the asthma symptoms.
- Monitoring the asthma so timely adjustments can be made.
- Educating the patient regarding the nature and management of the disease.

outcomes by helping the athlete to understand the rationale for using both of these therapeutic groups of drugs, to be compliant with the dosage regimen, to properly use inhalers, and to monitor the effectiveness of drug therapy.

This chapter will provide basic information concerning the asthma disease process, pharmacological information relative to asthma drugs, therapy guidelines for use of these drugs to treat asthma, and suggestions as to how the athletic trainer may assist the athlete to obtain better therapeutic outcomes from the asthma therapy and thus improve his or her performance.

For the athlete, a prime goal of asthma treatment is to enable him/her to compete without being hindered by the disease or by the therapy. This is also among the general goals of asthma therapy of the National Asthma Education and Prevention Program (NAEPP) as published in 1997 by the National Heart, Lung, and Blood Institute in *Expert Panel Report 2: Guidelines for the Diagnosis and Management of Asthma*. Box 9-1 lists the goals of asthma therapy reported in this document.

Achieving these goals requires cooperation and communication between the patient and the health care team. Consequently, it is important that the patient as well as health care professionals be active participants in the therapy process. The keys to achieving the therapy goals are listed in Box 9-1.

Pinpointing the appropriate medications and dosages is often a difficult task in asthma treatment. As discussed in this chapter, the severity of the disease differs among patients and thus the therapy should be tailored for each patient. It is therefore important for patients to accurately communicate to the physician the frequency and severity of the symptoms and to monitor the disease. Even when the appropriate drugs and dosages are prescribed, patient compliance with therapy is a significant problem because asthma is a chronic disease that necessitates long-term therapy, often with multiple drugs and/or multiple dosage units per day. Compliance is a problem in all subpopulations of asthmatics; overall approximately 50% of all asthmatics adhere to prescribed therapy. Inadequate prescribing of drug therapy adds to the number of patients receiving inadequate treatment for asthma. Consequently, suboptimal drug prescribing and poor compliance by patients are significant problems associated with asthma therapy.

Various substances can trigger asthma reactions, and these triggers differ among patients. An obvious strategy is to avoid or minimize exposure to these triggers, but as will be discussed, there are many potential triggers and thus avoidance of exposure to these triggers may be difficult. Appropriate monitoring can also help avoid the onset of some asthma attacks and can also provide information useful to evaluate the effectiveness of therapy. To keep asthma patients involved daily with these and other aspects of their disease requires active participation of health care professionals who can provide information and education to the patient. If patients know not only the "how," but also the "why" regarding treatment and monitoring, it may help them be persistent in the long-term management of the asthma.

FOUNDATIONAL CONCEPTS

There are several pharmacologic categories of drugs available to treat asthma. To understand the logic for using these drugs, it is helpful to understand the mechanism of the disease process, the symptoms of the disease, and the terminology used to classify the severity of the disease. Knowledge of the proper use of inhalers, spacers, and peak flow meters is also useful as these devices are important aspects of asthma management.

Disease Process

Asthma is a chronic inflammatory disease of the airways. The inflammation results in obstruction of the airways from bronchoconstriction, edema, and excessive mucus production. Symptoms include wheezing, coughing, and shortness of breath. The patient may experience a feeling of chest tightness. As the extent of inflammation increases, the severity of the symptoms typically also increases. Another characteristic of chronic inflammation is that it causes bronchial hyperresponsiveness to a variety of stimuli. This results in acute exacerbations of the inflammation with enhanced symptoms of wheezing, shortness of breath, and difficulty breathing, which can last for a few days. Although patients differ regarding their response to these stimuli, examples of stimuli include typical allergens (eg, dust, pollen, animal dander), exercise, tobacco smoke, cold temperatures, viral infections, nonsteroidal anti-inflammatory drugs (NSAIDs), chronic sinusitis, and gastroesophageal reflux.

The mechanism that results in the chronic inflammatory response and the accompanying hyperresponsiveness is not clear, although an *antibody-antigen* response is responsible for the allergen-mediated inflammation and may play a role in the mechanism for other stimuli as well. Regardless of the initiating cause, it is evident that there are many inflammatory chemical mediators that participate in the response. To understand the mechanism of action of several asthma medications, it is of particular importance to understand the process of mediator production through *arachidonic acid* metabolism (Figure 9-1). As discussed in Chapter 6, arachidonic acid metabolites are produced in virtually all cells. With respect to asthma pathophysiology, however, the products of the pathway catalyzed by 5-lipoxygenase play a key role. As Figure 9-1 illustrates, during an inflammatory response *phospholipase A$_2$* is activated in the lung mast cell and causes the release of arachidonic acid inside the cell. *Arachidonic acid* can be the substrate for *cyclooxygenase* (COX) to synthesize *prostaglandins* (PGs), or for 5-lipoxygenase to synthesize the *leukotrienes* (LTs). Leukotriene C$_4$ (LTC$_4$) synthase catalyzes the first step in the conversion of

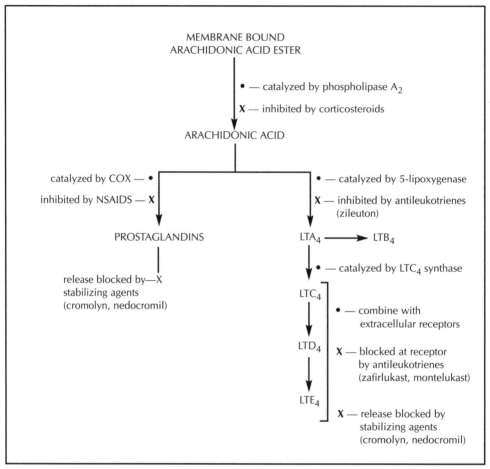

Figure 9-1. Biosynthesis pathways of arachidonic acid metabolites. Arachidonic acid is released from membrane-bound sites by the action of phospholipase A_2. If the arachidonic acid reacts with cyclooxygenase (COX), it is converted to prostaglandins; if it reacts with 5-lipoxygenase, it is converted to the leukotrienes. In either case, the arachidonic acid metabolites are released by the cell and will combine with the respective receptor on other cells to contribute to the symptoms of asthma. The sites of action are shown for the corticosteroids, leukotriene modifiers, and mast cell stabilizing drugs. • — Indicates reaction catalyzed by enzyme as designated. X — Indicates reaction inhibited by drug as designated (reprinted with permission from Houglum JE. Asthma medications: basic pharmacology and use in the athlete. *Journal of Athletic Training.* 2000; 35:179-187).

LTA$_4$ to produce LTC$_4$, which is then released by the *mast cells* and eventually converted to LTD$_4$ and LTE$_4$. The LTs activate LT receptors on bronchial smooth muscle, which causes vasodilation, increased vasopermeability, mucus secretion, edema, and marked bronchoconstriction. Regarding these effects, LTC$_4$ and LTD$_4$ are the most potent; LTE$_4$ is significantly less potent. Some cell types convert LTA$_4$ to LTB$_4$, which attract *eosinophils* and *neutrophils* to the site. Besides mast cells, other cell types such as *macrophages*, neutrophils, eosinophils, and *T lymphocytes* also contribute to the inflammatory process by producing arachidonic acid metabolites as well as other chemical mediators including *histamine, platelet-activating factor,* and *cytokines,* which contribute to the inflammatory process. Use of anti-inflammatory drugs interrupts one or more aspects of this process to decrease the damaging effects of chronic inflammation. Although the PGs contribute to the inflammatory response, they play a mixed role regarding the effect on bronchial smooth muscle, causing relaxation or constriction, depending on the specific PG.

Classifications

The specific drug therapy and dosages needed to control the symptoms of asthma vary from patient to patient depending primarily on the severity of the disease. The NAEPP has established guidelines for classifying asthma severity based on results of lung function tests and the frequency of symptoms prior to treatment (Table 9-1). The classifications are mild intermittent, mild persistent, moderate persistent, and severe persistent. The least severe classification, mild intermittent, exists if the patient has no more than 2 days per week with symptoms and no more than 2 nights' sleep interrupted with symptoms. The most serious, severe persistent, exists if the daytime symptoms are continual and the nighttime symptoms are frequent. All of the persistent categories require daily medication; only the mild intermittent category does not (Table 9-2).

Although the categorization of asthma severity is useful, patients often have symptoms that overlap categories. For example, a patient may have daytime symptoms of 3 to 6 times per week (mild persistent) but nighttime symptoms of more than once per week (moderate persistent). Patients should be placed in the category of greatest severity for treatment purposes.

The NAEPP has established guidelines for drug therapy (see Table 9-2) based on the classifications of asthma severity. The guidelines recommend that all patients use a quick-relief bronchodilator, and all patients with persistent asthma also use daily anti-inflammatory medication for long-term control of inflammation. As the severity classification increases, the guidelines call for an increase in dose and/or the addition of another long-term-control drug to the therapy. When therapy is initiated, however, aggressive therapy is recommended to control the symptoms, followed by an approach of a gradual decrease in drug therapy ("step down") to determine the least amount of medication necessary to maintain control.

In addition to the NAEPP classifications of severity of asthma, the following additional terminology identifies asthma based on some characteristic other than severity:

- Chronic asthma is the disease generally referred to as "asthma." It includes the chronic inflammatory condition already discussed.
- An acute asthma attack (exacerbation) is a sudden onset of symptoms that is generally caused from the hyperresponsiveness associated with chronic asthma condition. The onset of the acute attack may be due to exposure to known allergens or pollutants or from some unknown factor. The acute inflammatory response causes bronchoconstriction, excessive mucus production, and edema, resulting in the symptoms described previously (eg, wheezing, coughing, shortness of breath, difficulty breathing). These symptoms may be mild enough to ameliorate spontaneously, necessitate treatment with quick-relief (ie, rescue) medication, or be severe as to require emergency medical attention. Duration of an acute attack may be a few days.
- Exercise-induced bronchoconstriction (EIB) exists in 70% to 90% of patients with chronic asthma. Some patients may have EIB but do not have asthma-related symptoms at any other times. Onset of EIB symptoms typically occurs during exercise and for 20 to 60 minutes after exercise, with the maximum bronchoconstriction occurring within the first 5 to 15 minutes after exercise. Some athletes experience a subsequent refractory period of 2 to 4 hours in which additional exercise results in less bronchoconstriction. The refractory period may be a result of mast-cell mediators being depleted. As with chronic asthma, EIB symptoms can include wheezing, coughing, and shortness of breath. The loss of water and/or heat from the lung during exercise may contribute to the cause of EIB; avoiding exercise in cool, dry environments may reduce EIB.

Table 9-1. Classifications of Asthma Severity

Classification	Symptoms/Clinical Features Before Treatment	Nighttime Symptoms	Lung Function[1]
Step 4 Severe persistent	Continual symptoms Limited physical activity Frequent exacerbations	Frequent	FEV_1 or PEF ≤60% predicted PEF variability >30%
Step 3 Moderate persistent	Daily symptoms Daily use of inhaled short-acting β_2-agonist Exacerbations affect activity Exacerbations ≥2 times a week; may last days	>1 time a week	FEV_1 or PEF >60% to <80% predicted PEF variability >30%
Step 2 Mild persistent	Symptoms >2 times a week, but <1 time a day Exacerbations may affect activity	>2 times a month	FEV_1 or PEF ≥80% predicted PEF variability 20% to 30%
Step 1 Mild intermittent	Symptoms ≤2 times a week Asymptomatic and normal PEF between exacerbations Exacerbations brief (from a few hours to a few days); intensity may vary	≤2 times a month	FEV_1 or PEF ≥ 80% predicted PEF variability <20%

The presence of one of the features of severity is sufficient to place a patient in the category. An individual should be assigned to the most severe grade in which any feature occurs. The characteristics noted in this table are general and may overlap because asthma is highly variable. Furthermore, an individual's classification may change over time.

Patients at any level of severity can have mild, moderate, or severe exacerbations. Some patients with intermittent asthma experience severe and life-threatening exacerbations separated by long periods of normal lung function and no symptoms.

[1]Percent of person's best for peak expiratory flow (PEF) and percent predicted values for forced expiratory volume in 1 second (FEV_1).

Adapted from National Asthma Education and Prevention Program (NAEPP). Expert Panel Report II: Guidelines for the Diagnosis and Management of Asthma. Bethesda, Md: National Heart, Lung, and Blood Institute; 1997; and from National Asthma Education and Prevention Program (NAEPP). Expert Panel Report: Guidelines for the Diagnosis and Management of Asthma-Update on Selected Topics. Bethesda, Md: National Heart, Lung, and Blood Institute; 2002.

Table 9-2. Stepwise Approach for Managing Asthma in Adults and Children Age >5 Years

Asthma Classification	Daily, Long-Term Control Medications (preferred treatments are in bold)
Step 4 Severe persistent	• **High-dose inhaled corticosteroids <u>AND</u>** • **Long-acting inhaled β₂-agonists** <u>AND if needed,</u> • Corticosteroid tablets or syrup long-term (2 mg/kg/day, generally do not exceed 60 mg/day). (Make repeat attempts to reduce systemic corticosteroids and maintain control with high-dose inhaled corticosteroids.)
Step 3 Moderate persistent	• **Low-to-medium-dose inhaled corticosteroids <u>AND</u>** • **Long-acting inhaled β₂-agonists.** *ALTERNATIVE TREATMENT (listed alphabetically):* • Increase inhaled corticosteroids within medium-dose range <u>OR</u> • Low- to medium-dose inhaled corticosteroids and either leukotriene modifier or theophylline. IF NEEDED (particularly in patients with recurring severe exacerbations): • **Increase inhaled corticosteroids within medium-dose range and add long-acting inhaled β₂-agonists.** • Increase inhaled corticosteroids within medium-dose range and add either leukotriene modifier or theophylline.
Step 2 Mild Persistent	• **Low-dose inhaled corticosteroids.** *ALTERNATIVE TREATMENT (listed alphabetically):* • Cromolyn, leukotriene modifier, nedocromil, <u>OR</u> sustained release theophylline to serum concentration of 5 to 15 mcg/mL.
Step 1 Mild Intermittent	• **No daily medication needed.** • Severe exacerbations may occur, separated by long periods of normal lung function and no symptoms. A course of systemic corticosteroids is recommended.
Quick Relief All Patients	• Short-acting bronchodilator: 2 to 4 puffs short-acting inhaled β₂-agonists as needed for symptoms. • Intensity of treatment will depend on severity of exacerbation; up to 3 treatments at 20-minute intervals or a single nebulizer treatment as needed. Course of systemic corticosteroids may be needed. • Use of short-acting inhaled β₂-agonist >2 times a week in intermittent asthma (daily or increasing use in persistent asthma) may indicate the need to initiate (increase) long-term control therapy.

Step down: Review treatment every 1 to 6 months; a gradual stepwise reduction to treatment may be possible.

Step up: If control is not maintained, consider step up. First, review patient medication technique, adherence, and environmental control.

Adapted from National Asthma Education and Prevention Program (NAEPP). *Expert Panel Report II: Guidelines for the Diagnosis and Management of Asthma.* Bethesda, Md: National Heart, Lung, and Blood Institute, 1997; and from National Asthma Education and Prevention Program (NAEPP). E*xpert Panel Report: Guidelines for the Diagnosis and Management of Asthma—Update on Selected Topics.* Bethesda, Md: National Heart, Lung, and Blood Institute; 2002.

Figure 9-2. Examples of MDIs and DPIs (reprinted with permission from Houglum JE. The basics of asthma therapy for athletes. *Athletic Therapy Today.* 2001;6(5):18).

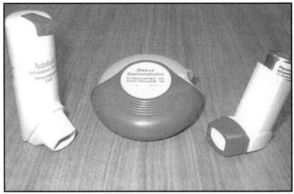

- Aspirin-induced asthma (AIA) occurs in 3% to 39% of patients with chronic asthma, depending on the subpopulation; the incidence increases with age and severity of chronic asthma. There is cross-hyperresponsiveness with the other NSAIDs so that patients who are sensitive to aspirin are likely to be sensitive to other NSAIDs. There is less cross-reaction with acetaminophen although as the dose increases above 650 mg, the likelihood of some cross-reaction increases. Even so, the symptoms of bronchoconstriction are typically milder with acetaminophen than with aspirin.
- Nocturnal asthma refers to symptoms of chronic asthma that interrupt sleep. Some patients experience more frequent occurrences of nocturnal asthma than others. The cause is unknown but may be due to varying exposure to some allergens due to changes in night-time ventilation, nighttime change in hormone levels, or other physiological changes such as gastroesophageal reflux.
- Atopic asthma occurs from immunoglobulin E (IgE)-mediated inflammatory response. *IgE* are antibodies located on the surface of mast cells in the airways. Patients with atopic reactions produce IgE as a result of exposure to common allergens such as cat dander, house-dust mites, cockroaches, fungal spores, and various pollens. When these antigens combine with the IgE, the mast cell releases chemical mediators such as LTs, PGs, and histamine. For many patients, atopic asthma is a significant component of the hyperresponsiveness associated with chronic asthma.

Inhalers and Spacers

Many asthma drugs are most effectively administered through inhalation because it quickly places the drug at the desired *site of action,* the lung. Because topical drug administration includes the mucous membranes, inhalation is considered topical application. Some pharmacokinetic parameters are eliminated by using inhalation, such as gastrointestinal absorption, the first pass effect, and systemic distribution to achieve the therapeutic effect.

The most common method for delivering asthma drugs by inhalation is by using a metered dose inhaler (MDI). The drug is in a pressurized container with a metering valve to control the amount of drug released during each use (Figure 9-2). A propellant is used to force the metered amount of drug from the inhaler each time the device is actuated. The drug exists as a solution or a suspended micronized powder in the inhaler, but is released from the inhaler as an aerosol for delivery into the patient's mouth. As the patient inhales deeply in a coordinated fashion with the actuation of the inhaler, the drug reaches the lung. Advantages of this method of drug delivery are that the drug is delivered more directly to the tissue, there are fewer systemic adverse effects, and a quicker response is obtained compared with the oral route.

Box 9-2. Summary of Advantages and Disadvantages of Metered Dose Inhalers

Advantages

- Some pharmacokinetic parameters are eliminated by using inhalation, such as gastrointestinal absorption, the first pass effect, and systemic distribution, to achieve the therapeutic effect.
- The drug is delivered more directly to the tissue.
- Fewer systemic adverse effects.
- Quicker response is obtained compared to the oral route.

Disadvantages

- Requires proper technique to be effective.
- Even with good technique <20% of the drug reaches the lung.
- Inconvenient as the MDI devices can be cumbersome and bothersome to use compared to taking oral medications.

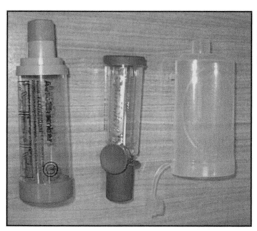

Figure 9-3. Examples of spacers (reprinted with permission from Houglum JE. The basics of asthma therapy for athletes. *Athletic Therapy Today.* 2001; 6(5):17).

Although there are advantages, there are also some disadvantages to the use of MDIs (Box 9-2). The primary concerns are that, even with good technique, generally <20% of the drug reaches the lung. Although this problem is somewhat accounted for in the canister dosage, inhalation technique can significantly vary the amount of drug reaching the lung. Proper technique requires the patient to follow a set of directions and requires a certain amount of skill to coordinate the activation of the MDI and the inhalation of the aerosol. Besides the potential for poor technique, another disadvantage of inhaler use is the inconvenience; carrying MDI devices can be somewhat cumbersome and using an inhaler is significantly bothersome for some patients compared to oral medications.

Spacers (Figure 9-3) can be used with the MDI to compensate for some of the disadvantages to inhaler use. Spacers are holding chambers that are attached to the MDI so that the drug is propelled into the spacer and thus travels through the spacer before being inhaled by the patient. This allows the patient an extra second or two before inhalation is necessary, making it easier for the patient to coordinate the activation of the inhaler with inhalation and thus improving the likelihood of better delivery of drug to the lung. It is primarily the smaller particles that have a chance of reaching the lung as they travel the furthest from the force of the propellant and are more readily carried into the lung during inhalation. Although some of the drug is exhaled, most of the remaining particles are the larger particles and, without the use of a spacer, they are deposited in the oropharynx. As the drug travels through the spacer, however, the particles of drug lose momentum so that fewer of the larger particles reach the patient's mouth. This provides a particular advantage when using inhaled corticosteroid, as the deposit of these drugs in the oropharynx contributes to hoarseness and oral candidiasis infections (thrush). These adverse effects can also be minimized by rinsing the mouth with water and spitting after use of inhaled corticosteroids.

The propellants used in MDIs have historically been chlorofluorocarbons (CFCs). These are the same type of gases that were used as refrigerants in air conditioners and refrigerators and now have been discontinued because of environmental policies. For the same reason, CFCs are being phased out in MDIs as non-CFC propellants (hydrofluoroalkanes) are developed. The new propellants must be approved by the Food and Drug Administration (FDA), as a change in propellant requires safety and efficacy studies. Patients being switched from CFC-propellant inhalers to hydrofluoroalkanes (HFAs) may require a dosage reduction as the HFAs generally deliver more drug to the lung. The spray of the HFA-delivery also feels less forceful.

Dry powder inhalers (DPIs) are also used for delivery of asthma medications to the lungs. Dry powder inhalers provide an alternative to the use of pressurized gases. As the patient inhales deeply, the process of inhalation through the inhaler draws the powdered drug into the lungs. The drug is contained in a capsule or other package form that the inhaler breaks open during use to allow the powder to be inhaled. The patient must be able to inhale deeply to provide enough suction to draw the drug into the lungs. Dry powder inhalers eliminate the need to coordinate inhalation with actuation of the propellant, which is a significant hindrance to adequate disease control in the elderly and very young patients, particularly. Dry powder inhalers cannot be used with a spacer, however.

A third type of inhaler is the breath-actuated MDI. The technique to operate this inhaler is somewhat of a cross between MDI and DPI; a propellant is used to expel the drug but it is not activated until the patient inhales. The breath-actuated MDI uses a lever to cock the mechanism, and the mechanism is released when the patient inhales through the mouthpiece. The breath-actuated MDI eliminates the need to coordinate the inhalation with actuation of the inhaler but, like DPIs, breath-actuated inhalers cannot be used with a spacer.

Regardless of the type of inhaler used, good technique is important to obtain adequate delivery of the drug to the lungs. The step-by-step procedure for good inhalation technique varies for MDIs compared with breath-actuated MDIs and DPIs. The procedure for use of typical MDIs is listed in Box 9-3.

Insufficient inhaler technique and poor compliance with prescribed therapy are common reasons for diminished therapeutic effectiveness and potentially diminished athletic performance and/or participation. Poor technique when using inhaled corticosteroids also leads to an increased incidence of hoarseness, cough, and oral fungal infection. Table 9-3 lists the trade names of some *MDI* and *DPI* devices; these are not trade names of the drugs but only the inhalation devices used to deliver the drugs.

Besides achieving appropriate technique, there are some other, but relatively minor, problems associated with inhaler use. For example, the nondrug components of inhaled suspensions can cause coughing. Inhalers and spacers must be kept clean to prevent accumulation of drug after repeated use. Moisture can cause problems for DPI by preventing the drug particles from flowing effectively, and cold temperatures can decrease the efficiency of the propellant gas in MDIs.

Nebulizers (Figure 9-4) are devices used to deliver drug to the lungs but these devices are larger than MDIs and DPIs. They are used primarily in hospitals and clinics, or in homes if the patient is unable to use inhalers. A few milliliters of liquid drug is placed in the nebulizer. An

Box 9-3. Procedure for Using a Typical Metered Dose Inhaler

Step	Action
1	Prepare the MDI according to directions on container (eg, suspensions must be shaken before use to obtain a consistent dose with each use).
2	Hold inhaler upright, tip head back slightly to facilitate flow of drug into the lungs.
3	Exhale slowly.
4	Place the inhaler (or spacer with inhaler attached) in mouth and seal lips securely around the mouthpiece of the inhaler (or spacer).
5	Press down on the inhaler to release the medication and at the same time take a slow, deep inhalation.
6	Hold the breath for about 10 seconds before exhaling.
7	If another puff is needed of a quick-relief inhaler, wait about 1 minute before taking the second puff. This will give time for the first puff to begin working and may improve the effectiveness of the second puff.
8	When using a corticosteroid, rinse mouth out with water.

Table 9-3. Inhaler Devices Used for Asthma Therapy

Inhaler Trade Name	Drug	Type	Comments
Autohaler	pirbuterol	MDI	Breath-actuated
Aerolizer	formoterol	DPI	Breath-actuated, single-dose capsule
Diskus	fluticasone and/ or salmeterol	DPI	Breath-actuated
Rotadisk	flutacasone	DPI	Breath-actuated
Rotahaler	albuterol	DPI	Breath-actuated, single-dose capsule
Turbuhaler	budesonide and/ or formoterol	DPI	Breath-actuated
Ventolin HFA	albuterol	MDI	Propellant contains HFAs, not CFCs

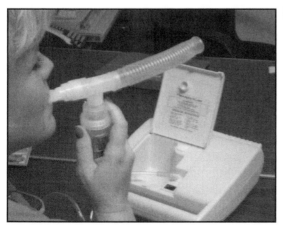

Figure 9-4. Example of a nebulizer.

Figure 9-5 Measurement of forced expiratory volume using a spirometer (reprinted with permission from Houglum JE. The basics of asthma therapy for athletes. *Athletic Therapy Today.* 2001;6(5):18).

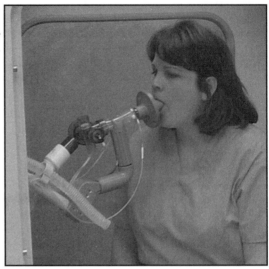

aerosol is created from the liquid by using either a stream of compressed air (jet nebulizer) or vibration (ultrasonic nebulizer) mechanism. The aerosol is inhaled by the patient by breathing normally through a mouthpiece during a 10- to 15- minute nebulizer treatment. Alternatively, the patient can breathe deeply and slowly with breath-holding to increase efficiency of drug delivery. Use of a face mask rather than a mouthpiece is less effective in delivering drug to the lungs because the nasal passage prevents some of the drug from reaching the lungs. The advantage of a nebulizer versus a MDI is that there is no actuation to coordinate with inhalation.

Pulmonary Function Tests

Pulmonary function tests provide a means of quantifying air flow to the lungs and thus are an objective measure of the severity of the asthma at the time of measurement (eg, during an acute exacerbation). Forced expiratory volume in 1 second (FEV_1) is one such test (Figure 9-5). The FEV_1 is determined using a forced expiratory *spirometer* and is a measure of the volume of air that can be exhaled in the first second after maximal inspiration. When compared with the normal values, the FEV_1 can be used to assess the severity of the asthma and, as indicated in Table 9-1, is one of the criteria used by NAEPP to classify asthma severity. The FEV_1 can be combined with other parameters, such as forced vital capacity (total volume of air that can be exhaled), as a means of diagnosis and monitoring of pulmonary disease.

The peak expiratory flow (PEF) is another pulmonary function test and is conducted using a *peak flow meter* (PFM). Peak expiratory flow is the maximum flow rate of forced expiration that the patient can achieve at that time. This is the most commonly used pulmonary function test by patients because PFMs are hand-held devices (Figure 9-6) that are easy to use and inexpensive. During a 2- to 3-week period when the patient's asthma is well-controlled, the patient's personal best PEF is determined so that subsequent values can be compared as a percentage of the personal best. Daily results from the PFM can be plotted to determine effectiveness of long-term therapy. The same PFM should be used each day for the most consistent results. If PEF decreases, it can be indicative of an imminent acute attack and the patient can make adjustments in therapy before the symptoms become prominent. The plan for adjusting therapy should be pre-established with the physician so that the patient knows what actions to take, particularly when

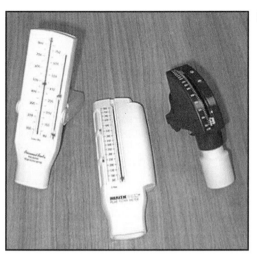

Figure 9-6. Examples of peak flow meters.

acute symptoms occur. For example, if the patient's personal best PEF is 600 and the patient begins to experience acute symptoms of bronchoconstriction, the patient uses the rescue medication as prescribed, checks PEF, and then takes the following actions as pre-established with the physician:

- If flow is >480 (>80% of personal best), maintain existing quick-relief therapy as directed by the physician and recheck PEF after each quick-relief dosage.
- If flow is 300 to 480 (50% to 80% of personal best), use additional rescue medication as predetermined and continue to monitor PEF until symptoms subside and PEF is at least 80% of personal best, and contact physician as soon as possible.
- If flow is <300 (<50% of personal best), use additional rescue medication immediately and go to the emergency room.

The exact plan of action may be different for each patient, but the point is that the patient should have a pre-established plan so that the PFM values can be used to appropriately adjust therapy. The athletic trainer must be aware of this plan. The NAEPP recommends patients with moderate or severe persistent asthma, or a history of severe acute exacerbations, have an action plan and consider using the PFM routinely to monitor the disease and the effectiveness of therapy.

Summary

Asthma is a chronic disease and it is an inflammatory disease. Consequently, for persistent asthma, treatment requires daily anti-inflammatory therapy to reduce the incidence of acute attacks and to decrease the long-term effects of chronic inflammation. Patients with chronic asthma are hyperresponsive to various allergens such as house dust-mites, cockroaches, pollen, animal dander, and cigarette smoke. The production and release of leukotrienes through the lipoxygenase pathway of arachidonic acid metabolism causes bronchoconstriction, mucus production, and edema, resulting in difficulty breathing, coughing, and wheezing. Most patients with chronic asthma also have exercise-induced bronchoconstriction, which can cause these symptoms during exercise and immediately following exercise, if not appropriately treated.

The severity of asthma is usually classified as mild intermittent, mild persistent, moderate persistent, and severe persistent based on the frequency of symptoms prior to treatment and the results of pulmonary function tests. One such test is the peak expiratory flow (PEF), which can be conveniently measured by the patient using a PFM. The use of a PFM can help patients with moderate and severe asthma monitor the severity of the asthma and determine the effectiveness of therapy.

Many asthma medications are administered as inhalants. MDIs are the most popular, but dry powder inhalers DPIs, and breath-actuated MDIs have become more readily available. Metered dose inhalers use a propellant to force the drug into the lung when the inhaler device is actuated. For adequate delivery of drug to the lungs, the use of an MDI necessitates a slow inhalation process at the same time the inhaler is actuated. The breath-actuated inhaler does not require the same degree of coordination as the metered dose is not released by the propellant until the patients inhales. The drug from DPI enters the lung as a result of the force of the inhalation and does not use a propellant. If proper technique is used, the MDI delivers sufficient drug to the lungs. If the patient cannot adequately coordinate slow inhalation with actuation, the DPI or breath-actuated MDI are alternatives. A problem with inhalers is that much of the drug is deposited in the back of the throat, which can contribute to increased incidence of hoarseness and thrush with inhalation corticosteroid use. Spacers can be used with MDIs to decrease the amount of drug deposited in the throat and increase the amount delivered to the lungs. Spacers are chambers into which an MDI is actuated so that the drug must travel through the chamber before it is inhaled. Larger particles of drug are not propelled far enough to make it out of the chamber so most of the drug that makes it into the airways is the smaller particles.

Poor compliance with therapy and improper inhalation technique are significant causes of poor therapeutic outcomes. The athletic trainer can assist the athlete in understanding the necessity for daily compliance with therapy and can provide instruction regarding proper inhalation technique to improve therapeutic outcomes.

Drugs to Treat Asthma

From a therapy standpoint, there are two main components of asthma to contend with: diminishing the chronic inflammation that is characteristic of the disease, and treating acute flare-ups that occur with varying frequency and severity among asthma patients. Drugs used to treat chronic asthma are referred to as long-term control medications, whereas drugs used to treat acute flare-ups are quick-relief or rescue medications. These two components of drug therapy are connected in the sense that patients with poorly controlled chronic asthma have a higher incidence of acute reactions and thus require more frequent use of quick-relief medication at higher doses.

From a pharmacological standpoint, there are two general categories of drugs that are used to treat the chronic and acute aspects of asthma: bronchodilators and anti-inflammatory medications. In each general category, there are also subcategories of drugs based on the pharmacological mechanism of action. Table 9-4 depicts this categorization and groups of drugs in each category that are discussed in this chapter. The bronchodilators act on the bronchial smooth muscle to cause it to relax, thus causing a larger airway opening. Anti-inflammatory drugs may act by several mechanisms but one prime focus is to inhibit the effects of the leukotrienes and other inflammatory chemical mediators.

Quick-Relief Drugs

The purpose of these drugs is to treat an existing acute attack (ie, "rescue therapy") or to prevent an imminent attack, such as prior to exercise. Consequently, these drugs are not taken on a routine daily schedule but rather on an as needed basis (ie, prn). The two types of quick-relief

Table 9-4. Categorization of Asthma Medications

By Therapeutic Use

Quick-relief therapy:
- Short-acting ß$_2$-agonists by inhalation
- Systemic corticosteroid by oral or parenteral
- Anticholinergics by inhalation

Long-term therapy:
- Corticosteroids by inhalation
- Long-acting ß$_2$-agonists by inhalation
- Leukotriene modifiers by oral
- Mast cell stabilizers by inhalation
- Methylxanthines by oral

By Pharmacological Activity

Bronchodilator drugs:
- Short-acting ß$_2$-agonists by oral or inhalation
- Long-acting ß$_2$-agonists by inhalation
- Anticholinergics by inhalation
- Methylxanthines by oral

Anti-inflammatory drugs:
- Corticosteroids by systemic or inhalation
- Leukotriene modifiers by oral
- Mast cell stabilizers by inhalation

drugs are the systemic corticosteroids and the bronchodilators, which include the *β$_2$-agonists* and *anticholinergic* drugs. According to NAEPP, every asthma patient should have a quick-relief inhalation β$_2$-agonist readily available.

β$_2$-Agonists

The most effective drugs for treatment of an acute asthma attack are the short-acting β$_2$-agonists administered by inhalation. Short-acting refers to the duration of action, but these drugs also have a short *onset of action.* There are long-acting (longer duration of action) bronchodilators available, but they should not be used for quick-relief therapy because they have a slower onset of action. Long-acting β$_2$-agonists are discussed in the section on drugs used for long-term control. The predominant *adrenergic* receptor in the bronchial smooth muscle is the β2-*receptor*. Other tissues such as skeletal muscle and liver also have β$_2$-receptors, whereas the heart and kidney have β$_1$-*receptors*. Agonists that combine with β$_2$-receptors cause bronchodilation in the lung, contraction (tremor) of skeletal muscle, and *glycogenolysis* and *gluconeogenesis* in the liver, which causes increased blood glucose. An advantage of using β$_2$-agonists by inhalation is that, not only does the drug reach the site of action quickly, but the principle adverse effects of β$_2$-agonists (ie, muscle tremor and hyperglycemia) are minimized. Regardless, however, muscle tremor tends to diminish with continued use, and hyperglycemia is very transient as the pancreas releases more insulin to compensate, although the diabetic may require an adjustment in insulin dosage.

The adrenergic receptor-type of prime importance in the heart muscle and kidney is the β$_1$-receptor. Activation of these receptors causes tachycardia and elevated blood pressure due to increased renin release by the kidney. Although the β$_2$-*agonists* are selective for the β$_2$-*receptor*, this selectivity is not absolute and some β$_1$-activity is possible, especially as the dose of the β$_2$-agonist increases. Consequently, β$_2$-agonists can exert some β$_1$-activity, causing elevated heart rate and blood pressure, but these too are minimized by using inhalation rather than oral β$_2$-agonists. Because there are several selective β$_2$-agonists that are effective bronchodilators for asthma treatment, there is no therapeutic rationale for using nonselective β-agonists (eg, isoproterenol, metaproterenol, epinephrine) as they will readily combine with β$_1$-receptors to cause a greater likelihood for adverse effects.

Table 9-5. Adult Dosages of Selected Quick-Relief Medications

Generic Name	Trade Name	Category	Dosage Form; Typical Adult Dosage
albuterol	Ventolin	ß₂-agonist, SA	MDI; 2 puffs (90 µg each) 3 to 4 times/day prn
ipratropium	Atrovent	anticholinergic	MDI; 2 to 3 puffs (18 µg each) 4 times/day
metaproterenol	Alupent	ß₂-agonist, SA	MDI; 2 to 3 puffs (650 µg each) 4 to 6 times/day prn
methylprednis-olone	Medrol	corticosteroid	oral; 40 to 60 mg/day for 3 to 10 days
pirbuterol	Maxair	ß₂-agonist, SA	MDI; 2 puffs (200 µg each) 3 to 4 times/day
prednisolone	Prednisolone	corticosteroid	oral; 40 to 60 mg/day for 3 to 10 days
prednisone	Prednisone	corticosteroid	oral; 40 to 60 mg/day for 3 to 10 days

SA = short-acting; prn = as needed for relief

There has been some controversy as to whether frequent, daily use of β_2-agonists decreases the bronchodilator effectiveness of these drugs. Daily use of long-acting β_2-agonists may somewhat diminish their *duration of action*, but not enough to negate the advantages of the bronchodilator effect. Regarding short-acting β_2-agonists, there is no therapeutic advantage to using them on a scheduled, daily basis.

Short-acting β_2-agonists are the drugs of choice for treatment of acute attacks (rescue therapy) on an as needed basis. When these drugs are used by inhalation, onset of action occurs within 5 minutes. Duration of action varies considerably but typically is 2 to 6 hours, with somewhat shorter duration being more likely if the drug is used for protection during exercise. These drugs react directly with bronchial smooth muscle to cause bronchodilation, regardless of the cause of the bronchial constriction. The usual dose is 1 to 2 puffs as needed for relief, preferably with about 1 minute between the puffs. This time between puffs allows for some bronchial dilation to occur from the first puff and may enhance the effectiveness from the second puff. To prevent exercise-induced bronchospasms (EIB), 1 to 2 puffs 5 to 15 minutes prior to exercise should offer sufficient protection for 2 to 4 hours. Administration of β_2-agonists by inhalation can be repeated during exercise *but the routine use of these additional doses during exercise is indicative of poor control of chronic asthma and thus long-term therapy (see below) should be reevaluated.*

The β_2-agonists are equally effective in producing bronchodilation at their respective therapeutic doses; the main difference is the duration of action. Typical adult dosages for β_2-agonists are shown in Table 9-5. A disadvantage of DPIs compared with MDIs is that some patients with an acute severe asthma attack may not be able to inhale with enough force to draw the drug into the lung.

Anticholinergics

Anticholinergic drugs are less effective than β_2-agonists for quick relief of acute attacks. Rather than stimulating β-*adrenergic* receptors for bronchodilation, anticholinergic drugs inhibit *cholinergic receptors* of the *parasympathetic* nervous system to cause bronchodilation. Anticholinergics are most effective in patients whose symptoms are due to excessive cholinergic stimulation. It is, however, not possible to identify these patients prior to treatment.

Although there are many anticholinergic drugs, most are older drugs (eg, atropine) that have too many adverse effects. A newer drug, ipratropium (Atrovent), is the only anticholinergic currently used to treat asthma. Although not free from adverse effects, ipratropium by inhalation has fewer adverse effects (eg, dry mouth, throat irritation, bad taste) but should not be used by patients who are allergic to peanuts.

> *Recall from Chapter 8 that anticholinergic drugs typically cause several adverse effects such as urinary retention, blurred vision, sedation, and constipation.*

Significant therapeutic effects occur within 5 minutes after inhalation of ipratropium, and additive effects are obtained when combined with β_2-agonists; consequently, ipratropium plus albuterol (Combivent) is available as a combination inhalation product. Ipratropium is used as a component of therapy to treat acute asthma, either by MDI or nebulizer, but is not included in NAEPP guidelines for long-term therapy of chronic asthma and has limited effectiveness to prevent EIB.

Systemic Corticosteroids

Systemic corticosteroids are used orally or by the parenteral routes to treat severe symptoms associated with an acute exacerbation (Table 9-5). The mechanism for these drugs is discussed later in this chapter, but in short, they inhibit the inflammatory response. A short course of therapy (3 to 10 days) is useful when short-acting β_2-agonists alone are not sufficient. Significant adverse effects are minimized with these short bursts of therapy. Some patients may experience mood changes and diabetics may observe a loss of glucose control. Significant adrenal suppression rarely occurs and thus discontinuation of the short therapy can be abrupt.

In situations where the acute exacerbations last longer and the use of systemic corticosteroids is continued, a tapering of the corticosteroid dose may be necessary.

> *Recall from Chapter 6 that adrenal suppression can occur as a result of extended systemic therapy with corticosteroids. This relatively constant exposure to the corticosteroids can cause the adrenal gland to decrease production of corticosteroid (ie, adrenal insufficiency) that may last for weeks to months after the corticosteroid drug has been discontinued. The extent of adrenal insufficiency depends on the daily dosage and the duration of corticosteroid therapy. The symptoms of adrenal insufficiency range from mild (nausea) to life-threatening. To avoid these symptoms after extended corticosteroid therapy, the dosage should be tapered according to established protocols. Abrupt withdrawal of extended corticosteroid therapy may also cause an exacerbation of the disease being treated.*

Long-Term Therapy

The purpose of long-term therapy is to reduce the incidence of acute exacerbations of the disease. Several categories of drugs are available for this purpose: corticosteroids, mast cell stabilizing drugs, leukotriene modifiers, methylxanthines, and long-acting β_2-agonists. All of these drugs except the long-acting β_2-agonists function principally by inhibiting the inflammatory process.

Inhalation Corticosteroids

Corticosteroids by inhalation are the mainstay of long-term therapy. They do not significantly affect acute bronchoconstriction, but when used on a daily regimen are very effective at reducing inflammation. This subsequently reduces the frequency and severity of acute attacks, improves control of nocturnal asthma, and provides protection from symptoms of EIB. Pharmacologically, corticosteroids are anti-inflammatory drugs with multiple mechanisms of action. Corticosteroids inhibit infiltration of leukocytes, inhibit the synthesis of *cytokines*, and increase the response of the β-*receptor* to β-*agonist* stimulation. In addition, a mechanism of

Table 9-6. Adult Dosages of Selected Long-Term Control Medications

Generic Name	Trade Name	Category	Dosage Form; Typical Adult Dosage
albuterol	Proventil Repetabs	ß$_2$-agonist, LA	Oral extended release; 4 mg every 12 hours
beclomethasone	Vanceril	Corticosteroid	MDI; 2 puffs (42 to 84 µg each) 3 to 4 times/day
budesonide	Pulmicort Turbuhaler	Corticosteroid	DPI; 1 to 2 inhalations (200 µg each) 2 times/day
cromolyn	Intal	Cell stabilizer	MDI; 2 to 4 puffs (800 µg each) 4 times/day
flunisolide	AeroBid	Corticosteroid	MDI; 2 puffs (250 µg each) 2 times/day
fluticasone	Flovent	Corticosteroid	MDI; 2 puffs (110 µg each) 2 times/day
fluticasone	Flovent Rotadisk	Corticosteroid	DPI; 2 inhalation (100 µg each) 2 times/day
fluticasone + salmeterol	Advair Diskus	Corticosteroid + ß$_2$-agonist, LA	DPI; 1 inhalation (250/50 µg, respectively 2 times/day
formoterol	Foradil	ß$_2$-agonist, LA	DPI; 1 inhalation (12 µg each) every 12 hours
montelukast	Singulair	Antileukotriene	Oral tablets; 10 mg once/day
nedocromil	Tilade	Cell stabilizer	MDI; 2 to 4 puffs (1.75 mg each) 4 times/day
salmeterol	Serevent	ß$_2$-agonist, LA	MDI; 2 puffs (21 µg each) every 12 hours
salmeterol	Serevent Diskus	ß$_2$-agonist, LA	DPI; 1 inhalation (50 µg) every 12 hours
theophylline	Theo-Dur	Methylxanthine	Oral extended release; 300 mg 2 times/day
triamcinolone	Azmacort	Corticosteroid	MDI; 2 puffs (100 µg each) 3 to 4 times/day
zafirlukast	Accolate	Antileukotriene	Oral tablets; 20 mg 2 times/day
zileuton	Zyflo	Antileukotriene	Oral tablets; 600 mg 4 times/day

LA = long-acting

prime focus is the inhibition of leukotriene production by inhibiting phospholipase (see Figure 9-1).

Table 9-6 includes several corticosteroids used by inhalation for long-term asthma therapy. These drugs have approximately equal effectiveness at equipotent doses, although the duration of action differs so that some corticosteroids (eg, budesonide and fluticasone) require fewer doses per day. One reason for poor adherence to therapy is the cumbersome nature of taking many doses per day of the corticosteroid. A product that requires fewer doses per day is therefore generally considered an advantage. According to NAEPP, inhalation corticosteroid is the recommended therapy for patients of all ages with persistent asthma. The dosage of corticosteroid is increased with increased asthma severity. Unlike quick-relief medications, which are used as needed, corticosteroids and other long-term medications must be taken on a regular daily schedule and may require up to 3 months of daily therapy before the maximum benefit with continued therapy is achieved.

The potential adverse effects with inhaled corticosteroids can be categorized as local and systemic effects. Although inhalation delivers sufficient drug to the lung for the therapeutic effect, most of the inhaled dose ends up in the oral cavity. The amount of corticosteroid that is deposited in the mouth and throat plays the major role in causing the local effects. These are primarily hoarseness, cough, and oral fungal (candidiasis) infection (thrush). The cough is likely due to additives in the MDI and may be reduced by using a DPI. The hoarseness and fungal infections are indicative of the amount of drug deposited in the mouth and throat. These effects can be minimized by using a spacer and by rinsing the mouth out with water after each use.

The systemic effects of inhaled corticosteroids are caused by the portion of the dose that is swallowed and the amount of drug that is absorbed into the blood from the lung. The systemic effects are minimized at lower dosages of inhaled corticosteroid use. The systemic effects of prime concern include growth suppression in children, decreased bone mineral density (BMD), and increased risk of cataracts. Although low to medium doses of inhaled corticosteroids may cause a small change in growth rate, the final adult height is generally unaffected. In other words, the growth suppression from corticosteroid inhalation therapy typically affects growth velocity rather than final adult height. Nonetheless, the potential long-term significance of the systemic effects must be evaluated in comparison to the long-term benefit of acceptable control of chronic asthma. When high-dose inhaled corticosteroid therapy is warranted in children, other long-term therapy should be used in conjunction with inhalation corticosteroids so that the inhaled corticosteroid dose can be reduced.

Regarding BMD, there is no significant effect of low to medium doses of inhaled corticosteroids on BMD in children. Some reduction in BMD correlating with dose of inhaled corticosteroid may occur in women, although the correlation with increased risk of bone fractures has not been established. Low to medium doses of inhaled corticosteroids do not increase the incidence of cataracts in children, although high cumulative lifetime doses may increase the incidence of cataracts in adults.

Long-Acting β-Agonists

As with the short-acting β_2-agonists, the long-acting β_2-agonists (see Table 9-6) are effective by inhalation, cause bronchodilation, and lack significant anti-inflammatory activity. Their onset of action, however, is slower than short-acting agonists and thus they cannot be used for rescue therapy. Another means of obtaining a longer-acting β-agonist effect is to use extended release oral tablets of short-acting β-agonists. The oral products are more convenient for the patient than inhalants but have the disadvantage of having more significant systemic adverse effects, including tachycardia and muscle tremors. Although more cumbersome to administer, inhalation long-acting β_2-agonists provide more direct contact with the target tissue and fewer adverse effects than oral β-agonists and therefore are used much more frequently.

Inhalation long-acting β_2-agonists can be administered as often as every 12 hours. They can be added to therapy as an alternative to increasing corticosteroid dosage; however, it may be too cumbersome and inconvenient for some patients to add a third inhaler to the corticosteroid and quick-relief medications. As an alternative, a fixed dose combination is available (Advair) that contains a corticosteroid (fluticasone) and long-acting β_2-agonist (salmeterol); this provides the convenience of one inhaler to simultaneously administer both drugs. Long-acting β_2-agonists are effective in reducing the use of short-acting β_2-agonists, decreasing nocturnal asthma, and improving protection from EIB. When using a long-acting β_2-agonist to prevent EIB, formoterol (Foradil) should be used at least 15 minutes prior to exercise, or salmeterol (Serevent) 30 to 60 minutes before exercise, and then not again for at least 12 hours. The long-acting β_2-agonist should not be used more frequently than twice per 24 hours; therefore, if the drug is being used twice a day as long-term therapy, it should not be used as an additional dose prior to exercise.

Mast Cell Stabilizing Drugs

Mast cell stabilizing drugs are inhibitors of the inflammatory process but are less effective than corticosteroids. Cromolyn (Intal) and nedocromil (Tilade) are the two mast cell stabilizing drugs currently available (see Table 9-6). These two are equally effective but only by inhalation. They are not effective as rescue therapy to treat acute attacks because they take 1 to 2 weeks to show noticeable improvement of chronic asthma, take about 4 weeks to achieve maximal effect, and do not produce bronchodilation. These drugs have a low incidence of long-term adverse effects and are virtually nontoxic. They are not preferred therapy but may provide an alternative to inhalation corticosteroids in children with mild persistent asthma, or be added to corticosteroid therapy to improve control of mild persistent asthma. Nedocromil can be used in children older than 5; cromolyn for all ages. Mast cell stabilizing drugs are effective to treat allergen-induced hyperresponsiveness and nocturnal asthma. They can also be used about 15 minutes prior to exercise to prevent EIB either alone or in combination with β_2-agonists when the use of a β_2-agonist alone is insufficient to prevent EIB.

As with the corticosteroids, there may be multiple mechanisms of action for mast cell stabilizing drugs, but a likely contributor to the mechanism is the ability of these drugs to inhibit the release of inflammatory mediators from bronchial mast cells. A stabilizing effect on the cell membrane prevents the release from the cell of inflammatory chemical mediators such as *leukotrienes, prostaglandins,* and *cytokines.*

Cromolyn and nedocromil are generally used 2 to 4 times per day. Very little drug is absorbed systemically so systemic adverse reactions are uncommon. Local adverse effects include minor throat irritation, which can be minimized by drinking water immediately after use, and a bad taste and headache associated with the use of nedocromil for some patients.

Leukotriene Modifiers

The leukotrienes are a group of chemical mediators principally produced during inflammation through the 5-lipoxygenase pathway from arachidonic acid (see Figure 9-1). LTC_4, LTD_4, LTE_4 are collectively referred to as the cysteinyl leukotrienes (cys-LTs) because cysteine is part of the chemical structure. The cys-LTs are synthesized from LTA_4 and are agonists for the cys-LT receptor, activation of which initiates bronchoconstriction. Another leukotriene, LTB_4, is also synthesized from LTA_4, contributes to the inflammatory response as a chemotactic mediator, but is not a cys-LT and thus does not combine with the cys-LT receptor.

The leukotriene modifiers (also called antileukotrienes) are subdivided according to which of two mechanisms define their activity. Leukotriene-receptor antagonists combine directly with the cys-LT receptor to inhibit the effect of the cys-LTs; montelukast (Singulair) and zafirlukast (Accolate) are leukotriene-receptor antagonists. Leukotriene-synthesis inhibitors are competitive inhibitors of 5-lipoxygenase and thus decrease the production of all the LTs; zileuton (Zyflo) is a LT-synthesis inhibitor.

The leukotriene modifiers are among the newest asthma medications. They are used orally, not by inhalation, and are for long-term therapy, not for quick relief. As evident from their mechanism, leukotriene modifiers are anti-inflammatory drugs, not bronchodilators. They improve lung function, decrease the incidence of asthma exacerbations, and decrease the frequency of need for rescue medication. However, leukotriene modifiers are generally considered less effective than inhaled corticosteroids. The NAEPP includes antileukotrienes as an alternative to therapy for some patients with mild persistent asthma. They may also be useful with corticosteroids to allow for a reduction in corticosteroid dose. Although not preferred, they provide an oral alternative in patients unable to use inhalation therapy, such as young children. The leukotriene modifiers may reduce bronchoconstriction after exercise but they should not be used as the only therapy for EIB; pretreatment with a β_2-agonist should be maintained.

A peculiarity with the use of leukotriene modifiers is that some patients are responders and some are not. The reason for this difference among patients is unclear but the extent to which the LTs contribute to the asthma symptoms may differ from patient to patient. For those patients in whom these arachidonic acid metabolites contribute significantly to the asthma response, leukotriene modifying drugs will have a larger impact. The contribution of the pathway may be a result of the extent to which the genes are expressed for the enzymes in the lipoxygenase pathway. In general, it appears that patients who experience aspirin-induced asthma also respond well to leukotriene modifier therapy.

The leukotrienes modifiers have relatively few adverse effects, although headache is one of the more common complaints. The most significant concern is the potential for liver damage with zileuton. An elevated blood level of liver enzymes, particularly alanine aminotransferase (ALT), is indicative of liver damage. Consequently, treatment with zileuton requires monitoring of liver function by measuring blood ALT levels each month for the first 3 months and then routinely but less frequently thereafter. Patients on zileuton or zafirlukast should be

> *Recall that ALT is a liver enzyme that is released into the blood when liver cells are damaged. Therefore, an increase in the blood ALT level implies liver damage.*

aware that the symptoms of liver toxicity include jaundice, fatigue, right upper-quadrant abdominal pain, nausea, lethargy, pruritus, and flu-like symptoms. The patient should discontinue the drug and contact the physician if these symptoms occur.

The incidence of *Churg-Strauss syndrome* is rare but has been noted with the use of leukotriene-receptor antagonist. This syndrome involves *vasculitis* that primarily affects the respiratory tract during its early stages and can progress to become life threatening. Most reported cases involved patients who had been receiving systemic corticosteroid therapy that was reduced after leukotriene-receptor antagonist therapy was added. This association with the reduced corticosteroid therapy suggests that the syndrome may have existed prior to antileukotriene therapy but was being masked by the anti-inflammatory effect of corticosteroids.

Zileuton (Zyflo) inhibits 5-lipoxygenase and thus reduces the production of all of the leukotrienes. It is approved for use as long-term therapy in adults and children over 12 years old. Zileuton is rapidly absorbed after oral administration regardless of the presence of food. Because of its relatively short half life (2 to 3 hours), the usual zileuton dosage is four times per day. As mentioned previously, ALT levels must be monitored throughout treatment, but particularly during the first 3 months of therapy. Zileuton is metabolized by *cytochrome P450 isozymes* and inhibits the metabolism of other drugs, notably theophylline and *warfarin*, which are also metabolized by the same isozymes.

> *Recall from Chapters 2 and 3 that drug metabolism by cytochrome P450 (CYP450) isozymes is quite common and that drug interactions involving these isozymes occur when one drug inhibits the metabolism of other drugs. In this case, zileuton, warfarin, and theophylline are metabolized by the same CYP450 isozyme. Zileuton inhibits the metabolism of theophylline and warfarin and therefore will increase the effect of the theophylline and warfarin, which may necessitate a reduction in the dosage of these two drugs.*

The relatively short duration of action, the necessity to monitor for liver toxicity, and the potential for drug interaction are significant disadvantages of zileuton.

Zafirlukast (Accolate) is effective as a long-term antiasthma medication for adults and children as young as 7 years old. It is absorbed from the gastrointestinal tract but the absorption is reduced significantly by the presence of food. To optimize absorption, zafirlukast should be taken 1 hour prior to or 2 hours after meals. Zafirlukast can also increase the effect of warfarin and may necessitate a reduction in warfarin dosage. Liver toxicity is a potential adverse effect. The half-life is longer than zileuton and requires only twice daily dosing.

Montelukast (Singulair) is an effective leukotriene-receptor antagonist. The absorption from the gastrointestinal tract is not affected by food. It is available as a chewable tablet and is approved for use in children as young as 2 years old. Montelukast has several differences compared with zileuton and zafirlukast—it does not have significant potential for drug interactions with theophylline and warfarin, liver toxicity has not been reported, and the dosing schedule is once per day.

Methylxanthines

The only methylxanthine used therapeutically to treat asthma is theophylline. Other methylxanthines of some notoriety are caffeine, and to a lesser extent, theobromine (a component of chocolate), which are best known for their central nervous system stimulant effects. Of the methylxanthines, theophylline has the most significant bronchodilator activity. There are likely multiple mechanisms that contribute to this activity. Two of these are the inhibition of *adenosine* receptors and the inhibition of *phosphodiesterases*.

Theophylline used to be a primary therapy for treatment of chronic asthma. It has significant drawbacks, however, that have caused it to be used much less frequently as other more effective asthma medications have become available (ie, corticosteroids, leukotriene modifiers, mast cell stabilizing agents, and β_2-agonists). One disadvantage of theophylline is the significant toxicity that necessitates blood level monitoring to maintain the blood concentration of theophylline within a relatively narrow *therapeutic window* (see Chapter 3). Another disadvantage is the moderate degree of therapeutic effectiveness compared with newer drugs. Theophylline decreases the incidence of acute attacks, including nocturnal asthma, prevents EIB, and is an alternative to corticosteroid therapy for children. Nonetheless, one or more of the newer drugs provide these same benefits with less concern for toxicity.

Adenosine is a compound that indirectly causes bronchoconstriction, possibly by enhancing the effect of inflammatory chemical mediators. Phosphodiesterases are enzymes that terminate the activity of the cyclic AMP (adenosine monophosphate) and cyclic GMP (guanosine monophosphate); inhibition of phosphodiesterases therefore enhances the activity of the cyclic AMP and GMP. Cyclic AMP and cyclic GMP are second messenger molecules inside the cell that initiate many regulatory processes of the cell, including contraction and relaxation of smooth muscle.

Theophylline is used orally and is available in immediate and sustained release formulations, but considerable interpatient variability in absorption exists among patients taking the sustained release formulations. Dosage is calculated on a mg/kg/day basis. Initial adverse effects include nausea, vomiting, nervousness, and insomnia, but these effects usually dissipate with continued use. Theophylline has a low therapeutic index; blood concentrations modestly above the normal therapeutic range have resulted in seizures, arrhythmias, and death. At the other end of the therapeutic window, levels below the normal range result in significantly reduced effectiveness, hence the need to adjust dosage based on routine monitoring of blood levels. Adding to the problem are the changes in the pharmacokinetics due to factors such as cigarette smoking, changes in kidney function from disease or age, and drug interactions.

Summary

Drug therapy for chronic asthma can be grouped broadly as drugs for quick relief and drugs for long-term therapy. Quick-relief drugs are used to treat existing acute attacks or to prevent exercise-induced attacks. Long-term therapy is used to decrease symptoms of chronic asthma, including the incidence of acute exacerbations of the disease. With the exception of corticosteroids, drugs that are used for long-term therapy are not used for quick relief and vice versa. Even in the case of corticosteroids, it is inhalation therapy that is the mainstay of long-term therapy, whereas a short course of systemic therapy is the primary mode of administration to treat acute exacerbations.

For quick relief, inhaled β_2-agonists, such as albuterol (Ventolin), are the most frequently used. These drugs have few adverse effects when used by inhalation and have an almost immediate onset of action. Systemic corticosteroids can be used for a few days to reduce the duration and severity of an acute exacerbation but do not provide the immediate bronchodilation effect obtained from β_2-agonists. When used several minutes prior to exercise, β_2-agonists are also effective in preventing EIB. Although administration of β_2-agonists by inhalation can be repeated during exercise, *the routine use of these additional doses during exercise is indicative of poor control of chronic asthma and warrants a reevaluation of long-term therapy.*

Long-term therapy is effective when used on a regular, daily basis and is not effective in treating an acute attack. The intent of long-term therapy is to reduce the incidence of acute attacks, including symptoms associated with nocturnal asthma and EIB. Improved control of chronic asthma is reflected in the reduced frequency with which quick-relief medication is needed. Besides the inhaled corticosteroids, other long-term medications include the inhaled mast cell stabilizing drugs, inhaled long-acting β_2-agonists, and oral leukotriene modifiers. Theophylline is also available orally but is used less frequently than the other agents because of the greater potential for significant adverse effects. Every patient with persistent asthma (mild to severe) should be using a long-term control asthma medication. Corticosteroids are the drugs of choice for all ages, although a leukotriene modifier or mast cell stabilizing drug are alternatives used for mild persistent asthma. As the severity of asthma increases, either the dose of corticosteroid is increased and/or another long-acting drug is added to therapy. Leukotrienes, mast cell stabilizing drugs, and long-acting β_2-agonists also help prevent the symptoms associated with EIB.

ROLE OF THE ATHLETIC TRAINER

Because asthma is a chronic disease, drug therapy is long-term and so is the need to monitor the effectiveness of drug therapy. Most asthmatics have EIB, which may hamper athletic performance if it is not adequately controlled. Because the most frequent causes of inadequate therapeutic outcomes are poor compliance with prescribed therapy and/or improper use of inhalers, spacers, or peak flow meters, the athletic trainer can play a key role in ensuring that drug therapy is optimized. The two principle areas for involvement by the athletic trainer are patient education and monitoring of asthma drug use and effectiveness. Some noteworthy points regarding therapy are:

- If the athlete does not know which medication is for long-term use and which is for quick-relief, it raises doubt as to whether the athlete is using the medications properly. Because the quick-relief β_2-agonists and the long-term corticosteroid therapy are both used by inhalation, the athlete could be confused concerning their relative use. However, as the functions of these two drugs and the dosing schedule for each are vastly different, a clear understanding of the proper use of the drugs is imperative to achieve suitable results. For example, the athlete should understand that the long-term medication provides no protective benefit if used immediately prior to exercise. Similarly, use of the long-term medication, such as inhalation corticosteroid, is much less effective if used sporadically. It is important to use the corticosteroid daily, even when there are no asthma symptoms. Doses are not to be skipped just because the athlete "feels better." Based on data from other patient populations, it is reasonable to expect that if athletes understand the proper use and purpose of the asthma medications, they will have improved compliance and enhanced effectiveness from the asthma therapy.

- Besides understanding the purpose of each drug, proper inhalation technique impacts the effectiveness of these drugs. Even with good technique, only about 20% of inhaled drug reaches the lung. Besides having good overall inhalation technique as described earlier in this chapter (see Box 9-3), other aspects of proper technique to watch for include:
  a. The athlete should have good coordination of inhaler actuation with inhalation. If not, either additional instruction and/or a spacer may be useful.
  b. If the athlete bends over to discretely take a puff of quick-relief medication, the amount of drug delivered to the lungs will be reduced. This may be the reason for additional puffs being required during exercise.
  c. To decrease the incidence of fungal infection, the athlete can decrease the deposit of corticosteroid in the mouth and throat through the use of a spacer and by rinsing the mouth out with water after inhalation of each corticosteroid dose.
  d. If a portion of the drug or propellant mist does not enter the mouth the athlete is likely not placing the inhaler properly in the mouth, possibly the teeth are partially blocking the flow of drug.

- If the athlete uses more than one 200-puff canister of quick-relief medication per month, asthma control is generally considered to be poor and re-evaluation of long-term therapy is likely necessary. Other criteria have been recommended by the NAEPP to classify the severity of asthma (see Table 9-1) and to use as a guide to the stepwise approach for managing asthma (see Table 9-2). Treatment should be aggressive enough to gain control of the symptoms, and then the athlete can be monitored and drug therapy gradually reduced to the least medication necessary to maintain control of the symptoms.

- The use of a quick-relief medication 5 to 15 minutes prior to exercise is an effective means to control EIB. If symptoms develop during exercise, additional puffs can be used. However, regular additional doses of quick-relief medication during exercise may be because the chronic asthma is inadequately controlled. A reassessment of long-term control therapy is recommended. The goal is to achieve a level of asthma management so that the disease has no impact on the athlete's performance. To that end, it may be necessary to increase the inhalation corticosteroid dosage or add a long-acting β_2-agonist, a leukotriene modifier, or mast cell stabilizer. The athletic trainer must be aware of the action plan and should notify the physician who will modify the treatment.

- If an athlete has AIA, the athletic trainer should be alert to the fact that there are many OTC medications that contain NSAIDs. Consequently, symptoms from AIA may occur if the athlete is self-medicating, or if NSAID-containing medications are used in the athletic training room. While looking for an OTC analgesic, the athlete may not realize that not only do brand name products such as Advil and Motrin contain ibuprofen, but so do others such as Ultraprin and Valprin. A similar problem exists with aspirin. Additionally, some cold and sinus remedies also contain NSAIDs (eg, Dristan Sinus, BC Sinus-Cold, and Advil Cold & Sinus). Although not considered a NSAID, acetaminophen does cause some degree of cross-reaction in asthmatics with AIA. About one third of asthmatics with AIA experience some degree of bronchoconstriction when treated with 1000 to 1500 mg of acetaminophen, although the symptoms are generally milder than with aspirin. Also, doses of <650 mg of acetaminophen result in only a small risk of bronchospasm. The ingredients of OTC products should be checked carefully for the amount of acetaminophen or content of any amount of NSAIDs.

- The athlete should avoid the factors that initiate symptoms. The precipitating factors vary among asthmatics but potential factors include allergens from pets, house-dust mites, fungal spores, viral infection, tobacco smoke, pollens, volatile chemicals, and physiological conditions such as chronic sinusitis and gastroesophageal reflux. Avoiding causative agents may improve the level of control of chronic asthma and reduce acute exacerbations. For example, depending on the causative agent, the athlete could exercise in an indoor, air-conditioned facility rather than outdoors during peak pollen season, require family members that smoke to do so outdoors, avoid contact with cats or dogs, or obtain appropriate treatment for contributing physiological conditions.

- Use of a PFM can be helpful for athletes who have moderate or severe persistent asthma. Use of a PFM provides a means of determining current status of airflow, anticipating the need for change in quick-relief medication, evaluating the improvement of airflow as a result of therapy, and making a decision as to course of action if airflow is reduced. To obtain the most effective use of a PFM, it is necessary to use it routinely, first to establish the athlete's personal best and then to monitor airflow as a percentage relative to the personal best. Results from a PFM provide a quantitative value as to the extent of airflow obstruction. A plan should be established with the physician, especially for athletes with moderate to severe asthma or a history of severe exacerbations. The athlete and athletic trainer should know what adjustments must be made if airflow drops below predetermined levels.

- Knowing when, where, and how to exercise can help reduce symptoms of asthma. For example:
  a. Athletes who are hyperresponsive to pollen should avoid outdoor exercise during midday when pollen counts are usually higher. Alternatively, it may be more advantageous to switch exercise routines to an air-conditioned indoor environment during peak pollen season.
  b. Exercise in cooler, drier air increases the likelihood of EIB, even following pretreatment with drugs; exercise in warmer, moist air decreases the likelihood of EIB symptoms.
  c. Submaximal warm-up activity for 15 to 30 minutes may delay symptoms of EIB.

As discussed in this chapter, there are several actions that athletic trainers can take to assist the athlete in maximizing the effectiveness of asthma drug therapy and minimizing the effect of asthma on athletic performance. These actions focus on monitoring the effectiveness of therapy and providing education to the athlete regarding the use and effects of asthma drugs and devices.

BIBLIOGRAPHY

Carlson AM, Stempel DA. A claims data analysis of patient acquisition of drug therapies for the treatment of asthma. *J Manag Care Pharm.* 1999;5:342-346.

Drazen JM, Israel E, O'Byrne PM. Treatment of asthma with drugs modifying the leukotriene pathway. *N Engl J Med.* 1999;340:197-206.

Halterm JS, Yoos HL, Kaczorowski JM, et al. Providers underestimate symptom severity among urban children with asthma. *Arch Pediatr Adolesc Med.* 2002;156:141-146.

Hopman WM, Owen JG, Gagne E. Assessment of the effect of asthma education on outcomes. *Manag Care Interface.* 1999;12:89-93.

Houglum JE. Asthma medications: basic pharmacology and use in the athlete. *Journal of Athletic Training.* 2000;35:179-187.

Houglum, JE. The basics of asthma therapy for athletes. *Athletic Therapy Today.* 2001;6:16-21.

Lee JH, Cassard SD, Dans PE, Wheelock C, Ober JD. Evaluating asthma medication use before and after an acute asthma-related event. *J Manag Care Pharm.* 2001;7:303-308.

National Asthma Education and Prevention Program (NAEPP). *Guidelines for the Diagnosis and Management of Asthma-Update on Selected Topics 2002.* Bethesda, Md: National Heart, Lung, and Blood Institute; 2002. NIH publication No. 02-5074.

National Asthma Education and Prevention Program (NAEPP). *Expert Panel Report II: Guidelines for the Diagnosis and Management of Asthma.* Bethesda, Md: National Heart, Lung, and Blood Institute; 1997. NIH publication No. 97-4051.

Settipane RA, Schrank PJ, Simon RA, Mathison DA, Christiansen SC, Stevenson DD. Prevalence of cross-sensitivity with acetaminophen in aspirin-sensitive asthmatic subjects. *J Allergy Clin Immunol.* 1995;96:480-485.

Sterné SC, Gundersen BP, Shrivastava D. Development and evaluation of a pharmacist-managed asthma education clinic. *Hosp Pharm.* 1999;34:699-706.

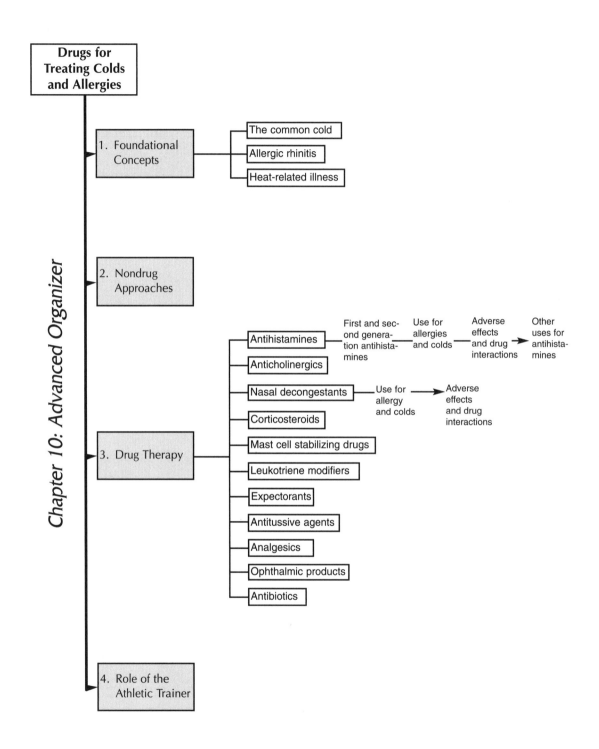

DRUGS FOR TREATING COLDS AND ALLERGIES

CHAPTER OBJECTIVES

At the end of this chapter, the reader will be able to:

- Describe the pathophysiology for the common cold and allergic rhinitis.
- Differentiate the signs and symptoms between the common cold and allergic rhinitis.
- Explain how over-the-counter (OTC) products used to treat the common cold and allergies can contribute to a heat-related illness.
- List several steps that can be taken to reduce the incidence of common colds and allergic rhinitis from occurring and/or spreading.
- Identify OTC medications for colds and allergic rhinitis that are combination products and choose the appropriate medication based on the patient is signs and symptoms.
- Explain the therapeutic use of antihistamines.
- Recall the adverse effects and common drug interactions for antihistamines and nasal decongestants.
- Differentiate between first- and second-generation antihistamines.
- Explain the mechanism of action for antihistamines and nasal decongestants.
- Explain the use of corticosteroids, mast cell stabilizing drugs, and leukotriene modifiers in the treatment of allergic rhinitis.
- Differentiate between an expectorant and antitussive.
- Recall the adverse effects for expectorants and antitussives.
- Explain the role of analgesics in the treatment of cold symptoms.
- Explain why antibiotics are not the medication of choice for treating the common cold and allergic rhinitis.
- Summarize the role of the athletic trainer for patients who are taking medications for colds or allergic rhinitis.

The common cold is one of the most frequent acute illnesses. Allergic rhinitis, affecting >15% of the population, is one of the most frequent chronic illnesses in the country. These conditions have some similarities in pathology and symptoms as well as aspects of drug therapy, but they also have some important differences that will be discussed in this chapter. Consumers spend billions of dollars annually on OTC medications to treat colds and allergies. These diseases cost an additional billions for prescription medications, hospital expenses, and lost work productivity. The frequent use of OTC medications to treat colds and allergies creates enhanced potential for *adverse effects*, drug interactions, and use of medications that may affect athletic performance. On

Table 10-1. Characteristics of the Common Cold and Allergic Rhinitis

Characteristic	Common Cold	Allergic Rhinitis
Cause	Virus	Hypersensitivity to allergens
Communicable	Yes	No
Coughing	Yes	No
Curative drug therapy	No	No
Duration	7 to 10 days	Seasonal or perennial
Histamine involvement	Minor	Major
Leukotriene, prostaglandin involvement	Yes	Yes
Nasal congestion	Yes	Yes
Nasal itching	No	Yes
Ocular inflammation	Infrequent	Frequent
Onset of symptoms	Gradual	Rapid
Potential for complications	Yes	Yes
Prevention strategies	Hand washing, avoid crowds during cold season	Avoid allergens as much as possible
Rhinorrhea	Yes	Yes
Sneezing	Occasional, forceful	Frequent, light
Sore throat	Yes	No
Therapy focus	Antihistamines, decongestants, expectorants, analgesics, antitussives	Antihistamines, decongestants, corticosteroids, leukotriene modifiers, ophthalmics

the other hand, effective use of drug therapy, coupled with nondrug measures, can minimize the effect of colds and allergies on the athlete's participation.

FOUNDATIONAL CONCEPTS

This section discusses the pathophysiology, causes, and symptoms of allergic rhinitis and the common cold. Several of these characteristics are similar for these two illnesses but many are quite different. A comparison of the characteristics for the common cold and allergic rhinitis are shown in Table 10-1.

The Common Cold

The common cold is caused by any one of >200 viruses. Two of the most common offenders are *rhinoviruses* and *coronaviruses*. The virus is passed from an infected person to a second person through airborne nasal discharge or, more commonly, from direct contact with the infected person's hand or an object recently handled (or sneezed on) by that person. Once the virus is on the second person's hand, it can be

There are many categories of viruses and many specific viruses within the categories. Rhinoviruses is one example of a virus category for which >100 specific viruses have been identified. Rhinoviruses are the most frequent cause of the common cold. There are several other categories of viruses that can cause the symptoms of the common cold (eg, coronaviruses).

readily transferred to the upper respiratory tract by direct contact with the nasal passage or eyes. Some viruses can remain viable for a few hours on inanimate objects or on the hands. The virus attaches to the human cell and eventually uses the biochemical process of the human cell to make more copies of itself. The mechanisms by which viruses infect human cells and propagate are much different than the mechanisms of bacteria and fungi, this antibacterial and antifungal drugs have no effect for the treatment of the common cold. Consequently, antibiotics (see Chapter 5) should not be used to treat these viral infections.

The viral infection of a common cold causes the release of various inflammatory mediators (eg, *prostaglandins, leukotrienes, kinins*) that result in increased mucous secretions and increased permeability and dilation of the blood vessels in the nasal passage, all of which contribute to nasal stuffiness. *Cholinergic* stimulation through acetylcholine release is also a significant contributor. *Histamine* plays a minor role in these events. Symptoms begin 24 to 72 hours after exposure to the virus and vary in severity depending on the specific virus. Symptoms typically begin with sore throat, followed by rhinorrhea (runny nose), nasal congestion, headache, body aches, occasional sneezing, and finally a cough that may persist longer than other symptoms. The common cold is usually self-limiting, lasting 7 to 10 days. Drug therapy can alleviate some of the discomfort associated with the infection but there is no cure for the common cold, hence the adage, "If you don't treat a cold it will last 7 to 10 days, but if you treat a cold it will last only 7 to 10 days."

> *When the neurotransmitter released by the parasympathetic fiber is acetylcholine, the response is referred to as a cholinergic response. The acetylcholine combines with the cholinergic receptor located on the surface of the cell to cause the response; in this case, increased mucus production.*

Complications sometimes develop as a result of a cold and these complications may extend the ramifications of the cold beyond 10 days. Two of the more common complications are ear infections, especially in children, and sinus infections. These occur as a result of inefficient drainage in the ear or sinuses, respectively. When these infections are bacterial in origin, they can be treated with antibiotics. Sometimes symptoms of other illnesses are mistaken for the common cold. For example, development of fever or nasal congestion and sneezing that lasts beyond 10 to 14 days may be indicative of allergic rhinitis or the development of a bacterial upper respiratory infection. A severe or persistent sore throat may imply a *streptococcal* infection. Another complication is exacerbation of asthma symptoms, a significant complication as breathing is already difficult. Treatment of asthma (see Chapter 9) may need to be more aggressive until the viral infection subsides.

Allergic Rhinitis

Allergic rhinitis is a hypersensitivity reaction in response to inhaled allergens. These allergens are also called *antigens* because they attach to *immunoglobulin E* (IgE) *antibodies* to initiate an allergic response. The extent of the hypersensitivity response will depend on the genetic predisposition of the patient and the extent of exposure to the allergen. There are two categories of allergic rhinitis, seasonal and perennial. Seasonal rhinitis (also called hay fever) is caused by inhalation of outdoor allergens, primarily pollen (eg, from weeds, trees, grasses) but also mold spores from

> *Recall from Chapter 9 that IgE is a type of immunoglobulin (ie, antibody) that combines with specific foreign substances (ie, antigens) that enter the body. The IgE are located on mast cells in the airways and on circulating basophils. When the antigen combines with the IgE, it causes the release of inflammatory chemical mediators from the mast cells and basophils. People with allergies have a lot of IgE specific for commonly encountered antigens such as pollen.*

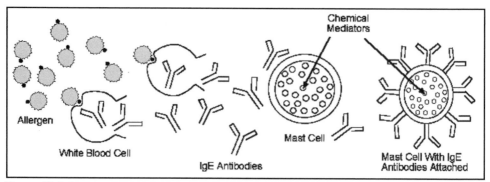

Figure 10-1. Sensitization to an allergen (modified from Dishuck J, Harrelson GL. Management and treatment of allergic rhinitis and sinusitis. *Athletic Therapy Today.* 2001; 6:6-10).

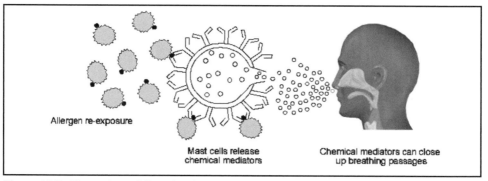

Figure 10-2. Allergic rhinitis IgE-mediated response to an allergen(s) (modified from Dishuck J, Harrelson GL. Management and treatment of allergic rhinitis and sinusitis. *Athletic Therapy Today.* 2001; 6:6-10).

decaying vegetation. Concentration of various pollens in the air changes with seasons and from one part of the country to another, but fluctuations also occur within each day. On the other hand, perennial rhinitis does not fluctuate with the seasons because it results primarily from contact with indoor allergens. House-dust mites, molds, pet dander, and cockroaches are common allergens. Consequently, symptoms of perennial rhinitis may exist sporadically or continuously depending on exposure to these allergens. The occurrence of seasonal allergic rhinitis is much more prevalent than perennial, affecting >35 million people in the United States.

Because allergic rhinitis is an IgE-mediated response, an initial exposure to the allergen is necessary, causing the production of IgE antibodies against that allergen (Figure 10-1). The IgE antibodies attach to mast cells located in the mucosa of the nasal passage (Figure 10-2). Upon additional exposures to the allergen, the allergen binds to the IgE, which results in the release of inflammatory mediators such as histamine, prostaglandins, leukotrienes, platelet-activating factor, and bradykinin (Figure 10-3). Histamine plays a major role in causing the symptoms of allergic rhinitis by combining with H_1 *receptors* (see below). The initial symptoms (early phase reaction) occur within minutes of exposure to the allergen and are largely due to the release of these mediators. Early phase symptoms include rhinorrhea, vasodilation of nasal capillaries, sneezing, and itching of the nose and eyes. Nasal congestion results from the increased mucus production and vasodilation. Activation of the parasympathetic cholinergic response also contributes to the mucus production. The patient tends to sniff frequently; experience more frequent, but less

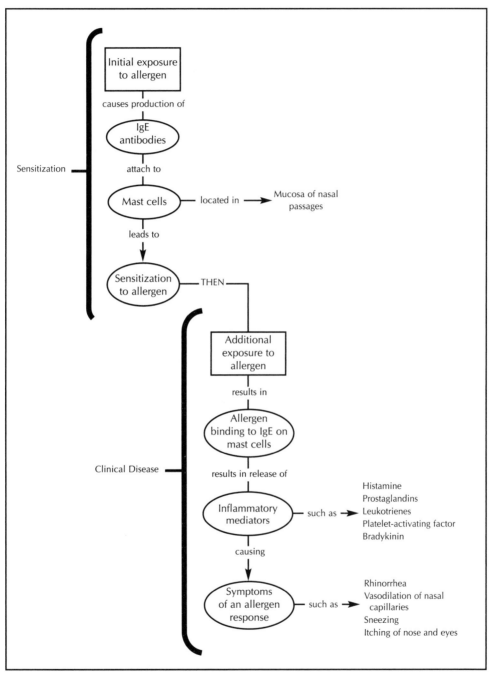

Figure 10-3. Manifestation of allergy symptoms.

severe, sneezes compared to a cold; and push the nose upward with the hand to alleviate the itch-ing.

Initial symptoms subside within 1 to 2 hours, but a late-phase response can occur several hours after exposure to allergens and results from the accumulation of inflammatory cells (eg, *basophils, eosinophils, mononuclear cells*) at the nasal mucosa. The presence of these cells con-tributes to sneezing, rhinorrhea, nasal congestion, and enhanced responsiveness to additional allergens, possibly due to the increased number of IgE-containing cells available to react with var-ious allergens.

Allergic rhinitis is a significant chronic disease, significant not only from the standpoint of frequency of occurrence in the population, but also regarding the impact on the patient. Persistent symptoms during allergy season, for example, can interfere with sleep, cause fatigue, affect social interaction, decrease performance at work, decrease ability to concentrate and learn in school, and limit ability to exercise. Overall quality of life can be notably diminished.

Heat-Related Illnesses

The topics in this chapter obviously do not include the treatment of heat-related illness but yet these conditions are worth mentioning because some drugs discussed in this chapter can con-tribute to the occurrence of heat-related illnesses (eg, heat cramps, heat exhaustion, and heat-stroke). These conditions result from an excessive loss of fluid and electrolytes or, in the case of heatstroke, the inability to adequately cool the body core temperature. Heatstroke is the most dangerous of these conditions and is a medical emergency. Any drug that increases loss of fluid or electrolytes or diminishes the normal cooling mechanisms of the body will have the potential to contribute to heat-related illnesses. Chapter 12 discusses diuretics and β-adrenergic blockers, which are prescription drugs that can contribute to heat-related illness. The current chapter, however, discusses commonly used OTC products used without medical supervision to treat the common cold and allergies. An adverse effect of some of these OTC drugs is that they can con-tribute to heat-related illness. Categories of drugs that can contribute to heat-related illness are:

- *α-adrenergic* agonists (nasal decongestants) constrict peripheral blood vessels and thus decrease the heat dissipated through these vessels.
- Antihistamines and other drugs that have anticholinergic effects (see Box 8-1) can decrease sweating and thus decrease a major cooling mechanism.
- Diuretics increase urine production and thus increase fluid loss.
- β-blockers decrease blood supply to skin, thus diminishing a cooling mechanism.

Summary

The common cold is caused by viruses that could infect anyone, whereas allergic rhinitis is a hypersensitivity reaction that affects genetically susceptible individuals. Both illnesses, however, cause an inflammatory response and an array of symptoms. For the common cold, these symp-toms are usually self-limiting whereas allergic rhinitis can be either seasonal or persist year around, with severity of symptoms ranging from mild to severe. Although a few of the symptoms of the common cold and allergic rhinitis are similar (eg, rhinorrhea and nasal congestion), there are many characteristics that differentiate these illnesses. Table 10-1 compared the characteristics of these illnesses. Quick onset of symptoms, the presence of itchy nose, watery eyes, and persist-ent sneezing are hallmark characteristics of allergic rhinitis and are among the characteristics that differentiate it from the common cold. Some drugs discussed in this chapter can decrease the effectiveness of the body's cooling mechanisms and thus contribute to the occurrence of heat-related illnesses.

Box 10-1. Ways to Reduce the Incidence of the Common Cold and Allergic Rhinitis

Cold

- Minimize the time spent in crowded locations
- Cover the nose and mouth when coughing and sneezing
- Wash hands frequently

Allergic Rhinitis

- Use weather channels to determine pollen count
- Limit outdoor activity during seasonal allergy seasons
- Keep windows closed and use air conditioning
- If possible, get rid on known allergen(s)
- Dust and vacuum frequently
- Use of a floor covering other than carpet can help reduce symptoms
- Use air filters that are designed to remove particulate matter

NONDRUG APPROACHES

Exposure to viruses is an everyday occurrence but there are some steps that can be taken to reduce the incidence and possibly the morbidity once infection with the common cold occurs (Box 10-1). Because one major means of transmission is by inhalation of airborne viruses, staying away from the coughing and sneezing of cold-sufferers seems obvious but is easier said than done. Crowded locations such as school or work cannot be totally avoided during the cold season, but minimizing time spent in crowded shopping malls or restaurants may be helpful. Covering coughs and sneezes is also obvious but not always practiced by cold sufferers. As the transfer of the cold virus often occurs by contact with the hands and then transfer to the recipient's eyes and nose, frequent hand washing can reduce infection.

When the symptoms of a cold appear, maintaining moisture in the throat and nasal passage helps reduce cough, throat soreness, and congestion. Increasing fluid intake, for example, reduces the viscosity of mucus so it is easier to move the mucus out of the throat and nasal passage. Sucking on hard candy can keep the throat moist and reduces the discomfort of a sore throat. Keeping the air moist with a vaporizer or humidifier is also helpful to maintain mucus viscosity and decrease throat dryness. As a nondrug measure to facilitate easier breathing, nasal strips are available that are applied on the nose to physically enlarge the nasal passage. The strips are also available with menthol, which may contribute to congestion relief.

Just as it is impossible to avoid exposure to all common cold viruses, it is also impossible for a person with allergic rhinitis to avoid contact with all allergens. There are several ways to minimize exposure (see Box 10-1). Seasonal allergy sufferers can limit their outdoor activity and use indoor exercise routines as much as possible during peak allergy season. Yard work can be limited to the time of day with the lowest pollen count, using weather channels to determine the pollen count. Windows can be kept closed and air conditioning used to reduce pollen indoors.

For the person with perennial allergic rhinitis, an obvious preventative measure is to get rid of the known allergens. Often this is associated with a family pet or house dust, which are not always easy to avoid. Nonetheless, minimizing exposure is the key. Pets can be restricted to certain rooms; not allowing them in the bedroom is helpful. Dust and vacuum frequently to reduce house mites as well as pet allergens. Because house-dust mites concentrate in carpets, use of floor covering other than carpet can reduce this allergen. Use air filters on the furnace that are designed to efficiently remove particulate matter.

DRUG THERAPY

There are several categories of drugs used to treat colds and allergic rhinitis. Some of these are used to treat both colds and allergies (*antihistamines, decongestants*), some are used primarily to treat colds (*antitussive, expectorants*), and some to treat allergies (*corticosteroids, leukotriene modifiers, mast cell stabilizers*). The latter group is also among the categories of drugs used to treat asthma, although the target tissue for allergic rhinitis is the nasal passage rather than the bronchial tissue, and thus nasal sprays are used rather than inhalers for administration of corticosteroids and mast cell stabilizers. The reason for this commonality of therapeutic agents is that the disease processes for both allergic rhinitis and asthma have symptoms that, at least in part, result from the release of inflammatory mediators produced from *arachidonic acid* (see Chapter 9). Also, *IgE*-mediated involvement is a component to the asthma disease process for many asthmatics. Not surprising, therefore, is that many patients with asthma also have symptoms of allergic rhinitis. The presence of these coexisting diseases complicates the drug therapy somewhat as both the nasal and bronchial symptoms must be treated.

There is what seems to be an endless array of products on the market to treat the common cold and allergic rhinitis. Table 10-2 lists some brand name OTC combination products. A glance through this table reveals that not only are there numerous combinations available but also the names are very confusing because many sound similar and the product name often gives little indication of the contents. Consider, also, that the patient has >250 brand name combination OTC allergy and cold/flu products from which to select, plus numerous generic brands. With all of these product names and combinations, it is easy to imagine that patients are confused about which product to select to self-medicate their symptoms.

Although use of a combination product can be more convenient, use of these products also lends to an enhanced potential for adverse effects that could be avoided. For example, a patient who needs an antitussive to treat a nonproductive cough at the end of a bout with the common cold may not need a decongestant or analgesic any longer but may select Alka-Seltzer Plus Cold & Cough Liqui-Gels to put an end to the cough. Depending on the patient, the pseudoephedrine and acetaminophen could cause adverse effects that would have been avoided with a single-entity product that contains only an antitussive (eg, Vicks 44 Cough Relief Liquid).

Antihistamines

Histamine is a mediator released primarily by *mast cells* and *basophils*, which store the histamine for quick release following the binding of an *allergen* to the *IgE* on the cell's surface. Histamine is found in several other tissues, including bronchial, intestinal, skin, and cerebrospinal fluid. Once released, histamine combines with the histamine receptor on the surface of other cells to initiate a response within that cell. Three histamine receptors have been identified—H_1, H_2, and H_3 receptors. The H_3 receptors are located in the central nervous system (CNS) but their function is not clearly understood and there are no drugs clinically available that are known to specifically block these receptors. The H_2 receptors are primarily found on stomach cells; activation causes an increased production of stomach acid. Drugs that inhibit the H_2 receptor (H_2 blockers) have been available since the mid-1970s and are used to treat ulcers (see Chapter 11). The H_1 receptors are found in the respiratory tract and near peripheral blood ves-

Table 10-2. Selected Over-the-Counter Combination Products for Treatment of Colds and Allergies[1]

Trade Name	Antihistamine	Decongestant	Antitussive	Analgesic	Expectorant
Allerest Maximum Strength Tablets	2 chlorpheniramine	30 pseudoephedrine			
Benedryl Allergy & Sinus Tablets	25 diphenhydramine	60 pseudoephedrine			
Sudafed Cold & Allergy Maximum Strength Tablets	4 chlorpheniramine	60 pseudoephedrine			
Dimetapp Children's Cough & Cold Elixir	1 brompheniramine	15 pseudoephedrine	5 dextromethorphan		
Robitussin Allergy & Cough Liquid	2 brompheniramine	30 pseudoephedrine	10 dextromethorphan		
Alka-Seltzer Plus Cold & Cough Liqui-Gels	2 chlorpheniramine	30 pseudoephedrine	10 dextromethorphan	325 acetaminophen	
Contac Severe Cold and Flu Maximum Strength Caplets	2 chlorpheniramine	30 pseudoephedrine	15 dextromethorphan	500 acetaminophen	
Tylenol Cold Complete Formula Tablets	2 chlorpheniramine	30 pseudoephedrine	15 dextromethorphan	325 acetaminophen	
Top Care Multi-Symptom Pain Relief Cold Tablets	2 chlorpheniramine	30 pseudoephedrine	15 dextromethorphan	325 acetaminophen	
Actifed Cold & Sinus Maximum Strength Tablets	2 chlorpheniramine	30 pseudoephedrine		500 acetaminophen	
Benedryl Allergy & Cold Tablets	12.5 diphenhydramine	30 pseudoephedrine		500 acetaminophen	

continued

Table 10-2. Selected OTC Combination Products for Treatment of Colds and Allergies[1] (continued)

Trade Name	Antihistamine	Decongestant	Antitussive	Analgesic	Expectorant
Benedryl Allergy & Sinus Headache Tablets	12.5 diphenhydramine	30 pseudoephedrine		500 acetaminophen	
Triaminicin Cold, Allergy, Sinus Medicine Tablets	4 chlorpheniramine	60 pseudoephedrine		650 acetaminophen	
Perogesic Extra StrengthTablets	12.5 diphenhydramine			500 acetaminophen	
Tylenol Severe Allergy Tablets	12.5 diphenhydramine			500 acetaminophen	
Alka-Seltzer Plus Cold & Flu Liqui-Gels		30 pseudoephedrine	10 dextromethorphan	325 acetaminophen	
Contac Severe Cold and Flu Non-Drowsy Caplets		30 pseudoephedrine	15 dextromethorphan	325 acetaminophen	
Sudafed Non-Drowsy Severe Cold Formula Maximum Strength Tablets		30 pseudoephedrine	15 dextromethorphan	500 acetaminophen	
Tylenol Cold Non-Drowsy Formula Tablets		30 pseudoephedrine	15 dextromethorphan	325 acetaminophen	
Vicks DayQuil Liquicaps Multi-Symptom Cold/Flu Relief Capsules		60 pseudoephedrine	20 dextromethorphan	500 acetaminophen	
Robitussin Cold, Multi-Symptom Cold & Flu Tablets		30 pseudoephedrine	10 dextromethorphan	325 acetaminophen	200 guaifenesin
Sudafed Cold & Cough Liquid Caps		30 pseudoephedrine	10 dextromethorphan	250 acetaminophen	100 guaifenesin

continued

Table 10-2. Selected OTC Combination Products for Treatment of Colds and Allergies[1] (continued)

Trade Name	Antihistamine	Decongestant	Antitussive	Analgesic	Expectorant
Novahistine DMX Syrup		30 pseudoephedrine	10 dextromethorphan		100 guaifenesin
Robitussin CF Syrup		30 pseudoephedrine	10 dextromethorphan		100 guaifenesin
Robitussin Cold, Cold & Congestion Softgels		30 pseudoephedrine	10 dextromethorphan		200 guaifenesin
Robitussin Cold Sinus & Congestion Tablets		30 pseudoephedrine		325 acetaminophen	200 guaifenesin
Advil Cold & Sinus Tablets			30 pseudoephedrine		200 ibuprofen
Alka-Seltzer Plus Cold & Sinus Tablets		5 phenylephrine		250 acetaminophen	
Dristan Cold Non-Drowsy Maximum Strength Tablets		30 pseudoephedrine		500 acetaminophen	
Phenapap		30 pseudoephedrine		325 acetaminophen	
Robitussin Severe Congestion Liquid Gels		30 pseudoephedrine			200 guaifenesin
Cheracol D Cough Formula Syrup			10 dextromethorphan		100 guaifenesin
Robitussin-DM Liquid			10 dextromethorphan		100 guaifenesin

[1]Values indicated per ingredient represent mg per dosage unit (eg, tablet, capsule) or per 5 mL for liquids.

Table 10-3. Examples of First- and Second-Generation Antihistamines

	Generic	Trade	Dosage	OTC/Rx
First-Generation	brompheniramine	Dimetapp Allergy	Capsules	OTC
	carbinoxamine	Histex CT	Extended release tablets	Rx
	chlorpheniramine	Chlor-Trimeton	Extended release tablets	OTC
	clemastine	Tavist Allergy	Tablets	OTC
	dexchlorpheniramine	generic	Extended release tablets	Rx
	diphenhydramine	Benedryl Allergy	Chewable tablets	OTC
	phenindamine	Nolahist	Tablets	OTC
	promethazine	Phenergan	Tablets	Rx
	triprolidine	Zymine	Liquid	Rx
Second-Generation	azelastine	Astelin	Spray	Rx
	cetirizine	Zyrtec	Tablets, syrup	Rx
	desloratadine	Clarinex	Tablets	Rx
	fexofenadine	Allegra	Tablets, capsules	Rx
	loratadine	Claritin	Tablets, syrup	OTC/Rx

sels. Antihistamines that block the H_1 receptor were on the market for decades prior to H_2 blockers and thus, historically, any reference to antihistamines without specifying the receptor type is generally understood to be referring to antihistamines that block the H_1 receptor. The remaining discussion of antihistamines in this chapter is in reference to H_1 antihistamines.

First- and Second-Generation Antihistamines

There are two categories of antihistamines (H_1), first-generation and second-generation. First-generation antihistamines have been available since the 1940s. The second-generation antihistamines were introduced in the 1980s; however, the second-generation antihistamines that were first introduced have since been withdrawn from the market due to the occurrence of cardiac arrhythmia, an adverse effect not observed with more recent second-generation antihistamines. Of the second-generation antihistamines that are currently on the market, the first was approved by the Food and Drug Administration (FDA) in 1993. Examples of frequently used first-generation antihistamines are diphenhydramine (Benadryl) and chlorpheniramine (Chlor-Trimeton). The most prominent adverse effect with these drugs is sedation. The second-generation antihistamines are less *lipophilic* and therefore do not cross the blood-brain barrier as readily as the first-generation compounds. Consequently, the primary characteristic that differentiates the first-generation from second-generation compounds is the significantly reduced incidence of sedation with the second-generation antihistamines. Examples of second-generation antihistamines, which are sometimes referred to as the nonsedating antihistamines, are fexofenadine (Allegra) and loratadine (Claritin). Other examples of first- and second-generation antihistamines are listed in Table 10-3.

The first-generation antihistamines have long been available OTC. In 2002, loratadine (Claritin) was the first of the second-generation products available OTC. One argument for this shift to OTC status was the fact that second-generation antihistamines have a lower incidence of adverse effects than first-generation antihistamines, which are already used as OTC products to treat allergic rhinitis.

All antihistamines are available as oral medications except azelastine (Astelin), which is a nasal spray (see Table 10-3). Some antihistamines are also available in liquid form as syrups or elixirs, and some come in extended-release dosage forms.

Use for Allergy and Colds

Histamine is considered a major contributor to the symptoms of allergic rhinitis, and consequently, antihistamines are a mainstay of therapy. Antihistamines decrease the rhinorrhea, itchy nose and eyes, and sneezing associated with allergic rhinitis. They do not decrease nasal congestion as significantly. This may be because other mediators also contribute to nasal congestion and, during the late-phase response, the accumulation of *immune cells* contributes to nasal congestion. Antihistamines are more effective when present prior to the release of histamine and, therefore, daily use of these drugs as a preventative is more effective than use after symptoms occur.

Histamine does not play a significant role in the symptoms of the common cold. Nonetheless, antihistamines are somewhat effective in reducing mucus production and drying the nasal passage, but the mechanism of action is not due to histamine antagonism. As discussed below, one adverse effect of anti-

> *Recall from Chapter 8 that anticholinergic effects include blurred vision, constipation, urinary hesitancy, dry mouth, and decreased sweating.*

histamines, particularly the first-generation antihistamines, is to cause anticholinergic effects. One *cholinergic* response is mucus production, and thus inhibition of this process becomes a benefit when treating the common cold, hence the inclusion of a first-generation antihistamine in many OTC cold products. However, the drying effect on the respiratory tract is a disadvantage when sinus drainage or movement of mucus out of the bronchial tree (ie, expectoration) is desired. *Consequently, first-generation antihistamines should be used with caution in patients with lower respiratory tract diseases (eg, asthma and chronic bronchitis).*

Adverse Effects and Drug Interactions

The adverse effect profile for the first-generation antihistamines is more notable than for the second-generation compounds. Sedation and anticholinergic effects are the prime concern. Some first-generation antihistamines have a greater effect (eg, diphenhydramine, clemastine) than others (eg, chlorpheniramine, brompheniramine). Not only is drowsiness a potential hazard while driving a vehicle, but it can also negatively impact performance at work, in school, and in athletics. Even if the person does not feel drowsy, cognitive abilities, including the ability to operate a motor vehicle, can be diminished. Because reaction time and perception are affected, athletic performance could also be affected. Drowsiness at nighttime can be an advantage to facilitate sleep, however, diminished cognitive function can continue even the morning following bedtime use. Concomitant use of other CNS depressants (eg, opioid analgesics, some anticonvulsants, antianxiety agents, and alcohol) will exacerbate the sedative properties. In some children and elderly patients, antihistamines can cause paradoxical CNS stimulation that results in insomnia, nervousness, irritability, and tremors. The incidence of sedation for the second-generation antihistamines varies from lower incidence at recommended doses (cetirizine, Zyrtec), to nonsedating even at higher than recommended doses (fexofenadine, Allegra).

Anticholinergic adverse effects are also more predominant with first- than with second-generation antihistamines. Again, there is some variation in the extent of these effects among the many first-generation compounds; for example, brompheniramine and chlorpheniramine have less of these adverse effects than diphenhydramine. The anticholinergic effects include dry mouth, urinary retention, blurred vision, tachycardia, reduced sweating, and constipation. These effects may be quite tolerable for most patients, but patients with pre-existing conditions such as cardiovascular disease, narrow-angle glaucoma, or urinary retention should avoid the first-generation products. Similarly, decreased sweating is not likely to be of significant consequence for most patients but it may be a contributing factor in the development of heatstroke in a predisposed patient who is exercising heavily in a hot, humid environment. The potential problems associated with the anticholinergic effects can be made worse if the antihistamine is combined with other drugs that also have anticholinergic effects (eg, drugs for motions sickness, certain groups of antidepressant drugs, gastrointestinal antispasmodics, and some drugs to treat Parkinson's disease).

Another adverse effect associated with first-generation antihistamines is that they can cause photosensitization in some patients, making them more prone to sunburn. Caution is advised with use in all patients; the use of sunscreens and appropriate protective clothing is recommended until the patient's response is determined.

Other Uses for Antihistamines

Besides being used to treat the common cold or allergic rhinitis, some antihistamines have other therapeutic uses. Histamine causes redness of the skin (urticaria) and itching (pruritus) as a result of atopic dermatitis (IgE-mediated hypersensitive response after systemic absorption of an allergen), contact dermatitis (eg, poison ivy), or eczema. Some antihistamines such as diphenhydramine (Benadryl), hydroxyzine (Vistaril), and promethazine (Phenergan) are used topically and/or orally for treatment of dermatitis.

The prominent sedative properties of diphenhydramine are used as an advantage to market antihistamines as OTC sleep aids (Nytol, Sominex). Diphenhydramine is effective for short-term use to treat insomnia. Some morning hangover is common and is a disadvantage as it may diminish the person's effectiveness in morning activities such as driving, completing tasks at work, or exercising/playing sports.

Some antihistamines are effective at preventing motion sickness and the nausea and/or vomiting associated with adverse effects of drugs. Drug-induced gastric irritation and motion sickness causes the release of acetylcholine, which stimulates the vomiting center in the CNS. Therefore, the anticholinergic

> *Scopolamine, an anticholinergic drug, not an antihistamine, is also useful to treat motion sickness and is available as a patch (Transderm-scop) for transdermal absorption.*

effect of antihistamines, especially when given prior to the offending drug or motion, can prevent the nausea and vomiting. Prescription and OTC agents are available such as promethazine (Phenergan), meclizine (Bonine), cyclizine (Marezine), dimenhydrinate (Dramamine), and diphenhydramine (Benadryl).

Anticholinergics

Because the *anticholinergic* effect of antihistamines can be advantageous in the treatment of the common cold and allergic rhinitis, it is not surprising that a drug in the anticholinergic category is available for treatment of these illnesses. Ipratropium (Atrovert) is available by prescription as a nasal spray. Systemic anticholinergics tend to have numerous adverse effects and thus are not used for these illnesses, but the spray minimizes the systemic adverse effects. Typical dosing is frequent, 2 sprays per nostril 3 to 4 times per day, and thus a disadvantage. The drug should not be used in patients who are allergic to peanuts because ipratropium may cause an allergic response. The inhaler dosage form of ipratropium is used to treat asthma (see Chapter 9).

Nasal Decongestants

Dilation of peripheral blood vessels in the nasal passage contributes significantly to nasal congestion. Decongestants are *α-adrenergic* agonists; they activate the *α-receptors* on the peripheral blood vessels of the nasal passage to cause constriction of those blood vessels and a decrease in mucosal edema. Because these drugs combine with one of the same receptors as the neurotransmitters of the sympathetic nervous system, and thus mimic these neurotransmitters, the nasal decongestants are also referred to as sympathomimetics.

> *Adrenergic refers to drugs that combine with the same receptors as the adrenergic neurotransmitters, norepinephrine and epinephrine, which are released by activation of the sympathetic nervous system. Therefore, α-adrenergic agonists combine specifically with the alpha-type of adrenergic receptor.*

Use for Allergy and Colds

Decongestants are used to relieve nasal stuffiness associated with the common cold and allergic rhinitis, both seasonal and perennial. The oral decongestant used in most OTC decongestant products is pseudoephedrine, available alone (Sudafed) or in many combination products (see Table 10-2) for the treatment of colds and allergies. It is available in several oral dosage forms, including capsules, tablets, syrups, and extended-release products. A few oral products contain phenylephrine. Phenylpropanolamine was a popular decongestant until 2000 when the FDA advised the removal of phenylpropanolamine from the market because of increased risk of hemorrhagic stroke in women taking these drugs.

Pseudoephedrine is absorbed readily from the gastrointestinal tract. *Onset of action* is <30 minutes and duration is about 4 hours. It does not have to be used prior to onset of nasal decongestion and thus can be used as needed or on a regularly scheduled basis.

Several decongestants are available for topical use as nasal sprays, inhalers, or drops. Nasal decongestants are more effective, faster acting, and produce fewer CNS stimulant and other systemic effects than oral decongestants. Nonetheless, their use should be limited to 3 to 5 days because of the potential to cause rebound congestion. Examples are tetrahydrozoline (Tyzine), desoxyephedrine (Vicks Vapo Inhaler), phenylephrine (Neo-Synephrine 4-Hour), ephedrine (Pretz-D), and oxymetazoline (Afrin 12-Hour Original, Neo-Synephrine 12-Hour).

> *Phenylpropanolamine was also used in weight loss products (ie, diet pills). Such use in OTC products had been controversial for years and contributed to the overall incidence of hemorrhagic stroke. No currently available OTC product has been proven to cause weight loss. Nonetheless, other adrenergic agonists, such as ephedrine, are promoted in products for this purpose. Considering that nondrug measures of diet and exercise can achieve weight loss, the risk of adverse effects from adrenergic agonists may outweigh the potential benefits for this use.*

As with other OTC products, the names are sometimes confusing because a few companies have several products that use the same brand name and are slight variations from one another in content or duration of action. For example, the following all contain 0.05% oxymetazoline as the decongestant: Afrin 12-Hour Original Pump Mist, Afrin 12-Hour Original, Afrin Severe Congestion with Menthol, Afrin No-Drip 12-Hour, Afrin No-Drip 12-Hour Severe Congestion with Menthol. Selection depends primarily on personal preference.

Adverse Effects and Drug Interactions

The most common adverse effect from pseudoephedrine is CNS stimulation that may cause insomnia, agitation, tremor, headache, or restlessness. Pseudoephedrine is marketed as a non-drowsy cold and allergy medication. Some products have pseudoephedrine in combination with first-generation antihistamines (see Table 10-2) as a means to counter the sedative properties of the antihistamine. Additional *adrenergic* effects can cause tachycardia, peripheral vasoconstriction, and altered glucose metabolism. The tachycardia and vasoconstriction can be of significance to patients who have existing hypertension or heart disease as these effects can exacerbate the disease. Consequently, oral decongestants should not be used in patients with these diseases and used in caution in patients with diabetes because of the potential to alter insulin requirements. Caution is also warranted even when topical nasal decongestants are used in patients with diabetes or cardiovascular disease. The peripheral vasoconstriction action of nasal decongestants can decrease the effectiveness of the body's natural cooling mechanism and therefore these drugs should be used with caution in patients who are in an environment conducive to heatstroke (eg, hot, humid, poor air circulation, heavy exercise).

Decongestants applied topically as intranasal sprays and drops generally have milder systemic effects. However, local adverse effects, such as local irritation and rebound congestion, are significant problems. Rebound congestion is a potential adverse effect with the use of decongestants applied topically to the nasal mucosa. The incidence of rebound congestion increases when nasal sprays and drops are used more than 3 to 5 days. In this condition, congestion becomes worse, and the effectiveness and duration of action of the decongestant diminishes with continued use of the decongestant. Patients with rebound congestion have a tendency to continue using the nasal decongestant in an effort to relieve the congestion, thus perpetuating the problem. If rebound congestion occurs, the topical nasal decongestant can be discontinued in one nostril at a time, and normal saline nasal spray used in that nostril to soothe the irritated mucosa. Use of an oral decongestant may also minimize the discomfort. It takes 1 to 2 weeks for the nasal mucosa to return to normal. Other potential problems associated with nasal decongestants are primarily local effects (eg, nasal burning, stinging, and dryness of the mucosa). *These local effects and the potential for rebound congestion with nasal sprays and drops make them less useful for perennial allergic rhinitis in which long-term therapy is needed.*

In terms of drug interactions, the one with the most devastating potential is the combination of any decongestant, including topical products, with monoamine oxidase inhibitors (MAOIs). Decongestants should not be used in patients who are using, or have used within the previous 3 weeks, MAOIs because hypertensive crisis can result. Another interaction is the combination of oral decongestants with caffeine. Use of caffeine is prevalent in soft drinks and coffee (see Table 13-4) and has CNS and cardiovascular effects similar to pseudoephedrine. These effects are additive when the two drugs are used together, and therefore, this combination can be particularly hazardous to patients with existing hypertension. The combination of caffeine and ephedrine has demonstrated a prolonged exercise time to exhaustion compared with placebo or either drug alone.

MAOIs are a group of drugs that are categorized therapeutically as antidepressant drugs, although they also have some other uses. Monoamine oxidase inhibitors inhibit the inactivation of sympathomimetics, enhancing their activity and causing a potentially dangerous exaggerated hypertensive response. Examples of MAOIs are phenelzine (Nardil) and tranylcypromine (Parnate).

Table 10-4. Corticosteroid Intranasal Products[1]

Generic Name	Trade Name	Dosage Form	Typical Adult Dosage (sprays/nostril)
beclomethasone	Beconase	Aerosol	1, bid to qid
beclomethasone	Beconase AQ	Spray	1 to 2, bid
budesonide	Rhinocort	Aerosol	1 to 2, bid
budesonide	Rhinocort Aqua	Spray	1 to 2, once/day
flunisolide	Nasalide	Spray	2, bid to tid
fluticasone	Flonase	Spray	2, once/day
mometasone	Nasonex	Spray	2, once/day
triamcinolone	Nasacort	Aerosol	1 to 2, once/day
triamcinolone	Nasacort AQ	Spray	1 to 2, once/day

bid = twice per day; tid = three times per day; qid = four times per day
[1]*All products are prescription only*

Corticosteroids

Topical use of *corticosteroids* as nasal sprays has become a primary therapy for control of allergic rhinitis. By inhibiting the production of inflammatory mediators (see Chapter 9), corticosteroids reduce all of the major symptoms of allergic rhinitis (eg, runny nose, itching, sneezing, and nasal congestion). They also reduce infiltration of inflammatory cells and inhibit symptoms of the late-phase reaction. The *onset of action* is slower for nasal corticosteroids than for antihistamines or decongestants. Some benefit is observed within 1 to 3 days, but maximal effect may take 2 to 3 weeks. Use of these corticosteroid products is most effective to prevent symptoms and thus it is beneficial to use them for 2 to 4 weeks prior to anticipated exposure as well as during exposure.

Adverse effects of nasal corticosteroids are relatively minor. Nasal irritation, headache, and pharyngitis occur in some patients. Localized infection of the nasal passage occurs only on rare occasions but necessitates discontinuation of the corticosteroid and/or treatment with an antibacterial agent. Significant systemic effects are rare.

Nasal corticosteroid products are available as aqueous sprays or as aerosol canisters with propellants. The aqueous sprays produce less drying and are less irritating to the nasal mucosa than the aerosols but produce more of a taste. Dosage regimens vary from 1 to 4 times per day, depending on the specific product and the response obtained. After a few weeks of therapy, the effectiveness should be assessed and the dosage regimen adjusted so that the lowest effective dosage is used. Table 10-4 lists some nasal products and typical adult dosage.

Oral corticosteroids are also used as short-term therapy (ie, up to 1 week) when symptoms are severe. An example of a typical regimen would be 20 mg of prednisone once daily for 7 days. As with use of systemic corticosteroids for any purpose, consideration should be given to other existing diseases that may be adversely affected by the corticosteroid (eg, hypertension, ulcers, and diabetes) (see Chapter 6).

Mast Cell Stabilizing Drugs

As with the corticosteroids, the mast cell stabilizing drugs are also used to treat asthma as well as allergic rhinitis and are discussed in Chapter 9. Their *mechanism of action* is to inhibit the release of inflammatory mediators from mast cells. Cromolyn (Nasalcrom) is available OTC as a nasal spray for treatment of allergic rhinitis. As with inhalation products for treatment of asthma, use of the nasal spray for rhinitis takes several days for a noticeable improvement, takes a few weeks or more for maximal effect, has a dosage regimen of multiple doses per day, and is most effective if dosing begins prior to onset of symptoms and then continues on a regular daily schedule. The advantages of cromolyn are the OTC availability and the lack of systemic adverse effects. The disadvantages are the frequent dosing schedule (3 to 6 times per day) and that the effectiveness is less than the corticosteroids. Nasal irritation occurs in some patients.

Leukotriene Modifiers

Leukotrienes are mediators released during inflammatory response that contribute to symptoms of asthma (see Chapter 9) and to the early and late-phase symptoms of allergic rhinitis. Leukotriene modifiers inhibit the effect of leukotrienes by one of two mechanisms: inhibition of the enzyme that produces them or competitive inhibition of the leukotriene receptor. Montelukast (Singulair), for example, blocks the leukotriene receptor. Montelukast was originally approved for asthma therapy but became available to treat seasonal allergic rhinitis in 2003. *Adverse effects* are infrequent but include headache and upper respiratory tract infection (eg, ear infection). The recommended dosage is the same as for treatment of asthma, one tablet orally per day at a dose of 4, 5, or 10 mg, depending on the age of the patient. Because the dosage form and regimen are the same for the treatment of allergic rhinitis and asthma, the drug can be of potential benefit in patients with both of these diseases.

Expectorants

An expectorant is a drug that decreases the viscosity of lower respiratory tract secretions so that they can be moved out of the respiratory tract more efficiently by coughing (ie, productive cough). Many cold and cough remedies contain an expectorant (see Table 10-2). For example, Novahistine DMX Syrup, Robitussin DM Syrup, and Sudafed Cold & Cough Liquid Caps all contain guaifenesin, the most commonly used expectorant. However, there is some question as to the usefulness of guaifenesin in these combination products because:

- An infection with the common cold (without complications) typically affects only the upper respiratory tract and the cough is nonproductive.
- Although recommended OTC dosages (200 to 400 mg every 4 hours) of guaifenesin are usually void of adverse effects, the therapeutic effectiveness at these dosages has not been established and thus is somewhat uncertain. High doses can cause vomiting, headache, drowsiness, and diarrhea.
- Use of first-generation antihistamines with expectorants is counterproductive regarding expectorant action because the anticholinergic action can dry mucous secretions and thus make the mucus more difficult to expectorate.

Nondrug measures to facilitate expectorant activity are to keep well-hydrated and to keep the air humidified.

Antitussive Agents

A frequent symptom of the common cold is coughing. *Antitussive* agents are cough suppressants. These drugs act in the CNS to increase the threshold for coughing. Cough is a reflex intended to mobilize mucus out of the respiratory tract and therefore should not be suppressed if it is productive. An antitussive is warranted, however, when a cough interferes with sleep or is unproductive. Usually viral respiratory infections are nonproductive. A rule of thumb is that it is appropriate to treat dry, hacking coughs with antitussives, and to treat productive coughs with an expectorant. Suppression of a productive cough could hinder the body's ability to fight the infection. Because the intended purpose of an expectorant is to move secretions from the respiratory tract, the combination of antitussives and expectorants in the same product is not logical; nonetheless, they are available.

The most common nonopioid antitussive is dextromethorphan. Characteristics of dextromethorphan are that it does not cause respiratory depression at therapeutic doses, it is available OTC, and it is effective at 10 to 30 mg every 4 to 8 hours. Dextromethorphan has a low incidence of adverse effects at normal antitussive doses but it can add to the CNS depressant effects of other drugs (eg, alcohol, antihistamines), and should not be used in combination with MAOIs. It should be noted that although dextromethorphan is the most common OTC antitussive, there is concern that it does have some abuse potential at higher doses. There are many reports of abuse, particularly among younger teens and pre-teens who do not have alcohol or other drugs readily available. Dextromethorphan remains OTC as scientific studies must be completed to confirm the abuse and physical dependence potential. Diphenhydramine (Benadryl) also has antitussive properties but is considered less effective and, as discussed earlier, has notable adverse effects.

The most frequently used opioid antitiussive is codeine (see Chapter 9). Hydrocodone is also effective but has a higher abuse potential. Codeine is more effective than dextromethorphan to treat severe cough. Usual adult dosages are 10 to 20 mg codeine every 4 to 6 hours. Codeine can produce euphoria and drug dependence but the likelihood is small at antitussive doses. Codeine can suppress respiration and thus should be used with caution in patients with respiratory disease such as asthma or emphysema. Respiratory depression is the cause of death in overdose situations; an opioid analgesic antagonist, naloxone (Narcan), can be use used to reverse this effect. Constipation is a common adverse effect. Codeine cough syrups are controlled substances (schedule V) and are available in mixtures containing various other drugs to treat colds (see Table 10-2). The laws of some states allow limited purchase of codeine-containing cough medications without a prescription.

In addition to systemic antitussive agents, cough drops are also used to relieve cough. These products contain dextromethorphan (eg, Robitussin Cough Calmers Lozenges) or menthol (eg, Robitussin Cough Drops), which has some local anesthetic action (see below) to suppress the cough and to sooth a sore throat. Sucking on hard candy also soothes the throat and offers relief.

Analgesics

Analgesics are often used as part of the treatment regimen for the common cold; in fact, they are a component of many cough and cold remedies (see Table 10-2). Relief of sore throat or headache pain is often the impetus for the use of analgesics, although they may also be used to reduce fever (antipyretic). Acetaminophen and ibuprofen (see Chapter 7) are the analgesics of choice for pain accompanying a cold. Aspirin is not recommended for children and teenagers because of the risk of Reye's syndrome when aspirin is used in conjunction with a viral infection. Most cough and cold remedies with an analgesic/antipyretic component have been reformulat-

Table 10-5. Selected Ophthalmic Products to Treat Ocular Symptoms of Allergic Rhinitis

Drug Category	Generic Name	Trade Name	OTC/Rx
Antihistamines	azelastine	Optivar	Rx
	emedastine	Emadine	Rx
	olopatadine	Patanol	Rx
Corticosteroids	dexamethasone	Decadron	Rx
	loteprednol	Lotemax	Rx
	medrysone	HMS	Rx
	prednisolone	Inflamase Forte	Rx
Mast cell stabilizers	nedocromil	Alocril	Rx
	pemirolast	Alamast	Rx
NSAID	ketorolac	Acular	Rx
Ophthalmic decongestants	naphazoline	Naphcon	OTC
	oxymetazoline	Visine L.R.	OTC
	phenylephrine	AK-Nefrin	OTC
	tetrahydrozoline	Vasine Moisturizing	OTC

ed to use acetaminophen. Normal adult dosages of acetaminophen range from 500 to 1000 mg, with a daily maximum of 4000 mg.

As an alternative to systemic analgesics, relief of sore throat can be attained through topically applied throat sprays or lozenges. Examples of lozenges that contain a local anesthetic are dyclonine (Sucrets Maximum Strength), menthol (Hall's Mentho-Lyptus), benzocaine (Vicks Children's Chloraseptic), or both menthol and benzocaine (Cepacol Maximum Strength). Camphor and menthol vapors have some antitussive and anesthetic action and thus are used as creams and ointments (Vicks VapoRub) for topical application to the chest and/or throat. A nondrug measure to relieve sore throat is merely to keep the throat moist by sucking on hard candy.

Ophthalmic Products

Itching, watering, and redness of the eyes comprise the ocular inflammation (allergic conjunctivitis) that is a significant component for many patients with allergic rhinitis. The systemic use of antihistamines or decongestants can help alleviate these symptoms. There are also many ophthalmic products available for treating these ocular inflammation symptoms. These products include drugs in the categories of corticosteroids, antihistamines, decongestants, mast cell stabilizers, and NSAIDs. Examples of ophthalmic products for treatment of allergic rhinitis are provided in Table 10-5. Each product is applied directly to the eye, most often as drops. Adverse effects are usually local in nature, such as stinging or burning of the eyes and blurred vision.

Antibiotics

Antibiotics are mentioned here to emphasize that they are effective only against bacteria and that neither the common cold nor allergic rhinitis are caused by bacterial infection. Many people have the mistaken impression that they should get "a shot of penicillin" to treat their cold when in fact antibiotics have no impact on viruses. Some patients, however, develop complications of bacterial infections as the symptoms of a cold or allergic rhinitis linger. Sinusitis and ear infections, especially in young children, are examples of bacterial complications that should be treated with antibiotics.

Summary

Second-generation antihistamines, decongestants, and nasal corticosteroids, used individually or in combination, have been the mainstay of treatment for seasonal and perennial allergic rhinitis. An oral leukotriene modifier has recently been approved as another option. Severe allergic rhinitis may require a few days of oral corticosteroids. Sedation and diminished cognitive performance are the most problematic adverse effects associated with the first-generation antihistamines.

The second-generation antihistamines do not readily cross the blood-brain barrier and thus have significantly reduced incidence of these adverse effects. Both groups of antihistamines are effective in blocking the H_1 receptor in the nasal passage and thus decreasing the occurrence of sneezing, rhinorrhea, and itching. Nasal corticosteroids inhibit the inflammatory response, including the impact of prostaglandins and leukotrienes. Topical use of corticosteroids in this fashion is the most effective therapy for allergic rhinitis and usually lacks systemic adverse effects. Other drugs such as pseudoephedrine (a decongestant), montelukast (a leukotriene modifier), or cromolyn (a mast cell stabilizer) can also be used to help alleviate the symptoms of allergic rhinitis.

First-generation antihistamines are used to treat the common cold, not because of the histamine blocking ability, but because of the anticholinergic effects that are attributed to these drugs. Anticholinergic response inhibits nasal secretions and causes a drying of the nasal passage. Decongestants are also frequently a part of the OTC regimen to treat a cold. These drugs constrict the blood vessels in the nasal passage to open the airways. However, because they also constrict other peripheral blood vessels and affect glucose metabolism, decongestants should be used cautiously in patients with hypertension, heart disease, or diabetes. Expectorants (decrease viscosity of secretions), antitussives (inhibit cough), and analgesics (relief of sore throat pain) are among the other OTC drugs that are available to treat the common cold.

ROLE OF THE ATHLETIC TRAINER

As is the case for many other diseases, inadequate therapy for allergic rhinitis can hinder the athlete's performance for longer than necessary. Although the duration of a cold is relatively short and self-limiting, serious complications can develop, which can significantly delay the athlete's return to normal activity level. Because both allergic rhinitis and the common cold are often self-medicated with OTC medication by the athlete, the potential exists for adverse effects from the OTC medication and/or drug interactions with other medications that the athlete is taking to treat other conditions. The role of the athletic trainer should focus on whether the athlete is taking the medications as prescribed (ie, right dose at the right time) and whether the athlete is experiencing sufficient response so that the negative impact of the disease and the therapy are minimized. Examples of therapy considerations of which the athletic trainer should be cognizant are:

- Does the athlete adhere to the dosage regimen prescribed by the physician? If effectiveness of therapy is not optimal, poor compliance to therapy is often the reason.
- Is the athlete experiencing symptoms that could be attributed to adverse drug effects? If symptoms are not readily explained by a diagnosed disease, suspect the drug therapy. Either the adverse effects of individual drugs or the drug interactions from combinations of drugs may be the cause. The most common adverse effects are drowsiness from first-

generation antihistamines and CNS stimulation with decongestants. If the athlete feels lethargic, use of these antihistamines during the day may be the cause. If the athlete is not sleeping well at night, use of decongestants too close to bedtime may be the cause. The athletic trainer should not discount the fact that the magnitude of the adverse responses vary from person to person and may be enhanced by drug interactions.

- Is the athlete competing at the level where nasal decongestants would be banned substances (see Chapter 14)?
- Is the athlete taking appropriate actions to avoid allergens that are contributing to the allergic rhinitis?
- If nasal corticosteroids are part of the therapy, is the athlete using appropriate technique to administer the nasal spray? Appropriate technique is to first clear the nasal passage of mucus, tilt head slightly forward, place the tip of the nasal spray into one nostril and point the tip away from the nasal septum while holding the bottle upright, block the other nostril, spray while breathing in slowly through the nose (ie, with mouth closed), hold breath for a few seconds, and then exhale through the mouth.
- Are the symptoms of a common cold lingering too long? If the symptoms are getting worse instead of better after 7 to 10 days, if sinus headache is reoccurring, or if fever develops that was not present earlier, complications may have developed that require medical attention.
- Is the athlete taking OTC combination products to treat cold or allergy symptoms that include more drugs than necessary? Single component products are available so that a decongestant is used only when congestion is present, an analgesic is included only when pain relief is desired, etc.
- Is the athlete who will be training in conditions that have a significant risk of heat-related illnesses also taking any drugs (OTC or prescription) that may contribute to these illnesses, particularly systemic decongestants and first-generation antihistamines? If such therapy cannot be modified without adding risk of exacerbation of existing disease, extra precautions should be taken (eg, lighter clothing, better air circulation, exercising during the cooler part of the day, and ensuring adequate fluid and electrolyte intake) to avoid heat-related illnesses.

Summary

For the athletic trainer, key roles regarding drug therapy are to be watchful that the therapy is appropriately effective and to educate the athlete regarding appropriate use of the medications. The starting point for the athletic trainer is to know what to look for and what questions to ask. If the symptoms of allergic rhinitis or common cold do not respond adequately to therapy, or if the therapy causes problematic adverse effects, there is likely to be a negative impact on the athlete's performance.

BIBLIOGRAPHY

APhA Special Report. *Self-Care of the Common Cold in Pediatric Patients*. Washington, DC: American Pharmaceutical Association; 2000.

Banerji S, Anderson IB. Abuse of coricidin HBP cough and cold tablets: episodes recorded by a poison center. *Am J Health Syst Pharm*. 2001;58:1811-1814.

DeSimone EM II. A review of oral (H1) antihistamines. *US Pharmacist*. 2001;August(Suppl):3-11.

Justice HJ, Hall EH, Howard K. Managing allergic rhinitis in children. *U.S. Pharmacist*. 2001;Sept(Suppl):3-13.

Larsen JS. Antihistamines and quality of life. *U.S. Pharmacist.* 2001;26:87-96.

Newer antihistamines. *The Medical Letter.* 2001;43:35.

Noonan WC, Miller WR, Feeney DM. Dextromethorphan abuse among youth. Letter to the editor. *Arch Fam Med.* 2000;9:791-792.

Over-the-counter (OTC) cough remedies. *The Medical Letter.* 2001;43:23-26.

Sampey CS, Follin SL. Second-generation antihistamines: the OTC debate. *J Am Pharm Assoc.* 2001;41:454-457.

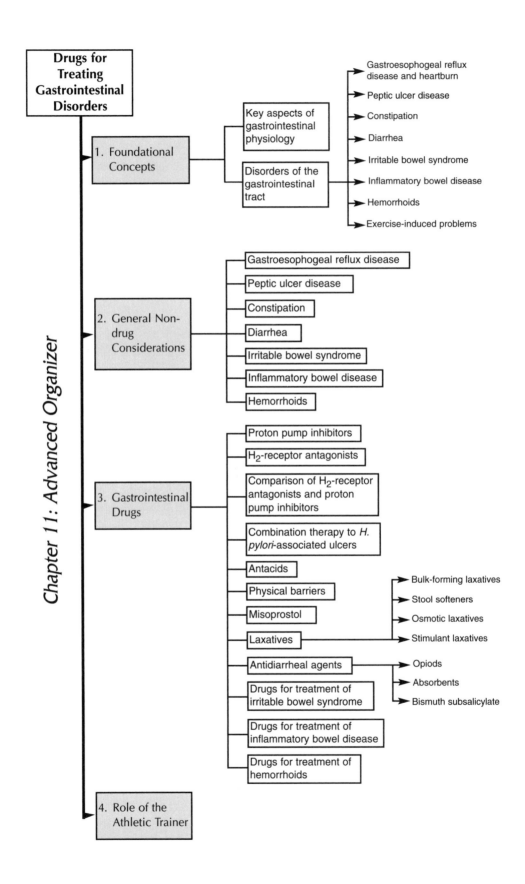

Drugs for Treating Gastrointestinal Disorders

Chapter 11: Advanced Organizer

1. Foundational Concepts
   - Key aspects of gastrointestinal physiology
   - Disorders of the gastrointestinal tract
     - Gastroesophogeal reflux disease and heartburn
     - Peptic ulcer disease
     - Constipation
     - Diarrhea
     - Irritable bowel syndrome
     - Inflammatory bowel disease
     - Hemorrhoids
     - Exercise-induced problems

2. General Non-drug Considerations
   - Gastroesophogeal reflux disease
   - Peptic ulcer disease
   - Constipation
   - Diarrhea
   - Irritable bowel syndrome
   - Inflammatory bowel disease
   - Hemorrhoids

3. Gastrointestinal Drugs
   - Proton pump inhibitors
   - H₂-receptor antagonists
   - Comparison of H₂-receptor antagonists and proton pump inhibitors
   - Combination therapy to *H. pylori*-associated ulcers
   - Antacids
   - Physical barriers
   - Misoprostol
   - Laxatives
     - Bulk-forming laxatives
     - Stool softeners
     - Osmotic laxatives
     - Stimulant laxatives
   - Antidiarrheal agents
     - Opiods
     - Absorbents
     - Bismuth subsalicylate
   - Drugs for treatment of irritable bowel syndrome
   - Drugs for treatment of inflammatory bowel disease
   - Drugs for treatment of hemorrhoids

4. Role of the Athletic Trainer

DRUGS FOR TREATING GASTROINTESTINAL DISORDERS

CHAPTER OBJECTIVES

At the end of this chapter, the reader will be able to:

- Explain the normal gastrointestinal (GI) physiological process and how drugs can affect this process.
- Explain the function of the proton pump in maintaining stomach acidity and how drugs affect the proton pump.
- Explain the pathophysiology and identify the signs and symptoms of gastroesophageal reflux disease (GERD), heartburn, and peptic ulcer disease (PUD) and recall how these conditions can be exacerbated.
- Explain the pathophysiology, signs and symptoms, and causes of constipation, diarrhea, irritable bowel syndrome (IBS), inflammatory bowel disease (IBD), and hemorrhoids.
- Summarize the effects of exercise on GI pathological conditions.
- Suggest nondrug interventions for the treatment of GERD, PUD, constipation, diarrhea, IBS, IBD, and hemorrhoids.
- Explain how proton pump inhibitors and H_2-receptor antagonists drugs affect GERD, PUD, and heartburn.
- Compare and contrast proton pump inhibitors and H_2-receptor antagonists categories of drugs.
- Describe a drug therapy regimen for the treatment of *Helicobacter pylori (H. pylori)*-associated ulcers.
- Summarize the mechanism of action, dosing regimen, and adverse effects of medications that are considered physical barriers in the treatment of GERD and PUD.
- Identify the different types of laxatives and recall their uses, mechanism of action, dosing regimen, and potential adverse effects.
- Identify common antidiarrheal medications and recall their mechanism of action, dosing regimen, and potential adverse effects and drug interactions.
- Identify the medications available to treat IBS and explain their mechanism of action.
- Explain the mechanism of action for drugs used to treat IBD and recall their potential adverse effects.
- Identify eight categories of hemorrhoidal medications and recall their mechanism of action and potential adverse effects.
- Summarize the role of the athletic trainer for patients who are self-medicating for GI symptoms or are on a physician-prescribed formal GI drug therapy regimen.

Figure 11-1. Stomach anatomy. During normal function, the lower esophageal sphincter (LES) prevents reflux of gastric acid and other contents into the esophagus, and the pylorus prevents unnecessary flow of gastric acid into the duodenum and also prevents entry of bile acids into the stomach (adapted from Lichtenstein GR. *The Clinician's Guide to Inflammatory Bowel Disease.* Thorofare, NJ: SLACK Incorporated; 2003.)

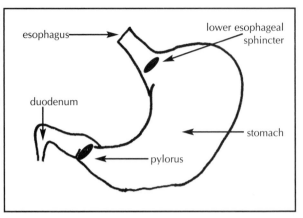

There are many GI disorders, with an array of varied characteristics. For example, the variation of some characteristics ranges from acute to chronic (traveler's diarrhea versus GERD); mild to incapacitating (heartburn versus IBS); fairly well understood to complex and poorly understood (PUD versus IBD); few therapy choices to many choices (diarrhea versus PUD). Consequently, it is beyond the intent of this book to discuss every GI disorder and appropriate therapy. The intent of this chapter is, however, to give the athletic trainer an overview of the most common GI disorders, their etiology, and the information regarding the most commonly used drugs for treatment of GERD, PUD, constipation, diarrhea, IBS, IBD, and hemorrhoids.

Many patients do not seek medical assistance for proper diagnosis and treatment of GERD, PUD, constipation, and diarrhea because, in part, there are many over-the-counter (OTC) medications available to treat these disorders. Because these are drugs that the athlete, like the general population, will be using with the least oversight by a health care professional, they are the focus of this chapter. The athletic trainer may be in a position to be the health care professional to provide some oversight in the form of basic advice regarding nondrug measures that may help alleviate symptoms, the appropriate use and potential effects from the drug therapy, or to refer the athletes with GI disorders to the appropriate health care professional for additional care.

FOUNDATIONAL CONCEPTS

The esophagus, stomach, and small intestine have several mechanisms to protect those tissues from being damaged and to keep them functioning properly. As a result of the harsh environment of acidity and digestive enzymes, an inappropriate diet, ingestion of certain drugs and chemicals, or the aging process, these mechanisms are compromised and result in GI disorders. A brief discussion of the GI disorders will be helpful to understand the mechanism of action and logic of the drug therapy. The focuses of this section are the cause and symptoms of these disorders. Common terminology is also defined.

Key Aspects of Gastrointestinal Physiology

From the mouth, the esophagus empties into the stomach (Figure 11-1) where the acidity can result in pH range of 1 to 5, depending on stomach contents. The lower esophageal sphincter (LES) provides a barrier between the stomach and the esophagus. This sphincter is usually constricted but relaxes during swallowing to allow the food to pass into the stomach. Because the

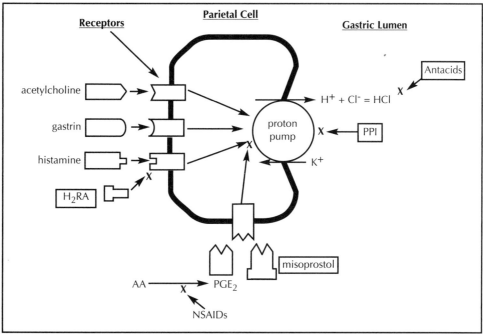

Figure 11-2. Production and inhibition of gastric acid. The parietal cell of the stomach is the source of acid production as it pumps protons (H+) into the gastric lumen to form hydrochloric acid (HCl). Acetylcholine, gastrin, and histamine bind to their respective receptors located on the surface of the parietal cell membrane, initiating a sequence of events inside the cell culminating in the secretion of protons by the proton pump. In a similar fashion, prostaglandin E_2 (PGE_2, see Chapter 6) binds to its receptor but causes a decrease in acid production as a mechanism to prevent excessive acid secretion. The drugs used to affect acidity are designated in ⬜ and their site of action designated by X. Proton pump inhibitors (PPIs), H_2-receptor antagonists (H_2RAs), and PGE_2 receptor agonists (misoprostol) decrease acid production whereas antacids neutralized the acid after it is released. The site of action of NSAIDs is also shown, which inhibit the protective effects of endogenous PGE_2.

esophagus does not have the same protective mechanisms as the stomach, one purpose of the sphincter is to prevent stomach acid and digestive enzymes from coming in contact with the esophageal tissue.

Gastric acid (hydrochloric acid) is released at a relatively low, baseline rate when food or other stimuli are not present. This baseline rate fluctuates, with greater production at night. The presence of food in the stomach causes the release of gastrin and acetylcholine, the latter also being released in response to the sight and smell of food. *Histamine* is also released by specialized stomach cells. The parietal cells of the stomach have receptors for histamine (H_2 *receptors*), *acetylcholine*, and *gastrin*. The binding of any of these three compounds to their respective receptor on the *parietal cells* (Figure 11-2) activates a process called the *proton pump* (also known as the H^+, K^+-ATPase), which actively transports hydrogen ions (protons = H^+) into the stomach to combine with chloride ions to form hydrochloric (HCl) acid. There are several mechanisms that help prevent excessive acid production. Two such mechanisms are the production of prostaglandins E_2 (PGE_2) and I_2 (PGI_2); PGE_2 inhibits acid secretion from parietal cells and PGI_2 increases secretion of protective mucus and bicarbonate buffer from epithelial cells.

One role of stomach acid in digestion is to activate the digestive enzyme *pepsin. Pepsinogen* is the inactive form of pepsin; it is produced by stomach cells and released into the stomach in response to autonomic regulation. The acid pH of the stomach catalyzes the conversion of pepsinogen to pepsin.

When food leaves the stomach, it enters the duodenum, the first segment of the small intestine, where most of the digestion and absorption of food (and drugs) occurs. The pyloric sphincter prevents intestinal enzymes and bile from entering the stomach and minimizes gastric acid movement into the small intestine. Damage to the duodenal mucosa can occur if gastric acid regularly passes into the duodenum. In the large intestine, normal bacterial flora has an important role because these bacteria break down waste products and produce some vitamins that are absorbed into the bloodstream. There are also a small number of potentially pathogenic bacteria and yeast that are present in the colon but, under normal circumstances, their numbers are too small to present a significant problem. Serious problems (diarrhea is a common symptom) can occur, however, if these pathogens are allowed to increase in number as a result of disease, diet, or drugs.

> *Drugs that combine with the acetylcholine receptor and have an action like acetylcholine are called cholinergic drugs. Because acetylcholine activates the parasympathetic nervous system, cholinergic drugs are also called parasympathomimetics.*

Peristalsis moves the contents through the small and large intestine. Mucus is produced to protect and lubricate the intestinal tract; local irritation and stress increase mucus production. The rhythmic movement of the intestinal smooth muscle and mucus secretion are increased by *parasympathetic* innervation and decreased by the *sympathetic* system. Consequently, *cholinergic* drugs will increase the rate at which the contents move through the intestine. If movement of intestinal contents is too fast, there is insufficient absorption of water and other intestinal contents from the intestine, and diarrhea results. Inhibition of the parasympathetic system (ie, anticholinergic drugs) causes constipation. Other mechanisms can also alter the normal absorption rate of water, electrolytes, and dietary contents and thus cause diarrhea or constipation. These include a change in the amount or type of bacteria in the intestinal flora, the presence of poorly absorbed substances (eg, magnesium ions), or inflammatory intestinal disease.

Disorders of the Gastrointestinal Tract

The GI disorders discussed in this section are primarily limited to those for which treatment is discussed later. The pathophysiology and mechanism of disease are discussed to an extent to facilitate an understanding of the approach to drug therapy.

Gastroesophageal Reflux Disease and Heartburn

Heartburn, also called acid indigestion, results from the contact of gastric acid, and to some extent bile and pepsin, with the esophageal mucosa. Heartburn feels like a burning chest pain primarily located behind the sternum but which may move upward toward the neck. Reflux of acid may cause spontaneous regurgitation of gastric contents to the throat, which can initiate bronchial constriction in patients with asthma. *Gastroesophageal reflux disease* (GERD) is a chronic condition that exists when heartburn occurs regularly (ie, more than twice a week). Because heartburn and GERD are often self-treated, it is difficult to accurately determine the incidence rate, but approximately one-third of adults experience heartburn symptoms at least once/month.

Repeated reflux for an extended period of time can result in reflux esophagitis or erosive esophagitis, which are associated with progressive inflammation and erosion of the esophageal

Box 11-1. Protective Stomach Mechanisms for Gastric Acid

- Secretion of the mucus barrier
- Secretion of the bicarbonate buffer
- Ability to repair damaged mucosal tissue
- Production of prostaglandins

mucosa. At least half of patients with untreated GERD have reflux esophagitis. *Barrett's esophagus* can occur as a result of years of reflux; this is a premalignant change in epithelial cells of the esophagus that significantly increases the risk of esophageal cancer. Approximately 10% to 20% of patients with chronic GERD will develop Barrett's and of these the incidence is 5% to 10% for the development of esophageal cancer.

The basic cause of heartburn is that the lower esophageal sphincter is inefficient in preventing the reflux of stomach contents into the esophagus; eventually, the presence of gastric acid and pepsin causes damage to esophageal tissue. A dysfunction of the pyloric sphincter can also allow some bile acid to enter the stomach and contribute to GERD symptoms.

The reflux of gastric acid, *pepsin*, and bile into the esophagus is most often due to spontaneous and transient relaxation of the sphincter. Reflux may also occur because of increased intra-abdominal pressure during straining, bending over, coughing, eating, or during pregnancy. Certain foods and drugs can directly irritate the esophageal mucosa, increase gastric acid production, or decrease the lower esophageal sphincter pressure, thereby decreasing sphincter effectiveness. Examples are chocolate, coffee, carbonated beverages, fatty foods, orange and tomato juice, tomato-based foods, spicy foods, garlic, onions, peppermint, spearmint, caffeine (from any source), anticholinergics, alcohol, aspirin, and other nonsteroidal anti-inflammatory drugs (NSAIDs). Fatty foods and large meals delay gastric emptying and increase the likelihood of reflux in patients who experience GERD. Factors that tend to protect the esophagus, such as the saliva buffering that coats the esophagus, diminish with age, and therefore damage to the esophagus occurs more often in the elderly. *Hiatal hernia* can also be the cause of GERD. This condition exists when the stomach partially sits in the chest cavity because of a weakness in the diaphragm. The severity of GERD depends on the amount and frequency of acid refluxing into the esophagus as well as the ability of the saliva to neutralize the acid. Long-term GERD can cause complications, including ulcer, cancer, or narrowing of the esophagus, which interferes with swallowing.

Peptic Ulcer Disease

Peptic ulcers are chronic erosion of the mucosa of the stomach (gastric ulcer) or small intestine (duodenal ulcer). Approximately 25 million Americans have *peptic ulcer disease* (PUD) during their lifetimes and there are about 6500 deaths annually from PUD-related complications (eg, GI bleeding). Abdominal pain is the most common symptom and may include burning or cramping, although some patients are asymptomatic. Pain often begins 1 to 3 hours after eating and is alleviated by food or antacids. Many patients have pain that awakens them from sleep. The most significant life-threatening problem associated with peptic ulcers is GI bleeding and *perforation.*

Gastric acid contributes to the cause of the peptic ulcer as well as the pain. There is usually an increased production of gastric acid associated with duodenal ulcers. However, the *ulcerogenic effect* of gastric acid occurs after one or more of the normal protection mechanisms have been compromised (Box 11-1). The defense mechanisms are compromised most frequently by use of

Box 11-2. Risk Factors That Increase the Occurrence of Peptic Ulcer Complications From Nonsteroidal Anti-Inflammatory Drugs

- Higher daily dosage
- Longer duration of daily use
- Advanced age of the patient, history of peptic ulcer
- Concurrent use of corticosteroids or anticoagulants

NSAIDs or by *Helicobacter pylori (H. pylori)* infection. There is also a significant causal relationship from cigarette smoking, but much less convincing correlation exists to directly connect diet and psychological stress as contributors.

Over half the people in the world may be infected with *H. pylori*, a gram-negative bacterium that has the ability to live between the mucus layer and the epithelial cells of the stomach. Transmission is by fecal to oral route such as through contaminated food or water. Mouth-to-mouth transfer is also possible. Only about 15% of the population infected with *H. pylori* eventually develop peptic ulcer, but almost everyone with non-NSAID-induced PUD are infected with *H. pylori*, and elimination of *H. pylori* significantly reduces the incidence of ulcer recurrence.

H. pylori has the ability to buffer hydrochloric acid in the organism's immediate vicinity and to cause damage to gastric mucosa by release of various enzymes and other factors produced by the organism. Other ramifications of the infection are an increased gastric acid secretion associated with duodenal ulcers and an altered immune response to the infection, which may contribute to the damage of gastric epithelial cells. Infection with *H. pylori* is the most common cause of duodenal and gastric ulcers.

> *Recall from Chapter 6 that synthesis of prostaglandins, thromboxanes, and prostacyclin (as a group referred to as eicosanoids) require the activity of an enzyme called cyclooxygenase (COX) and that there are two forms of the COX enzyme, COX-1 and COX-2. COX-1 is produced in virtually all tissues so that an appropriate level of eicosanoids exists to regulate normal functions. COX-2 is also produced for this purpose in some tissues, but the activity of COX-2 is greatly increased in response to pain and tissue injury. Prostaglandin production by stomach cells is a protection mechanism against the effects of stomach acid; NSAIDs diminish the protectant effect by inhibiting COX, particularly COX-1.*

NSAIDs are among the most commonly used prescription and OTC drugs and are the drugs most frequently associated with causing peptic ulcers. Repeated use of NSAIDs is the most common cause of PUD, particularly gastric ulcers, in patients not infected with *H. pylori*. Risk factors that increase the occurrence of complications from NSAID use are listed in Box 11-2. NSAIDs cause ulcers through topical irritation due to the acidic nature of most of these drugs, especially aspirin, and due to the systemic effect on prostaglandin synthesis. Additionally, these drugs may slow the healing process in existing peptic ulcers and contribute to GI bleeding as a result of their ability to inhibit platelet aggregation.

> *Recall from Chapter 6 that TXA$_2$ causes platelet aggregation but NSAIDs inhibit TXA$_2$ production in platelets. Aspirin has a more pronounced effect than other NSAIDs regarding this effect.*

Constipation

The "normal" frequency of bowel movements varies from one person to another and therefore the definition of constipation is not universal. Nonetheless, constipation is generally considered to exist if there are less than three bowel movements per week, if stools are hard and dry, if straining is necessary for bowel evacuation, or if there is a feeling of incomplete bowel evacuation. Although it occurs at any age, the incidence of constipation increases among those over 65 years old with about one-third of this population reporting constipation as a problem. Constipation is a symptom, not a disease itself.

The cause of constipation can be associated with endocrine diseases such as diabetes or hypothyroidism. The incidence of drug-induced constipation is most significant with the use of drugs that have *anticholinergic* effects (eg, *opioid analgesics, monoamine oxidase inhibitors, tricyclic antidepressants,* and *antihistamines*), and with calcium- or aluminum-containing antacids. Lifestyle, primarily related to diet and exercise, also influences bowel regularity. Dietary fiber increases the bulk of the fecal mass and stimulates peristalsis. Exercise increases abdominal muscle tone and facilitates the effect of gravity on bowel function. Sufficient water intake is also an important aspect to prevent dry, hard stools that can cause constipation. Water depletion from exercise must also be considered. As people get older, changes in diet, exercise, muscle tone, and therapeutic drug regimens may all be contributing factors to constipation. Another cause of constipation related to lifestyle is merely a conscious effort to prevent a bowel movement because of inconvenient timing (ie, busy lifestyle).

Besides a diminished frequency of bowel movements, other symptoms of constipation can include anorexia, headache, back pain, and abdominal discomfort. Further complications from constipation are primarily due to the need to strain during a bowel movement. Such an effort can eventually result in hemorrhoids, and patients with existing heart problems or hypertension can exacerbate those conditions while straining.

Diarrhea

Diarrhea is an increased frequency of bowel movements or decreased consistency of stool compared to the normal for that person. Two bowel movements per day could be normal for one person but considered diarrhea for another. As with constipation, diarrhea is not a disease but rather a symptom of an underlying condition. Most episodes of diarrhea are self-limiting but severe or chronic cases can be fatal, usually as a result of dehydration. Acute diarrhea usually lasts 1 to 3 days but could extend as long as 2 weeks. Chronic diarrhea lasts for a few weeks or more and requires more extensive medical attention to diagnose the cause, to monitor the patient's hydration and nutritional status, and to treat appropriately with both drug and nondrug measures. The focus of this discussion will be acute diarrhea.

The intestine absorbs almost 9 L of fluid per day, most of it from the small intestine. Diarrhea occurs because of a change in the normal processes of absorption or secretion of water and electrolytes from the intestine or a decrease in the amount of time to travel through the intestinal tract (ie, increased motility), which prevents fluid reabsorption. If the amount of water in the colon exceeds the amount that can be reabsorbed, diarrhea will result. This can occur for several reasons. Some illness such as acquired immunodeficiency syndrome, IBD, and IBS have diarrhea as part of the symptomatology. Some drugs cause diarrhea by directly affecting the intestinal content of water and electrolytes

> *Patients with lactose intolerance lack the digestive enzyme lactase. Therefore, lactose remains in the GI tract and becomes a nutrient for bacterial flora. By-products of enhanced bacterial metabolism cause cramps and diarrhea.*

(eg, antacids containing magnesium), disrupting the normal bacterial flora (eg, antibiotics, especially broad spectrum such as tetracyclines), damaging GI epithelial cells (eg, some anticancer drugs), or increasing GI motility with *cholinergic agonists* such as bethanechol (Urecholine), which is used to treat urinary retention. Some undigested foods have a laxative effect, such as foods that are very fatty or have high roughage content. Patients who are lactose intolerant will experience diarrhea from lactose-containing foods (eg, dairy products).

Most cases of diarrhea, however, are caused by bacterial, *protozoal*, and viral infections, often through contaminated food or water. For example, traveler's diarrhea is usually caused by various bacteria; the major causative agent differing from country to country. In the United States, *Campylobacter, Salmonella,* and *Escherichia coli (E. coli)* are often pinpointed as causative bacteria in food contamination. Some bacteria cause diarrhea by producing toxins whereas others directly affect the intestinal mucosal cells. Damage to epithelial intestinal cells decrease the absorption of solutes to cause an osmotic effect (ie, an increase in water content) in the GI tract. An inflammatory response to the infection decreases water absorption and increases mucus release into the intestinal lumen.

Most viral-induced diarrhea is from the 24-hour flu-type viruses that produce a sudden onset of diarrhea, which lasts 24 to 48 hours. *Giardia lamblia* is a common cause of protozoal diarrhea. It is transmitted by ingestion of fecal material from contaminated streams or lakes and is also prevalent among day care centers.

Symptoms of acute diarrhea include frequent, watery stools; abdominal cramps; fever; vomiting; and weakness. Symptoms may occur within hours or take a few days, depending on the cause. For example, infection with *Salmonella* will initiate symptoms within 12 to 24 hours and *E. coli* 8 to 72 hours, whereas it takes 2 to 4 days for the onset of symptoms from *Campylobacter* and 1 to 3 weeks for *Giardia*. Symptoms from most infectious diarrhea are self-limiting and last a few days, although *Giardia* may persist if not treated adequately. The most common complication of diarrhea is dehydration. Symptoms of mild dehydration are dry mouth and thirst. If dehydration progresses, additional symptoms may include dry mucous membranes, increased pulse, rapid breathing, lethargy, and confusion.

Irritable Bowel Syndrome

IBS is a common disorder in which the colon, for no apparent reason, is more sensitive to stimuli than normal. As a result, diet, hormones, and nerve impulses have an enhanced impact on the contraction of the large intestinal smooth muscle. For example, psychological or emotional stress (which may include anxiety or depression) and foods (eg, dairy products, onions, beans, broccoli, chocolate, alcohol, caffeine, dietary fat, and herbal teas) are common triggers. Onset of symptoms is often early adulthood and is typically initiated during a stressful event. For some patients, symptoms improve and disappear; for others they persist. IBS has also been referred to as spastic colon and colitis, the latter being particularly misleading as IBS is not an inflammatory condition and should not be confused with ulcerative colitis. There is no known underlying disease that causes the symptoms of IBS, nor does IBS eventually progress to another disease.

The most common symptoms of IBS are abdominal cramps and pain; gassiness; bloating; and either diarrhea, constipation, or diarrhea alternating with constipation. The diarrhea results from the increased frequency and force of smooth muscle contraction, and the constipation is caused by spasms that delay movement through the colon. The frequency and extent of these symptoms vary among patients from mild to disabling. Diagnosis is primarily based on the elimination of other causes of the symptoms.

Inflammatory Bowel Disease

Inflammatory bowel disease (IBD) is a term that refers to two similar diseases: *Crohn's disease* and *ulcerative colitis*. As the name implies, a major characteristic of these diseases is inflammation. Inflammatory bowel disease can affect people of all ages, but the onset of symptoms is usually between 15 and 25 years old and the incidence is about 5 per 100,000 population. Crohn's disease usually involves the small and large intestines but can affect any part of the digestive tract. All layers of the intestinal wall can be affected and the lesions are not continuous (ie, not confined to one area). Ulceration of intestinal tissue causes significant damage. Ulcerative colitis involves inflammation of the colon and rectum. Inflammation does not involve the full thickness of the bowel wall and the affected area is continuous. The cause of these diseases is unknown, but it is likely that genetic factors predispose patients to an autoimmune mechanism. So that, for example, antibodies produced in response to a microbial infection are antibodies of a genetically determined structure that happen to also attack the patient's own normal cells of the GI tract.

The symptoms of IBD include painful abdominal cramps and pain, fever, diarrhea, rectal bleeding, anemia, and weight loss. There are different levels of severity (mild, moderate, severe) among patients and the severity fluctuates over time for any given patient. In all cases, however, these diseases have pronounced symptoms and potential for complications involving other tissues (eg, eyes, joints, liver, and skin). The nature of these diseases necessitate that the patient be under the direct and careful supervision of a physician. Drug therapy is a necessary part of treatment but dietary modification and management of the resulting emotional stress are also a part of the treatment approaches. When drug therapy cannot control the symptoms, surgery is indicated to remove the affected portion of intestine. Surgery is usually curative for ulcerative colitis where the affected area is confined but recurrence is the norm for Crohn's disease.

Hemorrhoids

Hemorrhoids (or piles) are painful swelling at the anus of hemorrhoidal blood vessels. The vessels involved may be venous or arterial and may be internal or external; some patients have a combination of internal and external. Many factors have been attributed to the cause of hemorrhoids. Among these are pregnancy, constipation, diarrhea, straining with stool, heavy lifting with straining, prolonged sitting or standing, and heredity.

Mild symptoms of hemorrhoids include bleeding, itching, burning, and inflammation. More severe symptoms are increased bleeding, anal pain, protrusion outside the anal canal of hemorrhoidal or rectal tissue, seepage of fecal material, or blood clot formation within the blood vessel. Bleeding can occur with external hemorrhoids and almost always occurs with internal hemorrhoids, typically after defecation. Chronic blood loss can cause anemia. Symptoms similar to hemorrhoids are also a part of other anorectal diseases (eg, polyps and cancer), and therefore accurate diagnosis is necessary. As discussed below, there are many OTC products available to treat the various symptoms associated with hemorrhoids but large or protruding hemorrhoids are often surgically removed.

Exercise-Induced Problems

Some GI symptoms may be a result of, or exacerbated by, exercise. For example, diarrhea is a common problem among athletes, particularly participants in endurance sports. For long-distance runners, the persistent jarring of the intestinal tract during long-distance running or the diminished blood supply to the GI tract while the demand for blood to skeletal muscles is increased may play a role in causing diarrhea. Running may also aggravate pre-existing IBS in some patients. Diarrhea among early morning runners is a relatively common complaint. Gastroesophageal reflux disease occurs more frequently during exercise than at rest. Symptoms of GERD increase with increasing intensity of exercise, and exercise with more jarring is more problematic. Eating just prior to exercise can also contribute to symptoms of GERD.

Summary

Gastric acid is produced by the stomach and transported into the lumen by a proton pump mechanism (see Figure 11-2). Gastrin, acetylcholine, and histamine increase the release of gastric acid. The lower esophageal sphincter protects the esophagus from the damage by gastric acid. When the sphincter does not function properly, gastric acid can reflux into the esophagus and irritate the gastroesophageal mucosa, causing occasional heartburn or GERD if it occurs frequently. GERD-associated erosive esophagitis can also develop. Citrus fruits and juices, carbonated beverages, coffee, caffeine, alcohol, fatty and spicy foods, and NSAIDs exacerbate GERD symptoms. The most common symptom is chest pain located behind the sternum. Exercise, such as running that involves jarring of the abdominal organs, and exercise soon after eating, can contribute to GERD symptoms.

PUD encompasses gastric and duodenal ulcers. Chronic use of NSAIDs and the presence of *H. pylori* are the two causative agents linked to most PUD. Gastric acid contributes to cause and symptoms of PUD. Abdominal pain is a common symptom, especially 1 to 3 hours after eating. The potential for GI bleeding and perforation are also serious concerns.

Acute constipation is a common GI disorder, and although adverse effects of drugs are sometimes the cause, proper diet, exercise, and adequate fluid intake can prevent the problem in many situations. Diarrhea, on the other hand, may be caused by food, infection, drugs, or long-distance running in some athletes. Diarrhea and/or constipation are also among the most common symptoms of IBS, along with bloating, gassiness, and cramps. Patients with IBS are very sensitive to stimuli that cause these symptoms; common stimuli include certain foods and stress.

Inflammatory bowel disease refers to Crohn's disease and ulcerative colitis. Inflammation of various portions of the intestine, possibly due to an autoimmune mechanism, causes diarrhea, cramps, and pain. Other tissues (eg, eyes, joints, liver, and skin) may also be involved. Drug therapy, diet, and stress management are part of therapy but surgery is an option if these are insufficiently effective.

Hemorrhoids result from the swelling of hemorrhoidal vessels and can cause itching, burning, anal pain, and bleeding. Factors that precipitate hemorrhoids include pregnancy, poor bowel habits, heavy lifting and straining, sitting and standing for prolonged periods, and heredity.

GENERAL NONDRUG CONSIDERATIONS

There are a few nondrug measures that can be taken to help alleviate and reduce the recurrence of symptoms from the GI disorders discussed in this chapter. A change of lifestyle to incorporate these measures may be the most difficult aspect of therapy for some patients.

Gastroesophageal Reflux Disease

Treatment is aimed at alleviating the immediate symptoms, decreasing the frequency and/or acidity of the reflux, promoting healing of the esophageal mucosa, and preventing recurrence. Sometimes a combination of approaches is warranted to eliminate symptoms and facilitate healing. There are several nondrug measures that should be implemented to assist in accomplishing these treatment goals (Box 11-3).

Box 11-3. Nondrug Measures That Can Assist in the Treatment of Gastro-esophageal Reflux Disease

- Avoid foods that exacerbate symptoms such as fatty or spicy foods, onions (increase acid production), coffee, caffeine, alcohol, chocolate, citrus juices, tomato juice, carbonated beverages (increase pressure in the stomach and contributes to reflux), peppermint, and spearmint (decrease LES).

- Stop cigarette smoking.

- Elevate the head of the bed 6 to 8 inches by raising the legs at the head of the bed or by placing supports under the mattress. This improves clearance of acid from the esophagus. Merely adding pillows may increase reflux due to the sharper change in abdominal position.

- Avoid large meals or lying down within 3 hours after eating (eg, eating before bedtime).

- Minimize anything that increases abdominal pressure such as obesity, straining during bowel movements, and tight-fitting clothing.

- Eliminate as much as possible the use of drugs that have anticholinergic effects (eg, antihistamines, tricyclic antidepressants, and opioid analgesics), which will delay the movement of food from the stomach.

- Use a large amount of liquid when taking drugs that have a direct mucosal irritating effect such as NSAIDs, tetracycline antibiotics, iron, potassium supplements, and oral bisphosphonates such as alendronate (Fosamax) and risedronate (Actonel), which are used to treat osteoporosis. This helps to move the drug through the esophagus quicker.

- Avoid vigorous exercise for 2 to 3 hours after eating.

Peptic Ulcer Disease

PUD is not a self-treatment disease. Patients who have symptoms related to PUD should first obtain appropriate diagnosis. If use of NSAIDs is not a contributor to PUD, then infection with *H. pylori* is likely. Tests are available to confirm the presence of the organism. The treatment regimen will vary depending on the etiology of the disease. For example, eradication of *H. pylori* is the principle effort in treating PUD caused by this infection, whereas diminishing the effect of NSAIDs and inhibiting gastric acid production is the focus of therapy for NSAID-induced PUD. In either case, prescription drugs are a part of the most effective drug regimen. Regardless of the underlying cause, however, the goal for treating PUD is to alleviate pain, facilitate healing, and to prevent recurrence of the disease. Some specific nondrug measures that are helpful in accomplishing these treatment goals include eliminating the use of NSAIDs, avoiding foods that aggravate the patient's symptoms (eg, alcohol, caffeine, carbonated beverages, and spicy foods), and eliminating cigarette smoking. If use of NSAIDs cannot be eliminated,

> *As noted later in this chapter, magnesium has a laxative effect whereas aluminum has a constipating effect. Also, recall from Chapter 10 that first-generation antihistamines may have anticholinergic adverse effects, which include constipation.*

then either lowering the dose or switching to an NSAID that is more selective for *COX-2* (see Table 6-4) may decrease the problem. The use of corticosteroids in combination with NSAID therapy increases the risk of PUD and exacerbates existing PUD. Therefore, this combination should be avoided in patients with PUD, and other patients using these drugs concurrently should be monitored for PUD. The evidence is not clear whether oral corticosteroid therapy alone contributes to PUD but caution warrants that patients on corticosteroid therapy be watchful for the symptoms of PUD.

Constipation

There are several classes of drugs that are effective in the treatment of constipation, but therapy should also include lifestyle changes that can help alleviate the problem. Among these lifestyle changes are adequate fiber and fluid intake. Adult daily fiber intake should be 20 to 30 g. This can be achieved through high fiber foods such as bran cereals, fruits (especially apricots, dates, apples, prunes, and raisins), vegetables (especially green beans, peas, corn, broccoli, and carrots), and legumes. Plenty of fluid intake, primarily water, is also important, although the amount necessary varies depending on factors such as daily fluid loss (eg, sweating) and kidney function. Regular exercise can also help to maintain normal bowel function. Not to be overlooked is the contribution of drug therapy to the cause of constipation. In some cases, a change in therapy may be possible without sacrificing therapeutic outcomes (eg, switching from aluminum-containing *antacid* to one containing both aluminum and magnesium, or switching from a first-generation to a second-generation *antihistamine* for treatment of allergies).

Diarrhea

Acute mild to moderate diarrhea is by definition self-limiting and can usually be readily managed by combining drug therapy with nondrug measures. The goals of therapy are to relieve the symptoms and prevent fluid and electrolyte loss. Patients with severe or chronic diarrhea, however, should seek medical assistance so that the underlying cause can be determined and treated. This includes patients who experience diarrhea along with repeated vomiting, high fever, abdominal pain, or blood in the stools.

Regular diet may be suitable for patients with diarrhea, although avoiding foods rich in fat, simple sugar, spices, or caffeine may be advantageous as these could contribute to diarrhea. A priority in dietary management is to prevent depletion of fluids and electrolytes. Oral rehydration products are available that contain sodium and other electrolytes along with a low concentration of glucose (2.5%). The active transport of glucose during absorption from the GI tract also facilitates the absorption of sodium and water. However, the use of high concentrations of glucose (>10%) and other simple sugars can have an osmotic diarrhea effect and thus cause additional problems. Sports drinks that do not have high glucose concentrations (eg, Gatorade, Powerade, All Sport) may be used as a rehydration solution for mild diarrhea in older children and adults, especially if additional sodium is provided (eg, crackers).

If the cause of acute diarrhea can be identified, then removal of the causative agent is obviously a part of nondrug measures. For example, if the cause is lactase deficiency, then identifying and removing the source of lactose is appropriate. Diarrhea from the use of antibiotics, NSAIDs, or other drugs may warrant a change in drug therapy or reduction of the dosage.

Irritable Bowel Syndrome

The focus of nondrug treatment is management of diet, eating habits, and stress. Keeping a diary of foods eaten and symptoms experienced may help pinpoint specific foods that are exacerbating the disease. Introducing gas into the intestine can also contribute to symptoms and therefore it may be helpful to eliminate carbonated beverages and chewing gum (which causes swallowing of air). Smaller rather than larger meals can also reduce cramping and diarrhea.

Patients with constipation as a predominate symptom should increase dietary fiber and fluid intake. Other approaches that are effective in reducing symptoms are stress management and relaxation, including exercise, which is helpful for some patients.

Inflammatory Bowel Disease

The most notable nondrug measure for patients with IBD is to maintain proper nutrition. Inflammation of the GI tract can diminish the digestion and absorption of food in that portion of the digestive tract. Obviously, patients who have had surgical removal of affected portions of the GI tract will have a similar problem. Dietary supplements are generally sufficient to satisfy the nutritional needs. Among the supplements, iron may be needed if blood loss has been significant and folic acid should be given with sulfasalazine therapy (see below) as this drug diminishes absorption of folic acid. Patients with severe IBD may require *parenteral* nutrition.

Hemorrhoids

Because poor bowel habits can contribute to hemorrhoids, improvement in these habits is a good starting point for treatment. Avoiding constipation, diarrhea, straining with stool, and prolonged sitting on the toilet are all helpful. To prevent constipation, the patient may need to modify dietary habits, such as increasing fiber and fluid intake, and add exercise. Patients should also avoid heavy lifting or straining. Taking these actions will not alleviate existing symptoms but may reduce further aggravation of these symptoms. Use of a *sitz bath* for several minutes 2 to 3 times a day may provide some symptomatic relief.

Summary

Not surprising, diet and eating habits have an impact on the occurrence of symptoms for each of the diseases or conditions that affect the GI tract. Therefore, a common recommendation among the nondrug measures for treating these conditions is dietary modification. Fatty or spicy food, onions, coffee, alcohol, chocolate, citrus juices, and carbonated beverages are among the foods that can exacerbate symptoms of GERD. Many of these same foods are problematic for patients with PUD. Patients with constipation should increase the amount of high fiber foods in their diet and enhance their fluid intake. Diarrhea, on the other hand, requires the patient to guard against fluid and electrolyte loss. Certain foods may exacerbate symptoms of IBS but the causative foods differ somewhat from patient to patient. Patients can monitor their diet along with occurrence of symptoms to identify the foods that should be avoided. For IBD, rather than avoiding foods, nutritional supplementation is of greatest diet-related concern.

Drugs can also adversely impact these diseases. Drugs such as NSAIDs, tetracycline antibiotics, potassium, iron supplements, and oral *bisphosphonate drugs* can irritate the mucosa of the esophagus and enhance the pain associated with GERD. NSAIDs are also the major contributor to the drug-induced symptoms of PUD. Many drugs have the potential to cause constipation or diarrhea. In particular, however, drugs that have anticholinergic adverse effects and calcium- and aluminum-containing antacids can contribute to constipation; NSAIDs and some antibiotics are potential causes of drug-induced diarrhea.

GASTROINTESTINAL DRUGS

Most approaches to therapy for GERD and PUD are to neutralize the existing acidity of gastric acid, inhibit the secretion of the acid, physically block the effect of the acid on tissue, or to

Table 11-1. Proton Pump Inhibitors—Typical Adult Oral Dosage Regimens[1]

Generic Name	Trade Name	Peptic Ulcer Disease	GERD	GERD with Erosive Esophagitis	GERD Maintenance
esomeprazole	Nexium	na	20 mg	20 to 40 mg	20 mg
lansoprazole	Prevacid	15 to 30 mg	15 mg	30 mg	15 mg
omeprazole[2]	Prilosec	20 to 40 mg	20 mg	20 mg	20 mg
pantoprazole	Protonix	40 mg	na	40 mg	na
rabeprazole	Aciphex	20 mg	20 mg	20 mg	20 mg

[1]*All dosages are once per day, and except for maintenance therapy, duration is for 4 to 8 weeks.*

[2]*Also available OTC at 20 mg/day for 14-day treatment of frequent (≥ twice/week) heartburn; all others available only by prescription.*

na = not approved use by FDA.

increase the natural protective effects of mucus. Drugs that inhibit the secretion of gastric acid or chemically neutralize the acidity will cause an increase in gastric pH, which is an important factor to facilitate healing, and decrease the activation of pepsinogen to pepsin. The longer the period of time during the day that the pH is maintained above 4, the better the esophageal healing rate from GERD-induced damage. Chronic constipation and diarrhea may be caused from an underlying disease and thus a key part of treatment involves treating the underlying disease. Acute mild constipation and diarrhea, however, may be *idiopathic*, self-limiting, and respond adequately to OTC medications.

Not surprising, the site of action of many of the GI drugs discussed in this chapter is within the GI tract; many are not appreciably absorbed and thus their systemic effects are somewhat minimal. Even the GI drugs that work through a systemic mechanism (Proton Pump Inhibitors [PPIs] and Histamine-receptor antagonists [H$_2$RA]) have relatively few prominent adverse effects. Consequently, discussions of the pharmacological effects are relatively brief.

Proton Pump Inhibitors

PPIs are the most effective therapy for treatment of GERD, erosive esophagitis, maintenance therapy of GERD, and PUD. These drugs inhibit the H$^+$, K$^+$-ATPase (see Figure 11-2). This ATPase is an enzyme that secretes protons (ie, acidity) into the stomach in exchange for K$^+$ and therefore is also called the proton pump. As shown in Figure 11-2, the mechanism by which acetylcholine, gastrin, and histamine increase acidity is by activating the proton pump. Therefore, the effects of acetylcholine, gastrin, and histamine on acid secretion are inhibited by PPIs. These drugs irreversibly inhibit the ATPase enzyme and thus have a longer *duration of action*, making dosing once per day effective. Dosing is preferably about 30 minutes before a meal. Adult doses are shown in Table 11-1.

Recall from Chapter 2 that cytochrome P450 (CYP450) is a group of enzymes that are located in the liver and metabolize drugs.

All PPIs are inactivated by gastric acid, and thus the oral products contain an *enteric* coating that is dissolved in alkaline pH. Consequently, to ensure that the coating protects the drug, these products should not be crushed or chewed, and they should not be taken with meals because

Table 11-2. H$_2$-Receptor Antagonists—Typical Adult Oral Dosage Regimens

Generic	Trade	Heartburn	GERD	Peptic Ulcer Disease	Peptic Ulcer Maintenance
cimetidine	Tagamet	200 mg prn 1 to 2 times/day	400 mg qid or 800 mg bid	800 mg hs or 300 mg qid or 400 mg bid	400 mg hs
famotidine	Pepcid	10 mg prn 1 to 2 times/day	20 mg bid	40 mg hs or 20 mg bid	20 mg hs
nizatidine	Axid	75 mg prn 1 to 2 times/day	150 mg bid	300 mg hs or 150 mg bid	150 mg hs
ranitidine	Zantac	75 mg prn 1 to 2 times/day	150 mg bid	300 mg hs or 150 mg bid	150 mg hs

bid = twice a day; hs = at bedtime; prn = as needed; qid = four times a day

secretion of gastric acid is increased during this time. The PPIs are rapidly absorbed from the small intestine. They have half-life (t½) of about 1 to 2 hours; however, their effect lasts much longer because they have an irreversible effect on the proton pump molecules.

The incidence of adverse effects from PPIs is relatively low and are usually mild, but can include headache, dizziness, nausea, constipation, or diarrhea. These drugs are metabolized by cytochrome P450 enzymes and thus have the potential to decrease the metabolism rate (ie, increase the effect) of several drugs, including warfarin (an anticoagulant), phenytoin (an anti-convulsant), and benzodiazepines (anti-anxiety drugs), because the PPIs are well-tolerated, one has reached OTC status, omeprazole (Prilosec). This drug is available as a delayed release, once per day product for treatment of frequent (two or more days per week) heartburn and is meant to be taken as a 14-day course of treatment.

H$_2$-Receptor Antagonists

Histamine (H$_2$)-receptor antagonists (H$_2$RAs), also known as H$_2$-blockers, are competitive antagonists to histamine receptors on the stomach parietal cells (see Figure 11-2). Therefore, these drugs suppress gastric acid secretion and are effective in treating mild heartburn, GERD, and PUD. The H$_2$RAs are most effective in inhibiting basal and nocturnal gastric acid secretion as compared with the secretion stimulated by food or other triggers.

The H$_2$RAs can be used alone or combined with antacids. Table 11-2 provides examples and dosages for the H$_2$RAs. Lifestyle changes, along with a couple of weeks of treatment with these drugs, are usually sufficient to alleviate symptoms of mild heartburn. Increased dosages and longer treatment period are required to treat GERD. For example, dosages for ranitidine (Zantac) can range from 75 mg per day for up to 2 weeks for mild heartburn to 1200 mg per day for up to 12 weeks for erosive esophagitis associated with GERD. In general, the higher dosage regimen and more frequent dosing interval provide better healing rates. Not surprising, however, is that patients with less severe GERD experience higher healing rates when comparing any given dosage regimen.

The H$_2$RAs are all absorbed orally, some metabolism occurs in the liver but kidney excretion is the major means by which drug action is terminated. The incidence of adverse effects (eg, headache and diarrhea) is low for the H$_2$RAs and, as a result, they are available OTC for self-treatment of heartburn or mild GERD. These drugs are approximately equally effective and thus selection can be based on personal preference and/or cost. The one exception is regarding cimetidine (Tagamet), which, compared to the other H_2RAs, has a higher incidence of drug interactions, especially at higher doses. Cimetidine inhibits cytochrome P450 and therefore can increase the effect of other drugs that are also substrates for these enzymes. Examples include warfarin, phenytoin, and benzodiazepines.

Comparison of H_2-Receptor Antagonists and Proton Pump Inhibitors

Therapy with PPIs is more effective in treatment of moderate to severe GERD than treatment with H_2RAs. After 4 weeks of therapy, for example, healing rates are approximately 80% and 50% for PPIs and H_2RAs, respectively. Healing rates increase after 8 weeks of therapy but are again higher for PPIs. Patients with severe GERD who are placed on maintenance therapy to prevent relapse have a lower incidence of relapse with PPIs than patients on H_2RAs. The use of an H_2RA at bedtime as an addition to PPI therapy has been effective to resolve nighttime symptoms of GERD, which sometimes occur as a result of increased nocturnal secretion rates.

Both of these categories of drugs are effective for treatment of PUD, or as maintenance therapy for patients with recurrent ulcer symptoms. All of the H_2RAs are approximately equally effective in the treatment of PUD, as are all of the PPIs in comparison with each other. However, healing rates are somewhat higher, and relapse rates lower, with PPIs compared with H_2RAs. A PPI is generally recommended as a component of the three-drug regimen to treat *H. pylori*-associated ulcer (see below). Proton pump inhibitors are also the preferred treatment of gastric ulcers induced by NSAIDs or if the NSAID therapy must be continued despite the gastric or duodenal ulcer. As preventative therapy for patients taking NSAIDs and who are at risk for PUD (ie, elderly, PUD history, high dose NSAID, and concurrent use of corticosteroids or anticoagulants), PPIs or misoprostol (see below) are preferred. Use of H_2RAs may prevent NSAID-induced duodenal ulcers but is less effective in preventing gastric ulcers, which occur more frequently than duodenal ulcers from NSAID use.

Combination Therapy to Treat H. pylori-Associated Ulcers

Many combinations of drugs and varied dosage regimens have been used to treat ulcers associated with *H. pylori*. The intent of therapy is to treat immediate symptoms of PUD and to eradicate the infection as a means of preventing relapse. There is no treatment regimen that has attained universal acceptance as the ideal treatment. Rather, several different combinations of drugs and varied dosage regimens have demonstrated eradication rates of >80%. Use of just one drug does not achieve the same eradication rate nor is it as effective in preventing reoccurrence. For example, patients with *H. pylori*-associated PUD who are treated with H_2RAs alone have a recurrence rate of >85% within 1 year, whereas patients treated with *H. pylori*-eradication therapy have recurrence of 6% to 20%. Although two-drug regimens demonstrate a marked improvement in eradication rates compared to one-drug regimens, a variety of three-drug regimens are generally considered superior. The use of four-drug regimens has also been effective but introduces another layer of potential adverse effects and increases the likelihood of poorer compliance to therapy.

Table 11-3 lists some multiple drug regimens that are used. These combinations each include one or more antibiotics and either a PPI or an H_2RA. Chapter 5 discusses general principles regarding the use and effects of antibiotics, including specific aspects of therapy with penicillins and tetracyclines. Metronidazole is used to treat various *protozoal* infections but is also effective

Table 11-3. Examples of Drug Regimens to Eradicate *H. pylori*

	Drug Combination	Daily Dosage	Duration
1.	esomeprazole	40 mg once/day	10 days
	amoxicillin	1000 mg bid	10 days
	clarithromycin	500 mg bid	10 days
2.	lansoprazole	30 mg bid	10 to 14 days
	amoxicillin	1000 mg bid	10 to 14 days
	clarithromycin	500 mg bid	10 to 14 days
3.	lansoprazole	30 mg tid	14 days
	amoxicillin	1000 mg tid	14 days
4.	omeprazole	20 mg bid	10 days
	amoxicillin	1000 mg bid	10 days
	clarithromycin	500 mg bid	10 days
5.	omeprazole	40 mg once	14 days
	clarithromycin	500 mg tid	14 days
6.	rabeprazole	20 mg bid	7 days
	amoxicillin	1000 mg bid	7 days
	clarithromycin	500 mg bid	7 days
7.	ranitidine bismuth citrate	400 mg bid	28 days
	clarithromycin	500 mg tid	14 days
8.	bismuth subsalicylate	500 mg qid	14 days
	metronidazole	250 mg qid	14 days
	amoxicillin	500 mg qid	14 days
9.	bismuth subsalicylate	500 mg qid	7 to 14 days
	metronidazole	250 mg qid	7 to 14 days
	tetracycline	500 mg qid	7 to 14 days
10.	bismuth subsalicylate	500 mg qid	7 to 14 days
	metronidazole	250 mg qid	7 to 14 days
	tetracycline	250 to 500 mg qid	7 to 14 days
	omeprazole	20 mg bid	7 to 14 days

Generally the three- and four-drug regimens give higher eradication rates than two-drug regimens.

against anaerobic bacteria, including *Helicobacter*. Some adverse effects associated with the use of this antibiotic are nausea, vomiting, diarrhea, and a bad taste in the mouth. *Bismuth* has antibacterial effectiveness against *H. pylori* and is a component of several multiple drug regimens.

Antacids

The purpose of antacids is to neutralize some of the existing gastric acid and thus increase the gastric pH. Antacids are used for treatment of PUD, heartburn, or mild GERD although they are less effective than H$_2$RAs and PPIs to treat these conditions. The ability to neutralize acid is expressed as milliequivalents (mEq) of acid-neutralizing capacity (ANC). A dose of 40 to 80 mEq ANC is a reasonable starting dose. Typically, dosing is after meals and at bedtime; duration of use should not exceed 2 weeks.

The advantage of antacids is that they have a quick onset of action (5 to 15 minutes). The disadvantages of antacids are that they are significantly less effective in the treatment of GERD and PUD compared with other available drugs, have a short *duration of action* (<1 hour on an empty stomach), and have the potential for several adverse effects and drug interactions. The duration of action can be extended to 1 to 3 hours by use within 1 hour after eating, which delays gastric emptying and increases the time of contact with gastric acid. Nonetheless, the short duration requires frequent dosing to maintain continuous relief and also eliminates the possibility of effective suppression of gastric acid throughout the nighttime. Despite the significant disadvantages and the availability of more effective drugs, antacids remain popular for self-treatment of heartburn, GERD, and PUD. One of the more practical uses for these drugs is as an addition to acid suppression therapy (ie, H_2RAs or PPIs) on an "as needed" basis to provide relief of acute symptoms between doses of acid suppression therapy. Larger doses of some of these same products are used as laxatives.

Antacids are available as OTC products in many dosage forms, including suspensions, chewable tablets, and powders. The antacid components in these products are one or more salts of aluminum, magnesium, calcium, or sodium; the most common being aluminum hydroxide, magnesium hydroxide, calcium carbonate, and sodium bicarbonate (Table 11-4). As is often the case when there are so many similar OTC products available, the brand names can be confusing and even misleading. For example, Mylanta Gelcaps contain calcium carbonate and Mylanta Liquid contains aluminum hydroxide, whereas Mylanta Tablets and Mylanta Double Strength Liquid contain both aluminum and magnesium hydroxide.

Aluminum, magnesium, calcium, and sodium differ in their ANC, duration of action, and adverse effects. Aluminum salts decrease smooth muscle motility and thus cause constipation. Aluminum hydroxide has the lowest ANC but one of the longer durations of action. On the other hand, magnesium salts that enter the small intestine draw water into the intestine (osmotic effect) to cause diarrhea. Because aluminum causes constipation and magnesium causes diarrhea, these two are combined in many antacid products (see Table 11-4) in an effort to balance these effects; in reality, some diarrhea is often experienced. Some aluminum and magnesium are absorbed from the GI tract but are excreted by the kidney, thus accumulation of these ions is generally not a problem unless the patient has diminished kidney function.

Calcium carbonate and sodium bicarbonate (baking soda) have more ANC than aluminum and magnesium salts. However, when either of these two antacids react with gastric acid, they form carbon dioxide, which can cause belching and abdominal distention, both of which can increase esophageal reflux. Most of the calcium is not absorbed and can cause constipation. On the other hand, sodium bicarbonate is absorbed into the bloodstream. As with aluminum and magnesium salts, the calcium and sodium bicarbonate that are absorbed generally do not pose a problem. The exception is use of sodium bicarbonate, which can cause *metabolic alkalosis* in patients with reduced kidney function. The large sodium content may also be detrimental to patients who are trying to restrict their sodium intake. Therefore, sodium bicarbonate is not a preferred antacid and should not be used for an extended length of time.

The major potential for drug interactions is a result of the ability of the aluminum, magnesium, and calcium ions to bind to some drugs when they physically come in contact with them in the GI tract. The increase in gastric pH can also alter the solubility and absorption of some drugs and thus reduces their *bioavailability*. Examples are the binding of aluminum, magnesium, and calcium ions to tetracycline antibiotics to diminish their absorption, and the increase in gastric pH that reduces the absorption of some NSAIDs (including aspirin). *To avoid these problems, a general rule of thumb is that antacids should be used 2 hours apart from the oral administration of other drugs.*

Table 11-4. Selected Antacids

Trade Name	Aluminum Hydroxide[1]	Magnesium Hydroxide[1]	Calcium Carbonate[1]	Sodium Bicarbonate[1]
Amphojel (suspension)	320			
Amphojel (tablets)[2]	300			
Bromo Seltzer Effervescent Granules[3]				2781
Concentrated Phillips' Milk of Magnesia		800		
Extra Strength Maalox Suspension[4]	500	450		
Extra Strength Maalox Tablets[4]	350	350		
Maalox Antacid Caplets			1000	
Maalox Suspension	225	200		
Maalox Tablets	200	200		
Maalox Therapeutic Concentrate	600	300		
milk of magnesia (generic)		400		
Mylanta Double Strength Liquid[4]	400	400		
Mylanta Double Strength Tablets[4]	400	400		
Mylanta Gelcaps[5]			311	
Mylanta Liquid[4]	200			
Mylanta Tablets[4]	200	200		
Original Alka-Seltzer Effervescent Tablets[6]				1916
Phillips' Chewable		311		
sodium bicarbonate (tablets, generic)[7]				325
Tums			500	
Tums Ultra			1000	

[1]Content represents mg per dosage form or per 5 mL liquid.

[2]Also available as 600 mg.

[3]Also contains 325 mg acetaminophen.

[4]Also contains simethicone to reduce gas.

[5]Also contains 232 mg magnesium carbonate.

[6]Also contains 325 mg aspirin.

[7]Also available as 650 mg.

Physical Barriers

Sucralfate (Carafate) is more frequently used to treat peptic ulcers than GERD. It is the aluminum salt of sulfated sucrose. The acid environment of the stomach causes the sucralfate molecules to react with each other and become a viscous, sticky substance. The sucralfate adheres to epithelial cells to form a physical barrier of protection, especially in areas of damaged mucosa. Sucralfate also inhibits pepsin, binds to bile acids, and stimulates production of prostaglandins. Administration is recommended 1 hour prior to meals so that it is in sufficient contact with gastric acid and does not adhere to food components rather than to stomach epithelial cells and ulcer craters. Frequent dosing is required (four times per day) because the maximum duration of action is only 6 hours; a course of therapy is typically 4 to 8 weeks. As with antacids, sucralfate should be used 2 hours or more apart from other drugs to prevent potential drug interactions in the GI tract. Even with this 2-hour separation, the bioavailability of some drugs (eg, tetracycline, digoxin, ketoconazole, and the fluoroquinolone antibiotics) may be diminished; use of a different drug to treat PUD or GERD may be advisable for patients taking these other medications. Some patients experience constipation from the aluminum. Most of the sucralfate is excreted through the GI tract and thus systemic adverse effects are minimized.

Alginic acid is another drug that forms a physical barrier that may add protection from gastroesophageal reflux. Alginic acid is used in combination with various antacid combination products (eg, Gaviscon Tablets). When taken with a full glass of water, it forms a viscous foam that floats and provides a protective barrier to prevent reflux through the lower esophageal sphincter. This mechanism only works when the patient is in the upright position.

Misoprostol

Misoprostol (Cytotec) is a synthetic derivative of prostaglandin E_1 (PGE_1, see Chapter 6) and is used in conjunction with NSAID therapy to reduce the incidence of NSAID-induced ulcers. This drug adds back the protective effects of prostaglandins that the NSAIDs remove through inhibition of the COX-1 enzyme (see Figure 11-2). Misoprostol is a potent compound and hence the dosages are small, 100 to 200 μg 2 to 4 times per day with food. Adverse effects can be significant and include diarrhea, nausea, and abdominal cramps. A reduced dosage may be necessary in some patients to alleviate adverse effects. Misoprostol can cause uterine contractions, and thus is contraindicated during pregnancy or in patients in whom conception is a possibility.

Laxatives

The major categories of laxatives are bulk-forming, stool softeners, stimulant laxatives, and osmotic laxatives (Table 11-5). Selection of the appropriate laxative depends on the circumstances of the constipation. A bulk-forming laxative, for example, is more appropriate than a stimulant laxative for most patients with the need for more frequent use of a laxative. On the other hand, an osmotic laxative is more appropriate than a bulk laxative when a relatively quick evacuation of the bowel is desired. Some laxatives are also available for rectal administration as enemas (liquid applied into the rectum) or suppositories, which are usually cylinder or cone shaped semisolids made of a substance that melts at body temperature. Rectal administration offers an advantage if oral administration is undesirable (eg, due to nausea); however, there is some discomfort to the patient. Because the laxative reaches the colon immediately, the *onset of action* is shorter compared with oral administration (minutes versus hours). Patients with frequent or chronic constipation should see their physician to determine the cause and the appropriate treatment of the constipation.

Bulk-Forming Laxatives

Bulk-forming laxatives are generally nondigestible plant products such as psyllium (Metamucil) or semisynthetic cellulose material such as methylcellulose (Citrucel). These laxatives swell when in contact with fluid, forming a substance of gel consistency that stimulates peri-

Table 11-5. Examples of Over-the-Counter Laxatives

Classification	Generic Name	Trade Name	Dosage Form	Onset (h)
Bulk-forming	methylcellulose	Citrucel	Powder	12 to 72
	polycarbophil	Fiber-Lax	Tablets	12 to 72
	psyllium	Metamucil	Powder	12 to 72
Osmotic	magnesium citrate solution	generic	Solution	1 to 3
	magnesium hydroxide	generic milk of magnesia	Suspension	1 to 3
	polyethylene glycol solution	MiraLax	Solution	3 to 4
	sodium phosphate	Fleet Phospho-soda	Solution	1 to 3
	sodium phosphates	Fleet	Enema	<1
	glycerin	generic	Suppository	<1
Stimulant	bisacodyl	Dulcolax	Tablets	6 to 10
	bisacodyl	Fleet Bisacodyl	Enema	<1
	bisacodyl	Dulcolax	Suppository	<1
	cascara sagrada	generic	Tablets	6 to 8
	castor oil	Purge	Emulsion	2 to 6
	senna	Ex-lax	Tablets	6 to 10
Stool Softener	docusate	Colace	Capsules	12 to 72
	docusate	Therevac-SB	Enema	<1
	mineral oil	generic	Emulsion	6 to 8
	mineral oil	Fleet Mineral Oil	Capsules	<1

stalsis and travels readily through the GI tract, moving other intestinal contents with it at the same time. Consumption of at least 8 ounces of fluid per dose is important. Bulk-forming laxatives are the agents of choice for most patients with constipation and usually initiate a response in 12 to 72 hours. Systemic effects are rare because the laxative is not absorbed into the bloodstream. Bulk-forming laxatives can interfere with the absorption of some drugs (eg, tetracyclines, warfarin, and aspirin) when administered within 1 to 2 hours of the drug due to physical or chemical binding of the drug to the nonabsorbable laxative.

Stool Softeners

Stool softeners, such as docusate (Colace), are also called emollient laxatives. They are surfactants in that they reduce the surface tension to allow oil and water to mix, which results in softening of the stool and facilitates movement. Onset of action is 12 to 72 hours after oral use. These laxatives may be more useful in preventing constipation than treating it.

Mineral oil is usually categorized as a lubricant laxative because it coats the stool to facilitate easier movement; however, it also helps to keep the stool soft. It is not a preferred laxative and is the only lubricant laxative of practical use. Potential problems associated with use of mineral oil are aspiration into the lungs, anal leakage, and a decreased absorption of fat-soluble vitamins.

Osmotic Laxatives

Osmotic laxatives are agents that draw water into the intestinal lumen, which increases peristalsis. One group of osmotic laxatives is the saline laxatives. These are ions that are not appreciably absorbed from the GI tract, such as magnesium, sulfate, phosphate, and citrate. The onset of action is within a 1 to 3 hours and they are useful for an acute laxative effect rather than routine management of constipation. Laxative doses of magnesium hydroxide are larger than the antacid doses. Some magnesium ions are absorbed and therefore can lead to toxic levels of magnesium in the blood, especially in patients with reduced renal function. Abdominal cramps and nausea are potential adverse effects. As with antacid use, saline laxatives should be taken apart from other oral drug administration to avoid the potential for reduced absorption of the other drug.

Other examples of osmotic laxatives, but not saline-type, are Lactulose (Constilac) and polyethylene glycol (MiraLax). Lactulose is by prescription only and is a disaccharide that is not absorbed from the small intestine but is converted to organic acids in the large intestine, which then have an osmotic action to draw water into the lumen. Onset of action is 1 to 2 days and abdominal discomfort is common. Polyethylene glycol is not readily absorbed and also retains water in the intestine. It is recommended only for short-term use.

Glycerin is another osmotic laxative but is often referred to as a hyperosmotic because it has a local irritant effect along with the osmotic effect. It is absorbed orally and thus is not effective as a laxative by that route but is frequently used as a rectal suppository or enema. It causes a bowel movement in <1 hour and may cause a burning sensation during administration. Glycerin suppositories have been used for years in children and adults.

Stimulant Laxatives

The mode of action of the stimulant laxatives is a direct effect on the intestinal smooth muscle to increase motility. They may also cause an increase of water and electrolyte secretion into the intestine. Examples are cascara sagrada, senna (Ex-Lax), and bisacodyl (Dulcolax); all are available OTC and have an onset of action of 6 to 10 hours. They are not recommended for daily use but can be used occasionally for acute constipation or to evacuate the bowel prior to diagnostic procedures of the GI tract or prior to surgery. Castor oil (Purge) is also a stimulant laxative but has a shorter onset of action and has the potential to produce a strong peristaltic effect. The metabolism of castor oil in the small intestine produces an acid that is responsible for the stimulant effect. Abdominal cramps, which can be severe, are a common adverse effect of all of the stimulant laxatives.

Antidiarrheal Agents

There are only a few drugs available to provide symptomatic relief of diarrhea (ie, they do not resolve the underlying cause of the diarrhea). The exception may be bismuth subsalicylate, which has an antibacterial effect useful in the treatment of traveler's diarrhea.

Opioids

The principle opioids used to treat diarrhea are loperamide (Imodium), diphenoxylate (Lomotil), and difenoxin (Motofen).

> *Diphenoxylate (Lomotil) and difenoxin (Motofen) have similar effects because one is the metabolite of the other. The metabolism of diphenoxylate is an example of an active drug being converted by the liver to an active metabolite (see Chapter 2). In this case, the liver converts the active diphenoxylate to the active difenoxin:*
>
> *diphenoxylate ⟶ difenoxin.*

The antidiarrheal effect of these opioids is a result of their ability to combine with the μ-opioid receptor (see Chapter 7) on the GI smooth muscle, causing a decrease in motility. Although other opioids also diminish GI motility, these three drugs do not penetrate the CNS as readily as other opioids and therefore have significantly less potential for abuse and physical dependence. Among these three opioids, loperamide has the least abuse potential and thus is the only one that is not a controlled substance; difenoxin and diphenoxylate are schedule IV and V, respectively. A small amount of atropine (an *anticholinergic*) is added to diphenoxylate and difenoxin products to deter the use of higher doses for abuse purposes.

Because loperamide is very effective and has a low incidence of adverse effects, it is available OTC and thus is the most commonly used of the opioid antidiarrheals. It is used to treat acute nonspecific diarrhea (eg, traveler's diarrhea) as well as chronic diarrhea from various causes. For OTC use, the total daily dose should not exceed 8 mg. Loperamide is readily absorbed orally and is available in several dosage forms. Adverse effects can include drowsiness, dry mouth, nausea, vomiting, and constipation.

Although other opiates (eg, paregoric, opium tincture, and codeine) are effective in the treatment of diarrhea, they also have a higher incidence of adverse effects, potential for abuse, and they are controlled substances. Consequently, these products have a lower preference for use to treat diarrhea.

Absorbents

These compounds are nonselective in their ability to absorb other compounds and may be effective to treat nonspecific acute diarrhea. The most commonly used product is a combination of two absorbents, kaolin and pectin (Kapectolin). These compounds are not absorbed and therefore have negligible systemic effects. They may, however, interfere with the absorption of other drugs if administered close to the same time.

Polycarbophil (Fiber-Lax) and psyllium (Metamucil) are generally considered laxatives but may also be useful for mild diarrhea. Although the mechanism is not clearly understood, these products absorb water and may improve the viscosity of the stool. They have no known systemic toxicity but they may interfere with the absorption of some drugs if used concomitantly.

Bismuth Subsalicylate

Bismuth subsalicylate (Pepto-Bismol) is effective to treat mild, nonspecific diarrhea as well as mild to moderate traveler's diarrhea. The mechanism of its antidiarrheal action is not clear but the use of the drug is beyond its effectiveness at treating nonspecific diarrhea. The acidity of the stomach converts the bismuth subsalicylate to salicylic acid and bismuth oxychloride. The salicylic acid may have some local anti-inflammatory activity before it is absorbed into the blood. The bismuth remains in the GI tract where it has an anti-inflammatory and antibacterial effect. This antibacterial action contributes to the therapeutic effectiveness for treating bacteria-induced diarrhea (eg, traveler's diarrhea) and is also the reason for use in the multidrug regimen for the treatment of *H. pylori*-induced peptic ulcers (see Table 11-3).

Generally, bismuth subsalicylate is very safe and can be used up to eight times per day at the recommended dose. It can also be used four times a day to prevent traveler's diarrhea; hence, it is a widely used OTC antidiarrheal product. Nonetheless, it does have several potential adverse effects and drug interactions. Patients for whom use of aspirin is a precaution should not use bismuth subsalicylate. This would include patients who have aspirin-induced asthma, are taking warfarin, and children who have a viral infection such as the flu. Bismuth subsalicylate may also inhibit the absorption of other drugs given concurrently. Sulfides produced by bacteria in the mouth and intestine form bismuth sulfide, which causes a harmless darkening of the tongue and stool in some patients.

Table 11-6. Examples of Drugs Used to Treat Inflammatory Bowel Disease

Generic Name	Trade Name	Category
azathioprine	Imuran	Immunosuppressant
balsalazide	Colazal	Anti-inflammatory salicylate
cyclosporine	Gengraf	Immunosuppressant
infliximab	Remicade	Anti-inflammatory antibody
mercaptopurine	Purinethol	Immunosuppressant
mesalamine	Asacol	Anti-inflammatory salicylate
metronidazole	Flagyl	Antibiotic
olsalazine	Dipentum	Anti-inflammatory salicylate
prednisone	Deltasone	Anti-inflammatory corticosteroid
sulfasalazine	Azulfidine	Anti-inflammatory salicylate

Drugs for Treatment of Irritable Bowel Syndrome

The use of antidiarrheal agents and laxatives are a mainstay of drug treatment for IBS although treatment of coexisting depression or pain also has beneficial outcomes in many patients. Of the antidiarrheal agents, loperamide (Imodium) is used most often because it is OTC and has a low incidence of adverse effects. When constipation is a predominant symptom of IBS, bulk-forming laxatives are preferred, such as psyllium (Metamucil) or methylcellulose (Citrucel). If a bulk-forming laxative does not alleviate the problem, docusate (Colace) or an osmotic laxative (see Table 11-5) may be added.

Abdominal pain and depression are significant problems for some patients. A category of drugs referred to as tricyclic antidepressants are often effective for these patients. These drugs have been used for many years to treat depression but they also alleviate pain associated with IBS, an effect that is independent of the antidepressant effect. The mechanism for the pain relief is not clear. Although the tricyclic antidepressants have an *anticholinergic* effect that may contribute to the relief of bowel spasms, the benefit cannot be totally attributed to the anticholinergic effect. Examples of tricyclic antidepressants are imipramine (Tofranil), desipramine (Norpramin), and amitriptyline (Elavil). Tricyclic antidepressants should be used with caution in patients for whom anticholinergic effects are problematic (eg, glaucoma, cardiovascular disease, and urinary retention).

Drugs for Treatment of Inflammatory Bowel Disease

The seriousness and complexity of IBD (ulcerative colitis and Crohn's disease) requires that the drug therapy change as the symptoms change. Examples of drugs used to treat IBD are shown in Table 11-6. Therapy can be complex and include various anti-inflammatory agents, immunosuppressive therapy, and antibiotics. Additional drug therapy may also be necessary to treat systemic complications of the disease such as arthritis. No drug cures IBD, but the primary goal of therapy is to bring about remission, which may last a few years in some cases.

Mesalamine (Asacol) or one of its various chemical derivatives is frequently used to treat mild to moderate ulcerative colitis and Crohn's disease involving the colon. Mesalamine is a derivative of salicylic acid and 5-ASA is a synonym. It is available in oral dosage forms as well as enemas and suppositories for rectal administration. The anti-inflammatory activity of 5-ASA is primarily in the large intestine. The *mechanism of action* is unknown although inhibition of cyclooxygenase and/or lipoxygenase may play a part. Other derivatives of 5-ASA are olsalazine (Dipentum), balsalazide (Colazal), and sulfasalazine (Azulfidine). Of these, sulfasalazine has the most prominent adverse effect potential and includes headache, nausea, and fatigue. Patients should also know that sulfasalazine causes the urine to turn orange-yellow, a harmless effect. This drug may increase their sensitivity to the sun. Sulfasalazine inhibits the absorption of folic acid and therefore folic acid supplements are necessary during therapy.

The anti-inflammatory action of *corticosteroid* therapy is useful in treatment of moderate to severe ulcerative colitis and Crohn's disease. Oral corticosteroids such as prednisone (Deltasone) are effective for moderate to severe IBD, and rectally administered corticosteroids are useful when the affected area is at or near the rectum. Even with a short course of therapy (7 to 10 days) some adverse effects of corticosteroids can be expected, such as insomnia, mood changes, and nervousness. When the desired response is obtained, the corticosteroid is discontinued by tapering the dose. If corticosteroids cannot be tapered off without a relapse, surgery becomes a consideration.

Severe ulcerative colitis or Crohn's disease requires more aggressive therapy, including parenterally administered corticosteroid at higher doses, and thus hospitalization. Mesalamine derivatives are not effective to treat severe IBD. Cyclosporine (Gengraf), an immunosuppressive drug, is useful for treatment of ulcerative colitis and Crohn's disease that are unresponsive to corticosteroid. Additional immunosuppressive drugs and antibiotics that may be used to treat severe Crohn's disease are listed in Table 11-6. Use of these drugs may allow a reduction in corticosteroid dosage but yet achieve remission.

Mesalamine or one of its derivatives are standard treatment to maintain remission of IBD, although success is greater for ulcerative colitis patients. Azathioprine (Imuran) and mercaptopurine (Purinethol) are used to maintain remission in patients who do not respond to mesalamine or its derivatives. Corticosteroids are not effective in maintaining remission or changing the course of either disease. Consequently, dosage of corticosteroid should be tapered off when remission is obtained.

Drugs for Treatment of Hemorrhoids

The goal of treatment is to alleviate the symptoms of pain, itching, burning, and inflammation. There are several categories of drugs that are used to accomplish relief of these symptoms. Drugs in each category are available in OTC anorectal products, applied topically as creams, ointments, suppositories, solutions, and moist pads. By using topical dosage forms, the compounds are placed directly at the site of the problem. Although systemic effects are minimized when prescribed frequency of use is not exceeded, adverse effects are not eliminated as some systemic absorption occurs for several of these compounds.

Provided below is a list of the categories of hemorrhoidal treatments with a short description of their effects and generic names of some of the compounds in the category. Use of a bulk-forming laxative or stool softener may also be necessary to avoid constipation in some patients. Table 11-7 lists examples of products that contain these compounds.

- *Corticosteroids* are effective in reducing inflammation, itching, and swelling. Hydrocortisone is the most commonly used topical corticosteroid, and at 0.25% and 1% concentrations, it is the only one available OTC. Hydrocortisone is low potency and topical use does not cause systemic adverse effects.
- *Local anesthetics* provide temporary relief of itching, burning, and pain by blocking nerve impulses. Allergic reactions may occur and therefore patients should be instructed to discontinue the product if redness, swelling, and pain does not diminish or becomes worse. Examples are benzocaine, benzyl alcohol, dibucaine, pramoxine, and tetracaine.

Table 11-7. Examples of Anorectal Products for Treatment of Hemorrhoids

Trade Name	Active Ingredients	Dosage Form
Analpram-HC[1]	hydrocortisone acetate, pramoxine HCl	Cream
Anusol	starch, benzyl alcohol, soy bean oil, tocopherol acetate	Suppository
Fleet Medicated Wipes	hamamelis water, alcohol, glycerin, benzalkonium chloride, methylparaben	Pads
Hemorrhoidal HC[1]	hydrocortisone acetate	Suppository
Medicone	phenylephrine HCl, hard fat, parabens	Suppository
Pazo Hemorrhoid	ephedrine sulfate, camphor, zinc oxide, lanolin, petrolatum	Ointment
Preparation H	petrolatum, glycerin, shark liver oil, phenylephrine, cetyl and stearyl alcohols, EDTA, parabens, lanolin, tocopherol	Cream
Preparation H	shark liver oil, cocoa butter, corn oil, EDTA, parabens, tocopherol	Suppository
Proctocort[1]	hydrocortisone	Cream
Tronolane	zinc oxide, hard fat	Suppository
Tucks	witch hazel, glycerin, benzalkonium Cl, alcohol, parabens	Pads

[1] *By prescription only. All others are OTC.*

- *Astringents* relieve irritation and inflammation, decrease mucus, and coagulate protein in skin thus protecting underlying tissue. Examples are calamine, zinc oxide, and witch hazel (hamamelis water).
- *Vasoconstrictors* reduce swelling by constricting blood vessels and relieve local itching by slight anesthetic effect. Vasoconstriction occurs through an α-adrenergic effect (see Chapter 12) similar to the mechanism of nasal decongestants (see Chapter 10). Similar precautions and adverse effects exist for the use of vasoconstrictors for hemorrhoids as for nasal decongestants (eg, nervousness, tremor, precaution in patients with hypertension, diabetes). Examples are ephedrine and phenylephrine.
- *Antiseptics* have value as preservatives but there is no evidence that they prevent infection in the anorectal area. Examples are benzalkonium chloride and phenylmercuric nitrate.
- *Protectants* form a physical barrier on the skin, lubricate tissues to prevent irritation, and prevent loss of water from the tissue. Little or no systemic absorption occurs. Examples are aluminum hydroxide gel, lanolin, mineral oil, zinc oxide, cocoa butter, shark liver oil, bismuth salts, lanolin, petrolatum, glycerin, and hard fat.
- *Counterirritants* produce a feeling of cooling, tingling, or warmth and distract from pain and itching. Examples are menthol and camphor. Menthol can produce an allergic reaction, and therefore, patients should be instructed to discontinue the product if redness, swelling, and pain does not diminish or becomes worse.
- *Keratolytics* increase the rate of sloughing of epidermal surface cells so that medications may be more accessible to the underlying tissue. Examples are alcloxa and resorcinol.

Summary

Treatment of GERD focuses on neutralizing gastric acid or decreasing acid production. In either case, the amount of acid available for reflux into the esophagus is decreased, thus giving the esophageal mucosa time to heal. From the standpoint of healing rates, PPIs are the most effective therapy; examples are esomeprazole (Nexium) and omeprazole (Prilosec). Proton pump inhibitors have few and usually mild adverse effects. The H_2RAs such as ranitidine (Zantac) and famotidine (Pepcid) are also effective treatment for GERD and are all available by prescription and OTC for treatment of heartburn. The effectiveness among the PPIs is comparable, as is the effectiveness among the drugs in the H_2RA category. These two categories of drugs exert their effect via systemic action; therefore they must be absorbed into the bloodstream to reach their target sites in the specialized cells of the stomach. All of the drugs in these two categories are absorbed readily after oral administration.

Antacids are also used to treat GERD by virtue of their ability to neutralize gastric acid. However, although they have a quick onset of action, these drugs are less effective and have a shorter duration of action than either the PPIs or the H_2RA. Antacids can be used as an adjunct to other therapy. Among the more prominent problems associated with antacids is the potential for diarrhea with magnesium salts (Phillips' Chewable) and constipation with aluminum (Amphojel) and calcium (Tums) salts.

Treatment for PUD depends on the cause. If PUD is linked to the presence of *H. pylori*, then combination therapy to eradicate the bacteria is appropriate. Many effective combinations of antibiotics (eg, amoxicillin, clarithromycin, and tetracycline) and PPIs (eg, omeprazole) have been identified. If the PUD is NSAID-induced, removing the NSAID, or reducing the dosage, is appropriate, along with the use of drug therapy to treat the PUD. PPIs and H_2RAs are effective for treatment and maintenance therapy of PUD. Although healing rates are somewhat higher for PPIs, the cost of OTC H_2RAs is less, which may be a factor for some patients. PPIs or misoprostol (Cytotec), a synthetic prostaglandin derivative, are available to prevent PUD for patients who are at risk for PUD but must be maintained on NSAIDs.

Antacids (eg, Mylanta Tablets, Maalox Suspension) are less effective than PPIs or H_2RAs but are sometimes added to therapy. Sucralfate (Carafate) is also available. When used prior to meals, sucralfate offers protection by forming a viscous barrier between the epithelial cells and the gastric acid. Antacids and sucralfate may interfere with bioavailability of other drugs if administered concomitantly.

Acute constipation can be treated with any one of several categories of laxatives. Exercise, dietary fiber, and adequate fluid intake can all help prevent constipation. To treat constipation, dietary fiber can be added in the form of bulk-forming laxatives such as psyllium (Metamucil). Osmotic laxatives, such as milk of magnesia, are also effective and act by drawing water into the GI tract. For both types of laxatives, it is important that sufficient water be ingested at the time of the laxative dose. Bulk-forming laxatives take longer to act (12 to 72 hours) compared to osmotic laxatives (1 to 3 hours). Other mechanisms for laxative action are stool softeners and stimulants. Stool softeners, such as docusate (Colace), allow water to more readily mix with GI contents to keep the stool softer so it passes through the GI tract more readily; onset is 12 to 72 hours. Stimulant laxatives have a quicker onset (6 to 10 hours) but are not recommended for frequent use. They increase GI motility by acting on the smooth muscle; bisacodyl (Dulcolax) and senna (Ex-lax) are examples. Enemas and suppositories have the shortest onset of action (<1 hour).

Treatment of severe or chronic diarrhea necessitates the determination of the underlying cause. Management of acute mild to moderate diarrhea usually involves treatment of symptoms and maintenance of fluids and electrolytes. Loperamide (Imodium) is an OTC opioid and is a very effective and frequently used antidiarrheal agent. It acts on the smooth muscle to decrease GI motility. Drowsiness, dry mouth, nausea, and vomiting are potential adverse effects. Absorbent compounds, such as kaolin and pectin (Kapectolin), are not absorbed systemically and so have few adverse effects. Bismuth subsalicylate (Pepto-Bismol) is also frequently used although the mechanism is not clear. It is particularly effective for bacteria-induced diarrhea. The salicylate content is released when in contact with gastric acid and thus should not be used in patients who must avoid aspirin.

The focus of drug therapy for IBS is management of diarrhea or constipation. Loperamide (Imodium) is most frequently used for diarrhea; bulk-forming laxatives such as psyllium (Metamucil) are recommended for constipation. Tricyclic antidepressants are effective in relieving abdominal pain as well as depression in some IBS patients with these symptoms.

Treatment of IBD is more complex than IBS. Use of a salicylate derivate such as mesalamine (Asacol) is useful to treat ulcerative colitis and Crohn's disease. A corticosteroid, such as prednisone (Deltasone), is often effective as additional therapy for these diseases when of mild to moderate severity. Patients with severe IBD are hospitalized for treatment with higher doses of a corticosteroid and use of antibiotics or immunosuppressant drugs such as cyclosporine (Gengraf). Once remission is obtained, the aggressive therapy is discontinued and corticosteroid therapy is tapered off. Mesalamine or one of its derivatives is most often used to maintain remission; corticosteroids are not effective for this purpose. Crohn's disease is typically less responsive to drug therapy than ulcerative colitis, in part because Crohn's disease can recur in any part of the digestive tract whereas ulcerative colitis is limited to the rectum and colon.

The goal of therapy for hemorrhoids is to relieve the symptoms of itching, burning, pain, and inflammation. Many OTC products are available, often with several compounds present in one product, which attempt to alleviate these symptoms through various mechanisms. Using compounds that are local anesthetics, vasoconstrictors, counterirritants, physical protectants, or corticosteroids are among the approaches to relieve symptoms.

ROLE OF THE ATHLETIC TRAINER

There are a few unique aspects related to the symptoms and treatment of GI disorders that may impact the role of the athletic trainer. Many drugs are available OTC to treat various GI disorders and therefore athletes will self-diagnose and self-medicate, which may lead to inappropriate treatment. For example, an athlete who is using an OTC H_2RA to treat persistent and recurring symptoms of PUD may require *H. pylori* eradication treatment rather than continued H_2RA use, or an athlete may be trying to treat erosive esophageal GERD with heartburn doses of an OTC H_2RA. An athlete who is concerned about a persistent diarrhea may have an underlying GI condition or may be experiencing adverse effects from a drug such as an antibiotic. The athletic trainer should encourage the athlete to obtain accurate diagnosis, especially when symptoms persist or reoccur.

Another problem with self-diagnosis is that the athlete may observe some symptoms (eg, gastric pain) but not properly assess the significance of other symptoms. The athletic trainer should be aware that athletes with weight loss, bleeding, anemia, and difficulty swallowing should be referred to a physician as these are signs of more severe stages of GERD, PUD, and lower GI disorders. Also, chest pain below the sternum that occurs upon exertion or that radiates to the jaw or arm should not be interpreted as GERD, but requires immediate medical attention.

Once the athlete is properly diagnosed and treated, the athletic trainer can encourage the athlete to comply with therapy. If the therapy includes several doses per day of more than one drug, such as for *H. pylori* eradication treatment, it takes diligence to maintain the proper daily regimen throughout the entire course of therapy. For treatment of GERD and PUD, the dosage regimen and duration of treatment have a significant impact on the outcome.

Knowledge of nondrug measures related to GI disorders can allow the athletic trainer to provide additional useful information to the athlete. For example, is the athlete who periodically is bothered by constipation consuming sufficient water and fiber? Is an athlete with complaint of diarrhea consuming coffee or foods with high sugar content before running, or is there too much fiber in the diet? Athletes with GERD should be advised to not vigorously exercise too soon after eating, and athletes with PUD or GERD should be advised to avoid the most frequently used drugs—alcohol, caffeine, and nicotine (tobacco).

Fortunately, most of the drugs used to treat GI disorders have relatively few systemic adverse effects. Nonetheless, the potential for such adverse effects or drug interactions should not be overlooked. New complaints that arise even a few weeks after the addition of drug therapy could be the result of an adverse effect or drug interaction. The athlete can be encouraged to seek consultation with a pharmacist or physician for a review of the athlete's drug therapy to determine the likelihood that the new complaints are drug-related.

Because GI disorders are a very common group of disorders, and because OTC products are numerous and readily accessible for the treatment of these disorders, the opportunities exist for the athletic trainer to provide useful assistance and advice to the athlete regarding GI disorders and related therapy. The goal, after accurate diagnosis, is to attain proper management of the disease through appropriate drug therapy, as well as through nondrug measures, so that GI disorders do not hinder the athlete's performance.

BIBLIOGRAPHY

APhA Special Report. *Strategies for the Self-Treatment of Heartburn.* Washington, DC: American Pharmaceutical Association; 2001.

ASHP. Therapeutic position statement on the identification and treatment of *Helicobacter pylori*-associated peptic ulcer disease in adults. *Am J Health-Syst Pharm.* 2001;58:331-337.

Caro JJ, Salas M., Ward A. Healing and relapse rates in gastroesophageal reflux disease treated with the newer proton-pump inhibitors lansoprazole, rabeprazole, and pantoprazole compared with omeprazole, ranitidine, and placebo: evidence from randomized clinical trials. *Clin Ther.* 2001;23:998-1017.

Garnett WR, Yunker N. Treatment of Crohn's disease with infliximab. *Am J Health Syst Pharm.* 2001;58:307-316.

National Digestive Diseases Information Clearinghouse. Heartburn, hiatal hernia, and gastroesophageal reflux disease (GERD). Available at: http://www.niddk.nih.gov/health/digest/pubs/gerd/gerd.htm. Accessed March 2, 2003.

National Digestive Diseases Information Clearinghouse. Irritable bowel syndrome. Available at: http://www.niddk.nih.gov/health/digest/pubs/irrbowel/irrbowel.htm. Accessed March 25, 2003.

Over-the-counter omeprazole (Prilosec OTC). *The Medical Letter.* 2003;45:61-62.

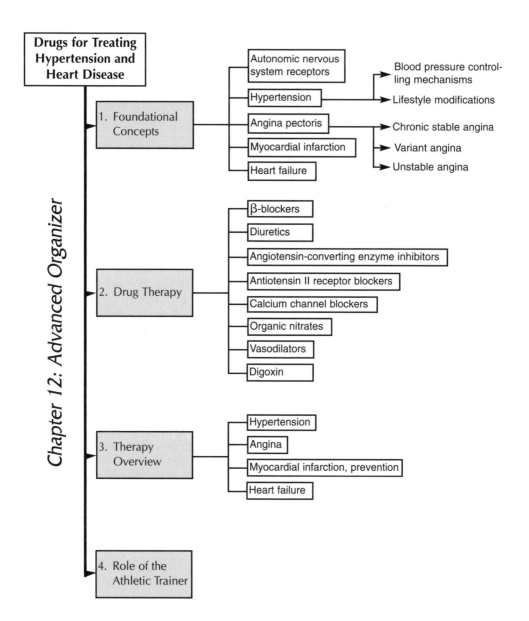

Drugs for Treating Hypertension and Heart Disease

Chapter 12: Advanced Organizer

1. Foundational Concepts
   - Autonomic nervous system receptors
   - Hypertension
     - Blood pressure controlling mechanisms
     - Lifestyle modifications
   - Angina pectoris
     - Chronic stable angina
     - Variant angina
     - Unstable angina
   - Myocardial infarction
   - Heart failure

2. Drug Therapy
   - β-blockers
   - Diuretics
   - Angiotensin-converting enzyme inhibitors
   - Antiotensin II receptor blockers
   - Calcium channel blockers
   - Organic nitrates
   - Vasodilators
   - Digoxin

3. Therapy Overview
   - Hypertension
   - Angina
   - Myocardial infarction, prevention
   - Heart failure

4. Role of the Athletic Trainer

DRUGS FOR TREATING HYPERTENSION AND HEART DISEASE

CHAPTER OBJECTIVES

At the end of this chapter, the reader will be able to:

- Explain the function of the two subdivisions of the autonomic nervous system, sympathetic and parasympathetic, and how they impact physiological process.
- Recall and describe the three major types of cholinergic receptors.
- Differentiate between sympathomimetic and parasympathomimetic types of drugs.
- Explain a classification system for hypertension and guidelines for managing hypertension based on this classification.
- Explain the important role that the renin-angiotensin-aldosterone system has in regulating blood pressure.
- Recall lifestyle modifications that can lower blood pressure and explain their therapeutic benefit(s).
- Describe the pathophysiology of angina, myocardial infarction, and heart failure.
- Differentiate the three types of angina.
- Explain the uses, mechanism of action, physiological effects, adverse effects, and drug interactions of beta blockers, diuretics, angiotensin-converting enzyme (ACE) inhibitors, calcium channel blockers, organic nitrates, and vasodilators in the treatment of cardiovascular conditions.
- Describe various considerations in the overall treatment plan for cardiovascular disease that can impact the effectiveness of drug therapy.
- Summarize the role of the athletic trainer for patients who are on drug therapy for cardiovascular disease(s).

This chapter discusses drugs used to treat several of the most prevalent serious cardiovascular diseases. Heart disease is the leading cause of death in the United States. These are also diseases for which exercise can improve symptoms and/or progression of the disease. Although patients may be diagnosed with just one of these diseases (eg, hypertension, angina, heart failure, myocardial infarction) there is a connection among them. For example, chronic hypertension increases the risk of angina, heart failure, and myocardial infarction; the presence of angina increases the risk of myocardial infarction; and myocardial infarction is one cause of heart failure. In this chapter, the drugs used to treat these conditions are discussed by pharmacological category (eg, β-blocker, calcium channel blocker, etc), and then reviewed briefly by therapeutic category (eg, antihypertensive, drugs for heart failure, etc). The complexity of the therapeutic regimen sometimes used to treat these diseases, along with the array of potential *adverse effects and drug interactions*, creates a challenge for the athletic trainer. However, a few useful principles are reiterated, which can guide the athletic trainer in assisting athletes who are receiving therapy for hypertension and heart disease.

FOUNDATIONAL CONCEPTS

Endogenous control mechanisms to maintain proper blood pressure and cardiac function require the intricate involvement of neurotransmitters from the autonomic and central nervous systems and the release of numerous hormones. The mechanisms of action of these neurotransmitters and hormones are also the *site of action* for drugs used to treat hypertension and heart disease. A discussion of some of these mechanisms is included in this section as a basis for understanding the cause of the disease (or symptoms) and the rationale for treatment regimens.

Autonomic Nervous System Receptors

The autonomic nervous system is the part of the peripheral nervous system that automatically controls body functions such as blood flow to organs and tissues, heart rate, respiration, digestive processes, and blood pressure. It has two subdivisions: the *parasympathetic* and *sympathetic* system. Usually a tissue response initiated by these two subdivisions will have opposite effects, so that, for example, activation of the parasympathetic system decreases heart rate whereas activation of the sympathetic system increases heart rate. Each of these subdivisions is a two-neuron fiber system (Figure 12-1). The first neuron (preganglionic fiber) begins in the spinal cord and terminates at the site of specialized nerve tissue called a *ganglion*. The cell body of the second neuron (postganglionic fiber) begins at the ganglion and ends at the tissue being innervated, typically smooth muscle or cardiac muscle. A small space (synapse) separates the pre- from the postganglionic fiber. The terms sympathetic and parasympathetic are anatomical terms; their differentiation is determined by several anatomical characteristics, such as the length of the pre- versus postganglionic fiber and the origin of the neuron from the spinal cord. The terms *cholinergic* and *adrenergic* are pharmacological terms that indicate the neurotransmitter released at the site.

Each nerve fiber releases a neurotransmitter. The preganglionic fibers of the sympathetic and parasympathetic systems release acetylcholine into the synapse at the ganglion. Acetyl*choline* is also released at the parasympathetic postganglionic fiber. Consequently, the parasympathetic system is referred to as the *choline*rgic nervous system. The neurotransmitter released at the tissue site by most of the sympathetic postganglionic fibers is norepinephrine. Another name for norepinephrine is nor*adren*alin; hence, the sympathetic system is also referred to as the *adren*ergic nervous system. When a neurotransmitter

> *Recall from Chapter 3 that transduction mechanisms are a sequence of reactions within the cell that are initiated as a drug or hormone combines with the appropriate receptor located on the surface of the cell.*

is released, it combines with the corresponding receptor, activates a *transduction mechanism* within the cell, and ultimately causes a tissue response (eg, smooth muscle contraction or relaxation).

Most tissues are innervated by sympathetic and parasympathetic fibers and, as previously mentioned, activation of these two fiber-types typically has opposite effects on the tissue. Table 12-1 lists the responses from the autonomic nervous system on selected tissues. Note that, in general, the stimulation of the parasympathetic system initiates processes that conserve energy or conduct "housekeeping" types of functions. These include digestion of food and increased rate

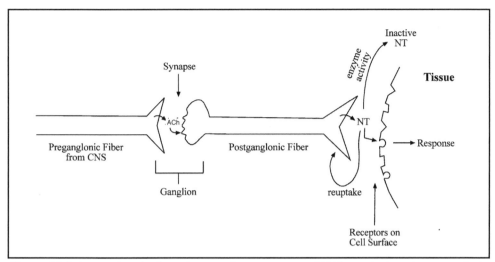

Figure 12-1. A nerve impulse from the central nervous system (CNS) travels along the preganglionic fiber, resulting in the release of the neurotransmitter acetylcholine (ACh) at the ganglion. Acetylcholine is the neurotransmitter at the ganglion for the sympathetic and parasympathetic fibers. Acetylcholine combines with the nicotinic receptor on the postganglionic fiber. The combination of the ACh with the nicotinic receptor causes the nerve impulse to be continued along the postganglionic fiber, which causes a neurotransmitter (NT) to be released at the site where the nerve fiber innervates the tissue. For sympathetic nerves, NT = norepinephrine (NE); for parasympathetic nerves, NT = acetylcholine. There are many types of receptors on the surface of each cell of the tissue. The NT binds to receptor for which it has an affinity, initiating a response inside the cell. The receptors to which NE binds are α- and β-receptors, and drugs that combine with these receptors are called adrenergic drugs. The receptors to which ACh binds are called muscarinic receptors and drugs that combine with this receptor are called cholinergic drugs. The binding of the NT (or agonist drug) to the receptor causes a response in the tissue; the binding of an antagonist drug (blocker) prevents the NT from binding to the receptor, and hence prevents the response from the NT.

Termination of action of the NT occurs by the reuptake of the NT into the nerve terminal or by inactivation of the NT by specific enzyme activity (eg, cholinesterase for ACh and monoamine oxidase [MAO] for NE). Drugs that inhibit these inactivating enzymes or reuptake mechanisms will prolong and/or intensify the effect of the NT, thereby indirectly mimicking the NT activity.

of excretory functions. In contrast, stimulation of the sympathetic system results in preparation for energy expenditure or for "fight or flight" functions. These include increased heart rate and decreased intestinal motility. In addition, a sympathetic preganglionic-like fiber innervates the adrenal gland to stimulate the release of epinephrine, which is released into the bloodstream. Release of epinephrine is increased as a result of excitatory response. Epinephrine causes increased heart rate, dilation of bronchial smooth muscle, and increased glycogen conversion to glucose (glycogenolysis). Although there is a low level of neurotransmitter release occurring all the time in each tissue, one subdivision of the autonomic nervous system dominates in each tissue (ie, it provides the autonomic tone for that tissue). As examples, sympathetic tone dominates in the cardiovascular system, whereas parasympathetic tone predominates in the digestive system.

The type of receptors that exist at any site will determine the response observed from neurotransmitters and from drugs that mimic neurotransmitters. There are two major types of adrenergic receptors: alpha (α) and beta (β). There are two major subtypes of these receptors, designated by 1 and 2 as subscripts. Table 12-1 shows the type of receptor that predominates in various tissues. Key tissue responses to especially note are the peripheral vasoconstriction (eg, skin

Table 12-1. Responses of Tissues to Autonomic Nervous System Activation

Tissue	Adrenergic Receptor	Adrenergic Activation (Sympathetic Activation)	Cholinergic Activation (Parasympathetic Activation)
Eye	α_1	Pupil dilation	Pupil constriction
Heart	β_1	Increased heart rate Increased contractility Increased conduction velocity	Decreased heart rate Decreased contractility Decreased conduction velocity
Blood vessels	α_1 β_2 β_2 β_1, β_2	Constriction in skin, mucosa, GI Dilation in skeletal muscle Dilation in liver, heart, lungs Dilation in kidney	– – – –
Kidney	β_1	Increased renin secretion	–
Bronchial muscle	β_2	Relaxation	Contraction
Intestinal motility Intestinal secretion	β_1	Decreased –	Increased Increased
Urinary bladder Urinary sphincter	β_2 α_1	Relaxation Contraction	Contraction Relaxation
Skeletal muscle	β_2	Increased glycogenolysis and increased contractility	–
Liver	α_1, β_2	Increased glycogenolysis and gluconeogenesis	–
Salivation	α_1	Increased (slightly)	Increased
Pancreas	α_1 β_2	Decreased insulin secretion Increased insulin secretion (slightly)	– –
Fat cells	β_1, β_3	Increased lipolysis	–

(–) Indicates no effect or may not be physiologically significant.

and mucosa) due to α_1-*receptor* activation, increased heart rate, and force of contraction due to activation of β_1-*receptors* in the heart, and dilation of the bronchial tube due to β_2-*receptor* activation in the bronchial smooth muscle. Activation of the α_2-*receptors* serves to inhibit the release of additional norepinephrine. Although α_2-receptors exist at some tissue sites, the action of drugs at these sites is minimal. However, some drugs (not discussed) are agonists at the α_2-receptor in the central nervous system (CNS) that decrease sympathetic outflow (ie, reduce the sympathetic response from CNS to the periphery), resulting in bradycardia and vasodilation, which are antihypertensive responses. An example is clonidine (Catapres).

There are three major types of *cholinergic receptors*: muscarinic, nicotinic ganglionic, and nicotinic neuromuscular (Box 12-1). The nicotinic receptors are so named because nicotine is an *agonist* at these receptors. Although there are some drugs that act as *agonists* or *antagonists* at the nicotinic ganglionic receptor, the use of these drugs is limited because they affect both the sym-

Box 12-1. Summary of the Three Major Types of Cholinergic Receptors

Muscarinic	Located in the tissue innervated by the postganglionic parasympathetic fiber, are used to increase or decrease the response of the parasympathetic nervous system.
	The terms "cholinergic" and "anticholinergic" are generally reserved for drugs that act at this receptor site.
Nicotinic Ganglionic	Drugs that combine with this receptor are limited because they affect both the sympathetic and parasympathetic systems and thus tend to have numerous adverse effects.
Nicotinic Neuromuscular	Drugs that combine with this receptor are also limited but some antagonists are used as skeletal muscle relaxants during surgery.

pathetic and parasympathetic systems and thus tend to have numerous adverse effects. Drugs that combine with the nicotinic neuromuscular receptor are also limited but some antagonists are used as skeletal muscle relaxants during surgery. Drugs that combine with the muscarinic receptor, located in the tissue innervated by the postganglionic parasympathetic fiber, are used to increase (agonists) or decrease (antagonists) the response of the parasympathetic nervous system. The terms *cholinergic* and *anticholinergic* are generally reserved for drugs that act at the muscarinic receptor site. Although drugs that act at the nicotinic receptors also either mimic or block the effects of acetylcholine at these sites, such drugs are usually specified as neuromuscular or ganglionic to differentiate them from the cholinergic muscarinic drugs.

Termination of receptor response occurs as a result of two general mechanisms: neurotransmitter reuptake back into the nerve terminal that released it and inactivation by enzymes (see Figure 12-1). Examples of enzymes are *cholinesterase*, which inactivates acetylcholine, and *monoamine oxidase* (MAO), which inactivates norepinephrine. Inhibition of these enzymes by drugs will cause the neurotransmitter to have a more intense and longer duration of action. For example, drugs that are *monoamine oxidase inhibitors* (MAOIs) can have an adverse effect of increased blood pressure because they increase the effect of norepinephrine at peripheral blood vessel sites.

> *Recall from Chapter 7 that MAOIs are drugs used to treat depression. These drugs are not first-line agents because they are notorious for adverse effects and drug interactions. Examples are phenelzine (Nardil) and tranylcypromine (Parnate).*

Drugs that mimic the sympathetic or parasympathetic nervous systems are referred to as *sympathomimetics* and *parasympathomimetics*, respectively. The mechanisms for mimicking these autonomic responses may be direct (receptor agonists) or indirect by inhibiting reuptake or inhibiting enzymatic inactivation of the neurotransmitter. Albuterol (Proventil) is an example of a direct β-agonist (see Chapter 9), whereas MAOIs are indirect acting sympathomimetics.

Hypertension

An estimated 50 million people in the United States have high blood pressure. Hypertension increases the risk of stroke, angina, myocardial infarction, heart failure, and kidney disease. Therefore, control of hypertension has obvious benefits in decreasing morbidity and mortality from these complications. Hypertension is more common among the elderly.

Table 12-2. Classification of Blood Pressure

Blood Pressure Classification	Systolic Pressure (mm Hg)		Diastolic Pressure (mm Hg)
Normal	<120	and	<80
Prehypertension	120 to 139	or	80 to 89
Stage 1 Hypertension	140 to 159	or	90 to 99
Stage 2 Hypertension	≥160	or	≥100

Adapted from National High Blood Pressure Education Program. *The Seventh Report of the Joint National Committee on Prevention, Detection, Evaluation, and Treatment of High Blood Pressure.* Bethesda, Md: National Heart, Lung, and Blood Institute; 2003. NIH publication No. 03-5233.

The classification of blood pressure in adults from the *Seventh Report of the Joint National Committee (JNC 7) on Prevention, Detection, Evaluation, and Treatment of High Blood Pressure* (2003) is shown in Table 12-2. According to this classification, what used to be considered normal blood pressure (120/80 mm Hg) is now included in the classification of prehypertension: systolic pressure 120 to 139 mm Hg and/or diastolic blood pressure 80 to 89 mm Hg. Also according to the JNC standards, stage 1 hypertension exists if either the systolic pressure is >140 mm Hg or the diastolic is ≥90 mm Hg, and stage 2 exists if the blood pressure is higher than the stage 1 values. Drug therapy should be initiated if blood pressure is ≥140/90, or ≥130/80 mm Hg for patients with diabetes or chronic kidney disease. Table 12-3 indicates the treatment approach as recommended in the JNC 7 report. Thiazide-type diuretics are recommended as the first drug with which to initiate therapy unless a compelling indication exists (eg, diabetes, chronic kidney disease, heart failure, or ischemic heart disease) to warrant other therapy. Initiating therapy with two antihypertensive drugs should be considered for patients with stage 2 hypertension, or blood pressure >20/10 mm Hg above the target pressure. An additional drug(s) is added if adequate control is not achieved; most hypertensive patients require two or more drugs for effective blood pressure control.

Blood Pressure Controlling Mechanisms

If the hypertension is known to be caused by the existence of a specific condition (eg, renal disease, adrenal tumor, pregnancy), it is secondary hypertension; if the cause is unknown, it is called primary or essential hypertension. Approximately 95% of patients have essential hypertension. It is presumed that most hypertension is multifactorial in origin, being caused by a combination of several environmental and genetic factors. Basically, any factor that increases peripheral vascular resistance will contribute to elevated blood pressure. These factors include increased peripheral vasoconstriction, obesity, and elevated fluid volume. An alteration in any of the many mechanisms that control blood pressure can contribute to hypertension. Some of these controlling mechanisms are listed in Box 12-2.

The *renin-angiotensin-aldosterone system* plays an important role in regulating blood pressure. *Renin* is an enzyme that is released by the kidney in response to a decrease in blood flow to the kidneys, drop in blood pressure, diminished sodium and water retention, or increased sympa-

Table 12-3. Management of Blood Pressure in Adults

Blood Pressure Classification	Lifestyle Modification	Without Compelling Indication	With Compelling Indications[1]
Normal (<120/<80)	Encourage	No antihypertensive drug indicated.	Drug(s) for compelling indications.[2]
Prehypertension (120 to 139/80 to 89)	Yes	No antihypertensive drug necessary.	Drug(s) for compelling indications.[2]
Stage 1 Hypertension (140 to 159/90 to 99)	Yes	Thiazide-type diuretics for most. May consider ACEI, ARB, BB, CCB, or combination.	Drug(s) for the compelling indications.[2] Other antihypertensive drugs (diuretics, ACEI, ARB, BB, CCB) as needed.
Stage 2 Hypertension (≥160/≥100)	Yes	Two-drug combination for most (usually thiazide-type diuretic and ACEI or ARB or BB or CCB).	

[1]*Compelling indications for which there are specific recommended drugs include heart failure, postmyocardial infarction, high coronary disease risk, diabetes, chronic kidney disease, and recurrent stroke prevention.*

[2]*Treat patients with chronic kidney disease or diabetes to blood pressure goal of <130/80 mm Hg.*
Drug abbreviations: ACEI = angiotensin-converting enzyme inhibitor; ARB = angiotensin receptor blocker; BB = β-blocker; CCB = calcium channel blocker.

Adapted from National High Blood Pressure Education Program. *The Seventh Report of the Joint National Committee on Prevention, Detection, Evaluation, and Treatment of High Blood Pressure.* Bethesda, Md: National Heart, Lung, and Blood Institute; 2003. NIH publication No. 03-5233.

thetic response through stimulation of β_1-*adrenergic receptors* on certain renal cells. Renin converts plasma *angiotensinogen* to *angiotensin*. Angiotensinogen is a glycoprotein that is continuously produced by the liver. Angiotensin I is a peptide comprised of 10 amino acids. Another enzyme, angiotensin-converting enzyme (ACE), catalyzes the conversion of angiotensin I to angiotensin II, which combines with angiotensin II receptors (Figure 12-2). Angiotensin-converting enzyme is present in cells of blood vessels and is therefore readily available to catalyze the formation of angiotensin II.

angiotensinogen ⟶ angiotensin I ⟶ angiotensin II ⟶ increase blood pressure
(in plasma)   renin   ACE

Angiotensin II has several effects that contribute to an increase in blood pressure and blood volume. It causes vasoconstriction by direct action on blood vessels and by the indirect action of increasing CNS sympathetic outflow and releasing epinephrine from the adrenal medulla. Angiotensin II also increases sodium and water retention by a direct action on the kidney and by indirect action through the release of *aldosterone* from the adrenal glands. *Aldosterone* is a miner-

Box 12-2. Controlling Mechanisms for Blood Pressure

- The central and sympathetic nervous systems contribute to the regulation of blood pressure. Excessive sympathetic response enhances the vasoconstricting effect through stimulation of the α_1-receptor on the arterioles and venules, and increases heart rate and contractility through stimulation of β_1-receptors. On the other hand, stimulation of α_2-receptors in the central nervous system (CNS) inhibits sympathetic outflow to decrease blood pressure.

- Calcium channels are pores on the surface of the cell membrane of the heart muscle, arteries, and arterioles. When the pores open, calcium ions are allowed into the cell, which leads to contraction of the vascular smooth muscle and cardiac muscle. In the heart muscle, activation of β_1-receptors leads to influx of calcium through the calcium channels, resulting in increased heart rate and force of contraction.

- Baroreceptors are an endogenous blood pressure sensing mechanism in the walls of some larger arteries. In response to rapid reduction in blood pressure, a feedback system stimulates the sympathetic nervous system to increase peripheral vasoconstriction and heart rate. An alteration of the effectiveness of these baroreceptors through disease, age, or genetics can contribute to hypertension.

- Excessive dietary intake of sodium increases blood pressure in some patients although the mechanism is unclear.

- Potassium plays a role in normal blood pressure maintenance to the extent that a deficiency of these ions can contribute to hypertension.

- Some medications cause increased blood pressure as an adverse effect by increasing peripheral vasoconstriction, increasing CNS sympathetic outflow, or increasing fluid volume. Examples include chronic alcohol use, corticosteroids, estrogens, MAOIs, antidepressants, NSAIDs, oral contraceptives, oral decongestants, and weight loss drugs.

- An abnormal renin-angiotensin-aldosterone system can result in increased sodium and water retention and/or increased vasoconstriction.

al corticosteroid that causes reabsorption of sodium and water by the renal tubule. As blood pressure begins to rise, the amount of renin released by the kidney decreases. In addition, angiotensin II acts as a feedback mechanism by inhibiting renin release. *In summary, an increase in renin activity will increase angiotensin II, which increases blood pressure by vasoconstriction and increased blood volume.*

Besides the effect on the *renin-angiotensin system*, ACE also catalyzes the inactivation of bradykinin. This peptide hormone has vasodilation properties that contribute to reducing blood pressure. *Therefore, inhibiting ACE will decrease blood pressure by diminishing the effect of renin and by increasing the effect of bradykinin.*

Although hypertensive patients may be asymptomatic, treatment of hypertension is important because chronic hypertension increases the risk of stroke, coronary heart disease, congestive heart disease, angina, myocardial infarction, transient ischemic attacks, retinopathy, and renal damage. Control of hypertension, therefore, decreases the occurrence of these conditions.

Lifestyle Modifications

All hypertensive patients, as well as people with prehypertension, should adopt lifestyle modifications as a part of therapy (Box 12-3). These modifications can lower blood pressure and can decrease the amount of antihypertensive medication needed to control the blood pressure.

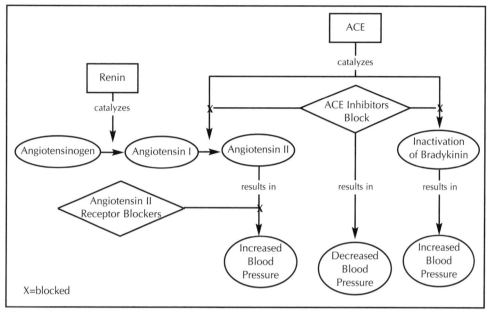

Figure 12-2. Effects of ACE on the renin-angiotensin system.

Box 12-3. Summary of Lifestyle Modifications to Lower Blood Pressure

- Eliminate cigarette smoking.
- Limit daily alcohol consumption.
- Weight reduction for patients above their desirable body weight.
- Reduction in dietary salt intake.
- Decrease in total fat intake.
- Maintain adequate dietary potassium.
- Regular aerobic exercise of mild to moderate intensity.

Among these modifications is elimination of cigarette smoking and limiting daily alcohol consumption (30 mL in men, 15 mL in women). Alcohol consumption and cigarette smoking increases blood pressure. Excess body weight contributes to hypertension, and therefore weight reduction should be a goal for patients above their desirable body weight; even a loss of 10 pounds can reduce blood pressure. Weight loss should be accomplished by a combination of diet management to reduce caloric intake and exercise.

A reduction in dietary salt intake can also reduce blood pressure in some patients. Processed food contributes to most of the salt intake for the average American diet. Limiting the total daily intake of sodium chloride (table salt) to about 6 g is helpful. Other dietary recommendations are to decrease total fat, particularly saturated fat intake, and maintain adequate dietary potassium. Potassium may protect against hypertension and improve blood pressure in hypertensive patients. Also, diuretic therapy can cause depletion of potassium and it is therefore important for these patients to be cognizant of their potassium intake. Selected fresh fruits and vegetables are among foods that are good sources of potassium (Table 12-4). Factors that do not appear to sig-

Table 12-4. Approximate Potassium Level in Foods

Food	<250 mg Per Serving[1]	250 to 500 mg Per Serving[1]	>500 mg Per Serving[1]
Apple	✓		
Apple juice		✓	
Apricots		✓	
Asparagus	✓		
Avocado			✓
Banana		✓	
Beans, baked/franks		✓	
Beans, kidney			✓
Beans, lima			✓
Beans, navy			✓
Blueberries	✓		
Broccoli		✓	
Cantaloupe		✓	
Carrots, cooked		✓	
Cauliflower, raw		✓	
Chicken		✓	
Corn	✓		
Dates			✓
Grapefruit juice		✓	
Ham		✓	
Hamburger		✓	
Hot dog	✓		
Kiwi		✓	
Milk, skim		✓	
Orange juice		✓	
Peach	✓		
Peanuts			✓
Peas	✓		
Pineapple juice		✓	
Pizza slice, pepperoni	✓		
Potato, baked + skin			✓
Potato, sweet		✓	
Raisins			✓
Rice	✓		
Salmon		✓	
Shrimp	✓		
Soup, split pea/ham		✓	
Soup, tomato		✓	
Soybean nuts			✓
Tomato		✓	
Tomato juice			✓
Tuna	✓		
Yogurt, plain			✓

[1]Serving size is 3 oz entree, 1 cup, 8 fluid oz, or per each where appropriate.

Box 12-4. Summary of the Three Forms of Angina Pectoris

Angina Type	Description	Therapy Focus
Chronic stable	• Also called exertional angina. • Due to partial occlusion of one or more of the coronary arteries, which is benign at rest but results in chest pain with increased activity due to the insufficient flow of oxygen to the heart.	Drug and nondrug interventions are intended to increase the amount of oxygen reaching the heart muscle and/or decrease the demand for oxygen.
Variant	• Also called Prinzmetal's angina or vasospastic angina. • Results from insufficient blood flow through a coronary artery but is caused from a coronary artery spasm.	Drug focus is to increase oxygen supply rather than to specifically reduce demand as the cause is not a result of increased demand.
Unstable	• Condition in which there is a change in the severity of pain or pattern of angina compared with what the patient has experienced previously.	Drug therapy focus is to increase oxygen delivery to the heart muscle, decrease demand for for oxygen, and alleviate persistent pain.

nificantly decrease hypertension are magnesium or garlic supplements, nor does the use of caffeine contribute to hypertension.

Exercise can also have a positive effect on hypertension. Regular aerobic exercise of mild to moderate intensity lowers blood pressure in patients with essential hypertension. The molecular mechanism for this antihypertensive effect has not been pinpointed, but it is likely that a reduction in cardiac output and/or peripheral resistance results. Moderately intense exercise, such as 30 to 45 minutes of brisk walking several days a week, can lower blood pressure. The initial exercise routine should be low intensity and short duration with a progressive increase in both parameters. The initial level and intensity of exercise as well as the target goal will vary depending on the severity of the hypertension, patient's age, and existence of other complicating diseases (eg, coronary heart disease, diabetes).

Angina Pectoris

Angina is a type of coronary heart disease (CHD) in which the coronary arteries are not able to supply sufficient oxygen to the heart muscle. Consequently, angina is also referred to as an ischemic heart disease. The major symptom of angina is a sudden pain that originates behind the breast bone and radiates to the left shoulder and arm. Pain or discomfort may also be felt in the neck and jaw. Pain occurs when the demand for oxygen to the heart muscle increases beyond what the coronary arteries can supply. There are three forms of angina pectoris: chronic stable, variant, and unstable (Box 12-4).

Chronic Stable Angina

Chronic stable angina, also called exertional angina, is the classic angina and is the most common form of angina (>6 million Americans). Atherosclerosis of one or more of the coronary arteries causes partial occlusion of the affected coronary arteries and thus restricts the amount of blood (hence oxygen) that can flow through those arteries. At rest there is sufficient oxygen reaching the heart muscle, but when the demand increases (eg, due to exercise for example), a portion of the heart does not receive enough oxygen to satisfy the demand, and pain results. The pain from exertional angina gradually subsides when the patient stops the exertion and rests. In contrast to an angina attack, if an artery becomes completely blocked, a myocardial infarction (MI) results, the pain lasts 20 to 30 minutes, and heart muscle cells that do not receive oxygen die if blood flow is not restored within a few hours.

Drugs to treat exertional angina are intended to increase the amount of oxygen reaching the heart muscle and/or decrease the demand for oxygen; the focus of nondrug measures is to accomplish the same thing. Loss of excess weight, smoking cessation, treatment of existing hypertension and hyperlipidemia, and a program of regular exercise are among the key nondrug measures.

Variant Angina

Variant angina (Prinzmetal's angina, vasospastic angina) also results in insufficient blood flow through a coronary artery but is caused from a coronary artery spasm. This spontaneous contraction of the smooth muscle of the artery causes reduced blood flow beyond that point and hence symptoms similar to chronic stable angina. However, Prinzmetal's angina symptoms can occur at any time, not specifically associated with exercise. The focus of drug therapy is to increase oxygen supply rather than to specifically reduce demand, as the cause is not a result of increased demand.

Unstable Angina

Unstable angina is a condition in which there is a change in the severity of pain or pattern of angina compared with what the patient has experienced previously (eg, if a patient with chronic stable angina experiences more frequent angina attacks, begins experiencing attacks even at rest, or if the intensity of the anginal pain increases noticeably compared with prior experiences). This suggests a change in the coronary heart disease status, such as the occurrence of a coronary emboli. The onset of unstable angina is a medical emergency since the risk of death is greater than with stable angina. The focus of drug therapy is to increase oxygen delivery to the heart muscle, decrease demand for oxygen, and alleviate persistent pain.

Myocardial Infarction

Coronary heart disease is the leading cause of death among men and women in the United States, and MI leads this list. As with angina, MI is an ischemic heart disease in that occlusion of a coronary artery prevents sufficient blood from reaching a portion of the heart muscle. With MI, however, the ischemia is persistent and progresses to cause death of some myocardial cells. The location and number of cells that die will determine the extent of loss of myocardial function. An MI is obviously an emergency situation and immediate goals include reducing myocardial oxygen demand, restoring coronary blood flow, preventing additional damage, and minimizing complications (eg, ventricular dysrhythmia and heart failure). Because an acute MI is an emergency and drug therapy is handled by emergency medical personnel and physicians, no discussion is included regarding therapy. The athletic trainer should realize that any patient who has symptoms of MI should immediately receive medical attention. Symptoms include chest pain or pressure, nausea, vomiting, profuse sweating, numbness or tingling in the arm, and shortness of breath.

Existence of atherosclerotic plaques, leading to thrombus formation and platelet aggregation, is the cause of the vast majority of MI. Not surprising, therefore, is that hyperlipidemia and hypertension are among the risk factors for MI, as are smoking and history of angina. Consequently, part of the drug therapy regimen includes treatment of these conditions.

Heart Failure

About 4.8 million Americans have *heart failure,* also know as congestive heart failure. The incidence increases with age with >70% of the patients being >60 years old. The 5-year survival rate is about 50%. The essence of the problem is that the heart cannot pump with enough force to adequately supply blood to the tissues. Factors that contribute to heart failure include hypertension, coronary heart disease, diabetes, valvular disease, obesity, high blood cholesterol, alcohol abuse, and the process of aging.

Initial treatment of acute MI includes immediate cessation of activity to decrease oxygen demand and providing supplemental oxygen. For rapid thrombolytic therapy, aspirin should be chewed and swallowed (160 to 325 mg) as soon as possible after the onset of MI symptoms unless the patient has an allergy or GI intolerance for aspirin. Morphine is the analgesic of choice because its cardiovascular effects reduce myocardial oxygen demand. Other therapies that are helpful in some patients within the first few hours after an MI are β-blockers, angiotensin-converting enzyme inhibitors, and either angioplasty or thrombolytic therapy such as alteplase (Activase), which are drugs that break apart an existing thrombus.

Heart failure develops over years. As failure begins, the ventricles fail to eject all of the blood and therefore the diastolic filling also increases. The heart enlarges as a result of excess blood in the chambers. When the heart muscle stretches, the compensating mechanism causes an automatic increase in contractility to increase cardiac output. There are limits, of course, to the compensatory mechanism, which are exceeded as heart failure continues. Other compensatory mechanisms also occur, such as an increased sympathetic tone and decreased parasympathetic effect. These autonomic nervous system effects cause an increased heart rate and contractility, which helps to increase cardiac output. Constriction of the blood vessels also occurs, which helps to maintain blood pressure to tissues but also increases the return of blood to the heart and increases the arterial pressure that the heart must pump against.

The *renin-angiotensin* system is also activated during heart failure, which increases *angiotensin II* and *aldosterone* levels. Aldosterone increases sodium and water retention; angiotensin II adds to an enhanced sympathetic tone by constricting systemic arterioles and veins to increase blood pressure. Decreased blood flow to the kidneys also contributes to water retention and eventual edema. As months or years of elevated aldosterone persist, it contributes to other aspects of the pathophysiology. For example, aldosterone increases the deposit of collagen within the heart, leading to cardiac fibrosis and eventual diminished function of the heart. This scenario of physiological changes eventually results in pulmonary and peripheral edema. Other primary symptoms of the condition include fatigue, exercise intolerance, shortness of breath, and tachycardia. Heart failure is a progressive disease, and consequently, there is a range of severity of these symptoms among patients. Heart failure is also referred to as congestive heart failure because of the pulmonary and peripheral edema, but the term is being used less frequently because some patients do not have symptoms of this fluid congestion. A widely used system of classifying patients regarding the severity of heart failure is the New York Heart Association Functional Classification (Table 12-5). In this classification, class I heart failure is the least severe and class IV the most severe.

Treatment of heart failure includes drug therapy, limiting sodium and excess fluid intake, reducing alcohol intake, losing excess weight, and exercising, depending on the severity of heart

Table 12-5. New York Heart Association Functional Classification of Heart Failure

Class I	Patient has no limitation of ordinary physical activity from undue fatigue, dyspnea, or palpitation.
Class II	Patient has slight limitation of physical activity. Normal physical activity produces fatigue, dyspnea, palpitations, or angina.
Class III	Patient has marked limitation of physical activity. There are no symptoms when patient is at rest but even mild activity causes symptoms.
Class IV	Patient experiences symptoms at rest and increased discomfort occurs with any physical activity.

failure. Regarding the exercise, note that patients with Class I and II heart failure (see Table 12-5) are physically active. In fact, low-intensity aerobic exercise on a regular basis has been demonstrated to improve symptoms and the quality of life in patients with stable heart failure. For safety reasons, patients need to progress slowly in an individualized exercise program and may require supervision during early stages of the exercise program.

DRUG THERAPY

Drug therapy for cardiovascular diseases generally requires long-term therapeutic regimens, often with multiple drug therapy to achieve desired therapeutic outcomes, along with routine monitoring of the disease to assess the effectiveness of the therapy. Some therapy is intended to alleviate acute symptoms whereas the focus of other therapy is to minimize the long-term effects of the disease. It may also be necessary in some patients to use other drugs to treat an underlying disease such as *dyslipidemia*, diabetes, or alcoholism. Consequently, it is likely that patients will be on multiple drug therapy for the cardiovascular disease, thus enhancing the likelihood of *adverse effects* and *drug interactions*.

β-Blockers

The number of *β-blocker* drugs has grown over the years to now encompass an array of more than a dozen drugs (Table 12-6). These drugs are *competitive inhibitors* of the *β-adrenergic receptors* and therefore are also called *β-adrenergic antagonists.* Blockade of these receptors causes a variety of effects, some beneficial and some not. Most of the therapeutic and adverse effects of these drugs can be explained by the activity at specific receptor sites. Not all β-blockers exhibit these effects to the same extent, in part because some β-blockers are relatively selective for β_1-adrenergic receptors (selective blockers) and other β-blockers are nonselective, combining significantly with both β_1- and β_2-receptors. Note that the selective β-blockers may elicit some β_2 response, particularly at higher doses. The primary effect of β-blockers with a brief discussion is provided (Box 12-5).

- Decreased heart rate and force of contraction as a result of blockade of β_1-receptors. When the level of adrenergic stimulation is low, the effect of adrenergic blockade will also be low. But when adrenergic agonist activity is high, such as during exercise or stress, the impact of an antagonist will be greater. As a result, β-blockers prevent the heart from over exertion but also prevent the automatic increase in cardiac output, resulting in exercise fatigue.

Table 12-6. β-Blockers

Generic Name	Trade Name	Dosage Range[1] (Total mg/day)
acebutolol[2]	Sectral	200 to 1200
atenolol[2]	Tenormin	25 to 100
betaxolol[2]	Kerlone	5 to 20
bisoprolol[2]	Zebeta	2.5 to 20
carteolol	Cartrol	2.5 to 10
carvedilol	Coreg	12.5 to 50
labetalol	Normodyne	200 to 1200
metoprolol[2]	Lopressor	50 to 450
nadolol	Corgard	40 to 320
penbutolol	Levatol	10 to 20
pindolol	Visken	10 to 60
propranolol	Inderal	40 to 480
timolol	Blocadren	20 to 60

[1]Adult oral dosage range for treatment of hypertension.
[2]Selective for β_1-receptors.

Box 12-5. Summary of Primary Effect of β-Blockers

- Decreased heart rate and force of contraction as a result of blockade of β_1-receptors.
- β-blockers slow the rate of impulses initiated by the SA node and the conduction velocity of the impulse through the AV node.
- Exercise fatigue may occur as a result of the β-blocker, preventing the heart from automatically increasing cardiac output.
- Reduced release of renin by the kidney as a result of β_1-receptor blockade, reducing the impact of the renin-angiotensin system.
- Bronchoconstriction from the blockade of β_2-receptors in the lung.
- Inhibition of glycogenolysis in the liver and muscle cells due to β_2-receptor blockade.
- Inhibition of sympathetic-induced activation of lipase in fat cells.
- Decreased peripheral vascular resistance as a result of long-term use of β-blockers.

- β-blockers slow the rate of impulses initiated by the SA node and the conduction velocity of the impulse through the AV node. Therefore, blockade of β_1-receptor is useful in treating certain tachydysrhythmias (abnormal rhythm in which the beats are too fast), including exercise-induced tachydysrhythmia.
- Reduced release of renin by the kidney as a result of β_1-receptor blockade, reducing the impact of the renin-angiotensin system.
- Bronchoconstriction from the blockade of β_2-receptors in the lung. This usually is of little consequence for patients with normal lung function. For patients with compromised lung function, however, this effect can be life-threatening. Consequently, nonselective β-

blockers are contraindicated in patients with asthma or chronic obstructive pulmonary disease (COPD); selective β_1-blockers must be used with great caution in these patients.

- Inhibition of *glycogenolysis* in the liver and muscle cells due to β_2-receptor blockade. Activation of glycogenolysis by sympathetic response (release of epinephrine from adrenal glands) mobilizes stored glucose from the liver during hypoglycemia. The epinephrine also elicits warning symptoms of hypoglycemia (eg, nervous feeling, tachycardia). Inhibition of this process by nonselective β-blockers is generally of little consequence for most patients, but it may delay recovery from hypoglycemia in patients who have insulin-dependent diabetes and may also mask the warning symptoms of hypoglycemia. Tachycardia usually accompanies hypoglycemia-induced sympathetic nervous system activation and is a warning sign of hypoglycemia but this helpful symptom is inhibited by all β-blockers.
- Inhibition of sympathetic-induced activation of *lipase* in fat cells. Activation of this enzyme causes the conversion of stored triglycerides to fatty acids and results in the release of fatty acids into the blood from fat cells. Although the exact mechanism is not pinpointed, and a third receptor (β_3) may be involved, nonselective β-blockers may affect the metabolism of triglycerides and fatty acids.
- Decreased peripheral vascular resistance as a result of long-term use of β-blockers. The mechanism is unclear but this is beneficial for treatment of cardiovascular disease.

Primary uses for β-blockers are to treat the chronic diseases of hypertension, angina, and heart failure. Therefore, useful characteristics of these drugs are that they are orally effective and require only once or twice per day dosing, either due to an inherent long half-life ($t\frac{1}{2}$) or due to an extended release formulation. The activity of some β-blockers is terminated primarily by liver metabolism (eg, metoprolol, propranolol, timolol), by excretion as active drug in the urine (eg, acebutolol, atenolol, nadolol), or by significant termination by both routes (eg, pindolol).

The β-blockers are approximately equally effective for treatment of hypertension, and thus selection of drug can be based in part on the most suitable *pharmacokinetic* parameters (eg, $t\frac{1}{2}$ as affected by liver and kidney function), cost, *adverse effects*, and existence of other diseases. These drugs are used either alone or in combination with other antihypertensive drugs. They decrease blood pressure in hypertensive, but not normotensive, patients. The mechanism for the antihypertensive response is not clear although a likely key factor is the ability of β-blockers to decrease peripheral vascular resistance after long-term use. Other mechanisms that may contribute to their use as antihypertensive therapy are the inhibition of the *renin-angiotensin* mechanism, decrease in cardiac output, and inhibition of reflex tachycardia that occurs with the use of vasodilators (see below).

Angina is also effectively treated with β-blockers. By decreasing the heart rate and contractility, the β-blockers decrease the oxygen demand and thereby decrease the frequency and intensity of anginal attacks. These drugs are effective for prevention of stable, not variant angina, when used on a daily basis. They also provide the benefit of inhibiting reflex tachycardia caused by nitroglycerin therapy (see below). If β-blocker therapy must be discontinued, gradual rather than abrupt withdrawal is necessary to prevent precipitation of anginal attacks or myocardial infarction.

Some β-blockers are effective in the treatment of heart failure. At one time, these drugs were contraindicated in patients with heart failure but they have been shown to slow the progression of the disease. Short-term use of β-blockers may not alleviate specific symptoms, but long-term use of the appropriate drug, beginning at a low dose, has shown to prolong life. Although the exact mechanism of this beneficial effect is not known, it is likely that a contributor is the ability of β-blockers to decrease the sympathetic response that is usually elevated in patients with heart failure. Metoprolol (Lopressor), carvedilol (Coreg), and bisoprolol (Zebeta) have demonstrated effectiveness for this use.

Table 12-7. Selected Diuretics

Category	Generic Name	Trade Name	Dosage Range[1] (Total mg/day)
Thiazide	chlorthalidone	Hygroton	12.5 to 50
	hydrochlorothiazide	Hydrodiuril	12.5 to 50
	indapamide	Lozol	1.25 to 5
	metolazone	Zaroxolyn	1.25 to 10
Loop	bumetanide	Bumex	0.5 to 10
	ethacrynic acid	Edecrin	25 to100
	furosemide	Lasix	40 to 240
	torsemide	Demadex	5 to 100
Potassium-sparing	amiloride	Midamor	5 to 10
	spironolactone	Aldactone	25 to 100
	triamterene	Dyrenium	50 to 150

[1]*Adult oral dosage range for treatment of hypertension.*

There are several other uses for selected β-blockers that are not as pertinent to this chapter but worth noting. Such uses include preventing migraine headache, treating acute panic symptoms, inhibiting some symptoms of pheochromocytoma (a catecholamine-secreting tumor), managing certain types of dysrhythmias, treating acute MI and preventing recurrences of MI, and treating glaucoma topically.

Some of the significant adverse effects are specific for patients who also have a coexisting disease. Because of the potential for bronchoconstriction (even with ophthalmic preparations), β-blockers should be avoided in asthmatics or limited to β_1-selective agents (eg, metoprolol, acebutolol, atenolol) if use of a β-blocker is necessary. Note that the cardioselectivity for β_1-receptors is lost as the dose increases. Similarly, due to the ability of β-blockers to mask the symptoms of hypoglycemia and to delay the recovery of hypoglycemia by *glycogenolysis*, the use of β-blockers in diabetics should be used with caution and limited to β_1-selective agents. Other adverse effects that are significant in some patients include bradycardia, insomnia, sexual dysfunction, depression, nightmares, increased levels of plasma triglycerides, reduced levels of HDL cholesterol, fatigue, and decreased exercise tolerance.

Diuretics

Diuretics are drugs that increase the excretion of sodium (Na^+) and chloride (Cl^-) ions. The amount of sodium chloride (NaCl) in the body is the major factor that determines the extracellular fluid volume, which then contributes to blood pressure. The more NaCl, the more extracellular fluid volume (and thus blood volume), and the higher the blood pressure. Accumulation of extracellular fluid in any tissue constitutes edema. The major uses of diuretics are to reduce edema and treat hypertension. Regarding these uses, there are three major categories of diuretics: thiazide diuretics, loop diuretics, and potassium-sparing diuretics (Table 12-7).

These categories differ in their specific site of action in the nephron of the kidney (Figure 12-3)—loop diuretics in the Henle's loop, thiazide diuretics in the early distal convoluted tubule, and potassium-sparing diuretics in the late distal convoluted tubule and collecting duct. Besides increasing the excretion of Na^+ and Cl^-, diuretics affect the exchange of other ions, potassium

Figure 12-3. Representation of nephron showing the sites of diuretic action. 1 = site of action of loop diuretics; 2 = site of action of thiazide diuretics; and 3 = sites of action of potassium-sparing diuretics.

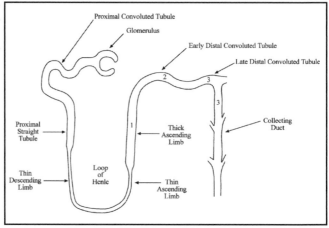

(K^+) being the one of prime concern. Thiazide and loop diuretics increase the excretion of K^+, whereas, as evident from the name, potassium-sparing diuretics prevent loss of K^+. The potassium-sparing diuretics have only a weak diuretic effect but are useful in combination with either a thiazide or loop diuretic to prevent hypokalemia (low blood potassium). The thiazide diuretics are the diuretics of first choice for treatment of hypertension; however, the loop diuretics are more potent and are used when a more pronounced diuretic effect is desired or when the thiazide diuretics are no longer sufficiently effective for the treatment of edema or hypertension.

Decrease in blood volume through *diuresis* is likely the mechanism for the initial antihypertensive activity. However, blood volume returns to nearly the initial level with continued use. A reduction in peripheral vascular resistance occurs with long-term use of diuretics and is likely the cause of continued antihypertensive activity. The mechanism for this long-term activity appears to be connected to low sodium levels as low dietary sodium is beneficial and high sodium is detrimental to the effectiveness of the diuretics. The loop diuretics also increase renal blood flow through a *prostaglandin-mediated* mechanism.

Of the potassium-sparing diuretics, amiloride (Midamor) and triamterene (Dyrenium) prevent potassium loss by directly inhibiting sodium-potassium exchange through sodium channels in the distal tubule. Spironolactone (Aldactone), however, produces its effect by inhibiting aldosterone, which indirectly decreases the sodium channels. In addition, the *aldosterone antagonism* decreases *cardiac remodeling*, a process that changes the shape, size, and effectiveness of the heart as a result of cardiac injury. Angiotensin II and aldosterone play a significant role in initiating the remodeling process, which contributes to the progression of heart failure. Consequently, spironolactone is recommended for the treatment of advanced heart failure and increases survival in these patients. The dosage of spironolactone for treatment of heart failure is lower (12.5 to 50 mg/day) than the dose needed for treatment of hypertension (50 to 100 mg/day).

Technically, the terms "thiazides" or "thiazide diuretics" refer to a group of diuretics that share a specific chemical structure and therefore also a common mechanism of action. Subsequent to the initial use of this term, several other diuretics with the same mechanism of action but without the thiazide structure were introduced. These diuretics are often jointly grouped as "thiazides and related diuretics" or "thiazide-type" diuretics. Because the differences are primarily in the chemical structure rather than pharmacological properties, for simplicity these two groups are referred together as thiazide diuretics in this text.

Diuretics may be used to treat edema associated with acute and chronic conditions, including congestive heart failure. These drugs are among the initial therapy recommended for treatment of hypertension. These diuretics are effective orally. The onset of diuretic action of the thiazide and loop diuretics is within 1 hour after oral ingestion. The potassium-sparing diuretics are not very water soluble and are therefore absorbed more slowly from the GI tract. Thiazide diuretics are usually the first choice to achieve diuresis, whereas loop diuretics have the potential to produce greater fluid loss than necessary. Thiazide diuretics are filtered at the glomerulus to reach their tubular site of action. Loop diuretics reach their tubular site by active transport, and therefore, are more effective in patients with heart failure as these patients typically have reduced glomerular filtration rate.

Concerning adverse effects, a major concern with long-term use of thiazide and loop diuretics is to prevent *hypokalemia*. Depending on the dose of diuretic and duration of therapy, patients using loop or thiazide diuretics may be advised to eat foods rich in potassium (see Table 12-4) or use potassium supplements. Alternatively, a potassium-sparing diuretic can be used concurrently with the loop or thiazide diuretic. Symptoms of hypokalemia include muscle fatigue and cramps, with eventual cardiac dysrhythmias. Because thiazide or loop diuretics are used to treat heart failure, and because digoxin is used to treat heart failure (see below), it is noteworthy that hypokalemia will cause toxicity from lower doses of digoxin. Consequently, potassium levels are monitored more closely for patients receiving digoxin and a diuretic.

Hyperkalemia is a concern with the use of potassium-sparing diuretics and therefore potassium supplements should not be used with potassium-sparing diuretics. Angiotensin-converting enzyme inhibitors also have a potassium-sparing effect and therefore are generally not used in combination with potassium-sparing diuretics. The potassium-sparing diuretic spironolactone (Aldactone) is chemically related to *androgens* and *progestins* and thus may cause gynecomastia and sexual dysfunction in men, whereas women may experience deepening of the voice, *hirsutism*, and menstrual irregularities. Adverse effects with thiazide and loop diuretics include increased plasma levels of *LDL cholesterol*, total cholesterol and total triglycerides, hyperglycemia, and sexual dysfunction. These are primarily a concern with higher doses of these diuretics (eg, 100 mg/day of hydrochlorothiazide). Use of nonsteroidal anti-inflammatory drugs (NSAIDs) with thiazide and loop diuretics can diminish the effectiveness of the diuretics. The mechanism for this is likely to include the NSAID inhibition of the *prostaglandin-mediated* improvement of renal blood flow, fluid excretion, and/or vasodilation. Thiazide diuretics have a sulfonamide component to their chemical structure and therefore should not be used in patients who are allergic to sulfonamides.

Angiotensin-Converting Enzyme Inhibitors

Angiotensin-converting enzyme inhibitors are very effective drugs for the treatment of hypertension, heart failure, and MI. By inhibiting ACE, these drugs decrease the production of angiotensin II and therefore diminish the effect of angiotensin II on vasoconstriction and *aldosterone* release. Angiotensin-converting enzyme inhibitors also prevent the breakdown of *bradykinin*, which, among other actions, increases the release of vasodilating *prostaglandins* (ie, ACE inhibitors prolong bradykinin's effect, which increases prostaglandin-mediated vasodilation). The result of ACE inhibitors is arterial and venous vasodilation, decreased systemic vascular resistance, increased sodium and water excretion, increased potassium retention, and increased blood flow to the kidney.

There are many ACE inhibitors on the market (Table 12-8). Captopril (Capoten) was the first to receive Food and Drug Administration (FDA) approval. All are effective antihypertensives,

Table 12-8. ACE Inhibitors and Angiotensin II Receptor Blockers

Category	Generic Name	Trade Name	Dosage Range[1] (Total mg/day)
ACE Inhibitor	benazepril	Lotensin	10 to 40
	captopril	Capoten	12.5 to 150
	enalapril	Vasotec	2.5 to 40
	fosinopril	Monopril	10 to 40
	lisinopril	Zestril	5 to 40
	moexipril	Univasc	7.5 to 30
	quinapril	Accupril	5 to 80
	ramipril	Altace	1.25 to 20
	trandolapril	Mavik	1 to 4
Angiotensin II Receptor Blockers	candesartan	Atacand	8 to 32
	eprosartan	Teveten	400 to 800
	irbesartan	Avapro	150 to 300
	losartan	Cozaar	25 to 100
	olmesartan	Benicar	20 to 40
	telmisartan	Micardis	40 to 80
	valsartan	Diovan	80 to 320

[1]Adult oral dosage range for treatment of hypertension.

with no particular clear-cut advantage of any one drug. These ACE inhibitors differ somewhat in their degree of oral absorption and potency, but recommended dosing accommodates for these differences. The activity of most ACE inhibitors is primarily terminated by renal excretion of the active drug, and therefore dosage adjustment may be necessary if renal impairment exists. Most of the ACE inhibitors are administered orally as a *prodrug* and thus rely on the liver to metabolize the drug to the active form. Captopril (Capoten) and lisinopril (Zestril) are exceptions. Because activation of the prodrug is dependent on liver function, diminished liver function can decrease the conversion of the prodrug to the active form. Typical oral dosing is 1 to 2 times per day.

The ACE inhibitors are effective alone or in combination with diuretics or β-blockers to treat hypertension. The vasodilation and reduced blood volume are major contributors to the antihypertensive effect. Unlike β-blockers, ACE inhibitors do not affect the automatic cardiac and *baroreceptor* responses and therefore do not cause significant exercise intolerance. They also do not cause sexual dysfunction, fatigue, bronchoconstriction, *hypokalemia*, or hyperglycemia as do β-blockers or diuretics. The lack of these effects provides an advantage for the use of ACE inhibitors for the treatment of hypertension in patients who also have diabetes or asthma. The potassium retention aspect of ACE inhibitors is an advantage to prevent hypokalemia when combined with thiazide diuretics. In fact, use of potassium supplements and potassium-sparing diuretics should be avoided with ACE inhibitors unless blood tests reveal the existence of *hypokalemia*. The antihypertensive effect of ACE inhibitors is greater in some patients than others. Patients with high renin blood levels respond better to ACE inhibitors, but patients with normal *renin* levels may also respond, presumably due to a decreased rate of *bradykinin* inactivation, a higher level of angiotensin II produced in local tissue sites, or due to greater tissue responsiveness to normal angiotensin II levels.

Angiotensin-converting enzyme inhibitors have become an important part of the therapy for heart failure. Therapy with these drugs relieves symptoms and delays progression of the disease. Use of ACE inhibitors provides a multi-pronged approach: dilation of arterioles improves cardiac output; venous dilation reduces pulmonary and peripheral edema; inhibition of aldosterone increases sodium and water excretion to reduce edema; and inhibition of the angiotensin II-mediated effect on cardiac remodeling and dilation of arterioles to the kidneys improve renal function, which also reduces edema.

Treatment of MI is another approved use of some ACE inhibitors; their use with acute MI decreases mortality. Therapy is begun immediately and may be continued long-term if necessary.

Although most patients generally tolerate ACE inhibitors quite well, some adverse effects can be problematic. A persistent dry cough occurs in 5% to 20% of patients, which may require discontinuation of the ACE inhibitor. The cough develops, at least in part, from the accumulation of bradykinin. It occurs more frequently in women than men and dissipates over several days after discontinuation of the ACE inhibitor. For patients being treated for heart failure with ACE inhibitors, pulmonary edema should be eliminated as the cause of the cough before the ACE inhibitor is discontinued; diuretic therapy should diminish the cough if pulmonary edema is the origin.

Another bradykinin-linked adverse effect is *angioneurotic edema*, a rare condition in which rapid swelling in the nose, throat, and larynx may lead to death if not treated; it occurs more frequently in African Americans than in Caucasians. Other adverse effects that may warrant discontinuation of therapy are skin rashes, loss of taste, and taste disturbances that occur in 4% to 10% of patients. First-dose hypotension is common with ACE inhibitors, especially in patients who are sodium- or volume-depleted or in patients on diuretics. Consequently, patients should be started with a low dose ACE inhibitor and diuretics should be discontinued 2 to 3 days prior to initiating ACE inhibitor therapy.

Drug interactions with ACE inhibitors occur with antacids and NSAIDs. Antacids can interfere with the absorption of ACE inhibitors and should not be taken concurrently. NSAIDs can decrease the antihypertensive effect by inhibiting the bradykinin-induced antihypertensive (ie, vasodilation) effects. Concurrent use of diuretics may cause first-dose hypotension (see above). To prevent hyperkalemia, potassium supplements and potassium-sparing diuretics should be avoided with ACE inhibitors unless hypokalemia is identified.

Angiotensin II Receptor Blockers

Angiotensin II receptor blockers (ARBs) are a relatively new category of drugs approved for use to treat hypertension, obtaining FDA approval in 1995. In contrast to ACE inhibitors, which decrease the production of angiotensin II, ARBs combine with the receptor site to prevent the response of angiotensin II after it has been produced. Therefore, ARBs have pharmacological effects similar to ACE inhibitors: vasodilation and increased sodium and water excretion through suppression of aldosterone release. Angiotensin II receptor blockers, however, do not affect *bradykinin* metabolism, and therefore, the incidence of some adverse effects is significantly reduced in comparison with ACE inhibitors.

There are several ARBs approved for treatment of hypertension (see Table 12-8). They have approximately equal antihypertensive effectiveness. The *dose response curve* (see Chapter 3) for these drugs is quite flat, which means that increasing the dose does not cause much increase in response. The *pharmacokinetics* are somewhat dissimilar for the drugs within this category: the plasma half-lives range 2.5 to 24 hours; major routes of plasma clearance of *active drug* vary from liver metabolism, to bile excretion, and renal elimination; and depending on the drug, liver metabolism results in the drug being converted from inactive to active, from active to inactive, or from active to more active.

For treatment of hypertension, ARBs are as effective as ACE inhibitors in lowering blood pressure. Angiotension II receptor blockers provide an alternative to the ACE inhibitor for patients who experience the bothersome cough. Angiotensin II receptor blockers have shown effectiveness in treatment of heart failure and to treat MI. More data are necessary to verify the long-term effects and to compare therapeutic effectiveness of ARBs relative to other antihypertensives.

Adverse effects from ARBs are minimal. In comparison with ACE inhibitors, the cough, *angioneurotic edema*, first-dose hypotension, and taste disturbances are greatly reduced or nonexistent with ARBs. *Hyperkalemia* is only a concern if ARBs are combined with potassium-sparing diuretics, potassium supplements, or in patients with renal disease.

Calcium Channel Blockers

Calcium channels are the gates that control the flow of calcium into the cells of arterial smooth muscle and cardiac muscle. Influx of calcium results in contraction of these muscle cells, which causes peripheral vasoconstriction, increased heart rate and force of contraction, and cardiac arteriole vasoconstriction. Blocking these channels with *calcium channel blockers* (CCBs) causes the opposite effects: peripheral vasodilation, decreased heart rate and force of contraction, and dilation of arterioles of the heart. There are two types of CCBs: those that affect the calcium channels of the heart and vascular muscle and those that are selective for only vascular smooth muscle.

The CCBs are approved for treatment of hypertension (Table 12-9) and some are also approved for treating chronic stable and vasospastic angina. They are absorbed readily after oral administration, but first-pass liver metabolism significantly diminishes the amount of active drug that reaches the active site. Typical dosages account for the *first-pass effect* but patients with liver dysfunction may need a lower dosage due to a diminished impact on first-pass metabolism. Elderly patients may also require dosage adjustment due to diminished hepatic function.

Peripheral arteriole vasodilation reduces blood pressure. Dilation of the arterioles of the heart increases blood and oxygen to the heart muscle, coupled with the reduced arterial blood pressure, are of obvious benefits in treating angina. The effect on heart rate and contractility reduces the oxygen demand on the heart and is beneficial for treating both hypertension and angina. Rapid vasodilation can occur with CCBs, resulting in reflex tachycardia (a *baroreceptor* reflex effect), which is counterproductive for treatment of both angina and hypertension. This tachycardia is offset by cardiac effects of nonselective CCBs: verapamil (Calan) and diltiazem (Cardizem). Nifedipine (Procardia) and all of the other CCBs currently available (nifedipine-like CCBs) are much more selective for the calcium channels of vascular smooth muscle than heart muscle. Consequently, the selective CCBs do not have the cardiac effects to offset the reflex tachycardia and therefore some antihypertensive benefit is lost. Some of the nifedipine-like CCBs (also called dihydropyridines from their chemical structure) have a greater reflex tachycardia response than others in this group but can be combined with a β-blocker to prevent the reflex tachycardia. Alternatively, slow release dosage forms can be used so that the drop in blood pressure is gradual, thus minimizing the *baroreceptor reflex*. CCBs do not have an effect on exercise tolerance.

Table 12-9. Calcium Channel Blockers

Generic Name	Trade Name	Dosage Range[1] (Total mg/day)
amlodipine[2]	Norvasc	2.5 to 10
diltiazem[2,3]	Cardizem SR	120 to 360
felodipine	Plendil	2.5 to 10
isradipine	DynaCirc CR	5 to 20
nicardipine[2]	Cardene SR	60 to 120
nifedipine[2]	Procardia XL	30 to 120
nisoldipine	Sular	10 to 60
verapamil[2,3]	Calan SR	120 to 480

[1]*Adult oral dosage range for treatment of hypertension.*
[2]*Also approved for treatment of chronic stable and vasospastic angina.*
[3]*Besides blocking calcium channels in vascular smooth muscle, also blocks calcium channels in the heart = nonselective.*

Adverse effects are related to the vasodilation and smooth muscle relaxation effects. For example, facial flushing, headache, gingival hyperplasia, and edema of lower extremities are adverse effects common to all the CCBs. Additionally, CCBs decrease the contraction of intestinal smooth muscle, which results in constipation. Bradycardia from verapamil (Calan) and diltiazem (Cardizem) can occur but is of little consequence unless the patient also has certain heart diseases (eg, *heart block*, heart failure), in which case a *nifedipine-like* CCB is preferred because they do not affect heart muscle. Although β-blockers reduce reflex tachycardia from *nifedipine-like* CCBs, use of β-blockers with verapamil (Calan) or diltiazem (Cardizem) should be avoided because they have similar effects on the heart and therefore if used together will increase the potential for heart block.

Organic Nitrates

Nitroglycerin is the prototype organic nitrate. Although it has been used since the 1800s, it remains the most frequently used drug to treat acute angina attacks. The principle effect of nitroglycerin is to dilate peripheral vascular smooth muscle. This primarily involves veins, although arterioles are affected to a lesser extent. Vasodilation reduces the blood returning to the heart and therefore decreases the oxygen demand by the heart; a beneficial effect in a patient experiencing stable (exertional) angina. The relaxation of vascular smooth muscle by nitroglycerin also alleviates spasms of those muscles, and hence nitroglycerin is also useful for the treatment of variant angina.

Nitroglycerin is very potent (0.3 to 0.6 mg for relief of acute attack) and very lipid soluble; both being attributes that are conducive to the use of sublingual and transdermal dosage forms. Regardless of the dosage form, the plasma half-life of nitroglycerin is very short, about 5 minutes. Sublingual administration is the most common route for treatment of acute angina with nitroglycerin. The sublingual tablets are inexpensive and dissolve very quickly under the tongue, provided the patient does not have a dry mouth. Onset of action is within 3 minutes and duration is <1 hour. Patients should take the first dose as soon as possible when pain begins. If relief is not obtained with three sublingual tablets over 20 minutes, the patient should seek emergency care. Sublingual tablets can be used 5 to 10 minutes prior to exertion as a short-term preventative of anginal attacks. Nitroglycerin is chemically unstable and will lose effectiveness as it is exposed to light and moisture. Therefore, tablets should be stored in tightly closed glass containers, protected from light and moisture and should be discarded after 6 months. Sublingual tablets are not effective orally (by swallowing) because of significant first pass metabolism.

Recall from Chapter 2 that the oral route refers to the drug being swallowed. Recall also from Chapter 2 that nitroglycerin taken orally is subject to the enzymes in the intestinal cells and the liver before reaching the general circulation (ie, first-pass metabolism). Therefore if sublingual nitroglycerin tablets are swallowed, the nitroglycerin is inactivated before it can reach the site of action.

A burning sensation under the tongue is indicative of active nitroglycerin, although some patients, especially elderly, may lack sufficient sensation to experience the burning.

Other dosage forms for treatment of acute angina are buccal tablets and translingual spray. The buccal tablets are placed between the lip and gum or cheek and gum. These tablets provide onset within 2 minutes, but sustained effect for 3 to 5 hours. Buccal tablets provide relief of acute attacks, but compared with sublingual tablets they provide more sustained relief for longer periods of exercise tolerance. The translingual spray provides a metered dose of nitroglycerin onto or under the tongue with onset and duration similar to sublingual tablets.

Nitroglycerin is also available in sustained release tablets and capsules, transdermal systems, and ointments, which provide the drug for a longer time frame. Larger doses (2.6 to 13 mg/dosage unit) are used for the tablets and capsules, not only to provide drug for a longer time but also to accommodate for the first-pass hepatic metabolism. Onset is 20 to 45 minutes and duration is up to 8 hours. The many transdermal systems make nitroglycerin available in various patch devices and allow a continuous release of nitroglycerin. The doses of transdermal patches are designated as release rates (eg, 0.2 mg/h); the higher the release rate, the higher the blood concentration of nitroglycerin achieved. Nitroglycerin ointment is also placed on the skin for a transdermal effect. Doses of ointment are measured as inches of ointment squeezed from the tube. The ointment is spread over an area of skin on the chest or back.

The *onset of action* of the sustained release and transdermal nitroglycerin products are too slow to be used to treat acute attacks but they are used to prevent angina attacks. A significant concern regarding the daily use of nitroglycerin is the development of tolerance, referring to a diminished effectiveness of the nitroglycerin as a result of frequent or continuous exposure to the drug. Tolerance can develop after 1 day of continuous exposure, especially at higher doses of nitroglycerin. The cause of tolerance is not clear. To prevent tolerance, each day should include 8 to 12 hours in which no nitroglycerin (or other nitrate drug) is administered. For example, the transdermal patch could be removed at night. When the patch is reapplied, onset of action occurs in about 1 hour.

Adverse effects from daily nitroglycerin use are generally manageable. Headache is common, sometimes severe, but subsides after several days of treatment. The rapid vasodilation causes reflex tachycardia through the *baroreceptor reflex*. Tachycardia is counterproductive in the treatment of angina and therefore a β-blocker or a CCB that suppresses the heart (verapamil or diltiazem) can be used to prevent reflex tachycardia. *Orthostatic hypotension* (postural hypotension) is also a potential problem associated with vasodilation. Dizziness, with potential for fainting, occurs upon standing because of blood pooling in the veins from nitrate-induced vasodilation. This pooling prevents a sufficient transient increase in blood pressure needed upon standing. Concurrent use of alcohol or CCBs, which also have a vasodilation effect, can accentuate the *orthostatic hypotension* response. Use of sildenafil (Viagra), a drug to treat erectile dysfunction, within 24 hours of nitroglycerin or any other organic nitrate can result in potentially fatal hypotension.

Other organic nitrate drugs are also available for the treatment of angina. These are available as oral, chewable, or sublingual dosage forms for prophylaxis of angina attacks and/or treatment of acute attacks. The adverse effects, potential for tolerance, and drug interactions are similar for these drugs as for nitroglycerin. Examples are isosorbide mononitrate (Imdur) and isosorbide dinitrate (Isordil). They offer no particular therapeutic advantage over nitroglycerin.

Vasodilators

As discussed in this chapter, ACE inhibitors, CCBs, and organic nitrates all have a vasodilation component to their mechanism of action. There are other categories of drugs that also cause peripheral vasodilation as a major component of their mechanism. These other vasodilators are used to treat hypertension, but they are not the first-line or second-line drugs for most patients because they exert a lesser impact on the symptoms or disease process, or because the frequency or severity of adverse effects is more pronounced. Consequently, vasodilators as a category of drugs are only briefly mentioned here to provide a more complete picture of the drugs available to treat hypertension.

These vasodilators fall into three general categories: α_1-adrenergic blockers, centrally acting α_2-adrenergic agonists, and direct-acting vasodilators. The α_1-adrenergic blockers combine with the a-receptors on the peripheral blood vessels to prevent *adrenergic-stimulated* vasoconstriction; prazosin (Minipress) is an example. Activation of the α_2-*receptor* in the CNS indirectly affects the peripheral nervous system by decreasing sympathetic outflow (ie, reduces the CNS controlled sympathetic response), thereby reducing the response at the *α-adrenergic receptor*. An example of a centrally acting α_2-adrenergic agonist is clonidine (Catapres). Minoxidil (Loniten) is a direct-acting vasodilator; it does not function selectively through adrenergic receptors but acts directly on the vascular smooth muscle to cause vasodilation.

Digoxin

Digoxin (Lanoxin) is a member of a group of drugs called cardiac *glycosides* but is the only one in this group commonly used therapeutically. The major use for digoxin is to treat heart failure. The therapeutic benefit stems primarily as a result of digoxin's ability to increase the force of contraction. As a result of the positive *inotropic* response, cardiac output increases, exercise tolerance improves, urine output increases, edema decreases, and renin release is decreased, which subsequently reduces the response from angiotensin II and aldosterone. These effects help to alleviate symptoms of heart failure but digoxin does not improve survival.

The mechanism for digoxin centers on the drug's ability to inhibit the enzyme called Na^+, K^+-ATPase. (Note: This ATPase has a different function than the one in the stomach cells discussed in Chapter 11.) Inhibition of this enzyme results in an accumulation of calcium ions within the cell, which increases the force of contraction. The concentration of potassium plays an important role in the therapeutic effect and toxic effect of digoxin. Potassium competes with digoxin for the same ATPase enzyme binding site, and therefore an increase in potassium concentration decreases the response from of digoxin, and a decrease in potassium will increase digoxin effects. Consequently, *hyperkalemia* minimizes digoxin effectiveness whereas *hypokalemia* can cause digoxin toxicity, both effects occur without a change in the digoxin dosage. Monitoring of potassium blood levels is therefore a part of digoxin therapy.

Two key characteristics of digoxin are that it has a low *therapeutic index* and that many factors affect the *pharmacokinetic* and *pharmacodynamic* parameters. Significant changes in these parameters may warrant a dosage adjustment of digoxin to maintain optimal effectiveness. As already mentioned, blood potassium levels can affect the response from digoxin. Considering that diuretics are also frequently used as a component of heart failure therapy, and that some diuretics can cause *hypokalemia* (eg, thiazide and loop diuretics), caution is warranted to prevent a problem when diuretics and digoxin are combined.

Digoxin is excreted mostly unchanged in the urine. As urine output increases with increased cardiac output, the dose of digoxin may need adjustment as it is excreted at a faster rate. Drug interactions occur with a variety of drugs that alter the absorption or renal excretion of digoxin, or change the conduction of impulses in the heart to either potentiate or antagonize the cardiac effects of digoxin. Examples of drugs that increase an effect of digoxin are erythromycin, tetracyclines, β-blockers, CCBs, and *sympathomimetics*. Examples of drugs that decrease an effect of digoxin are antacids and *cholestyramine*.

Because of the potential for the effectiveness of digoxin to be modified by drug interactions, changes in potassium blood concentration, and changes in kidney function, it is standard procedure to monitor the patient's digoxin blood concentration and/or signs of cardiac toxicity. Adverse effects that may be early signs of toxicity are anorexia, nausea, vomiting, fatigue, blurred vision, or the appearance of halos around objects. Cardiac toxicity includes a variety of dysrhythmias that can progress to heart failure. Closer monitoring of digoxin blood levels and adverse effects typically occurs: at the beginning of therapy; if there is a change in dosage; if there are signs of toxicity; if symptoms of heart failure increase; or if a drug with the potential for drug interaction is added to the patient's drug therapy.

Typical dosage range for maintenance digoxin therapy is 0.125 to 0.5 mg/day in a single dose of an oral tablet. Digoxin has a long half-life ($t\frac{1}{2}$ = 1.5 to 2 days), and consequently, it takes at least 6 days (4 $t\frac{1}{2}$) for a stable blood level to be obtained when initiating therapy or adjusting the dose unless a loading dose is given. Oral absorption of digoxin tablets varies from

> *Recall from Chapter 3 that a loading dose is one or more doses that are higher than the maintenance dose and administered at the beginning of therapy for the purpose of more quickly achieving the desirable blood level.*

70% to 80% among most patients. Digoxin is also available as liquid-filled, soft capsules (Lanoxicaps), which provide a somewhat higher rate of absorption. The higher absorption rate necessitates a downward adjustment in dosage with the capsule compared with tablets; the major disadvantage is higher cost.

Summary

For the treatment of hypertension and heart disease, there are several categories of drugs with numerous examples within each category. Knowledge of the mechanism of action of these drug categories provides a means of understanding the uses and many of the common adverse effects. Some key points are:

- β-blockers decrease the heart rate and force of contraction and therefore prevent the heart from overexertion. The selective *β₁-blockers* are more specific for the heart than nonselective *β-blockers* and thus have fewer adverse effects. Uses include the treatment of hypertension, angina, MI, and heart failure. The potential for significant adverse effects resides primarily with patients with coexisting diseases of asthma or diabetes. Exercise intolerance is also a common adverse effect.

- Diuretics decrease the workload of the heart by decreasing blood volume and peripheral vascular resistance. These drugs are used to treat hypertension and edema associated with heart failure. *Hypokalemia* is a common adverse effect associated with thiazide and loop diuretics but the addition of potassium supplements or potassium-sparing diuretics can offset the problem. Unrelated to the diuretic effect, spironolactone is also effective in treating heart failure.
- Angiotensin-converting enzyme inhibitors prevent the formation of *angiotensin II* and thus inhibit the peripheral vascular constriction and fluid retention effects of angiotensin II. Angiotensin-converting enzyme inhibitors are useful for the treatment of hypertension, heart failure, and MI. A persistent cough is a common adverse effect that sometimes warrants discontinuation of the drug. Angiotensin-converting enzyme inhibitors do not pose the problems to diabetics and asthmatics as do β-blockers and they are also useful in combination with diuretics for their potassium-sparing effect.
- Angiotensin II receptor blockers have a usefulness similar to ACE inhibitors because both categories of drugs interfere with the *renin-angiotensin system.* The ARBs do not cause the cough and have less significant potassium retention effects compared with ACE inhibitors.
- Calcium channel blockers decrease the contraction of myocardium and vascular smooth muscle. Selective CCBs only affect vascular smooth muscle. Because CCBs cause vasodilation, reflex tachycardia can occur with the selective CCBs unless a β-blocker is used concurrently. Uses for CCBs are primarily for treatment of hypertension and angina.
- Nitroglycerin is the drug of choice for treatment of acute angina attacks. This drug reduces the oxygen demand on the heart by causing peripheral vasodilation. Sublingual tablets produce an effect within 3 minutes but also are of short duration. Adverse effects are short-term, a burning sensation under the tongue, and headache being the most common. Transdermal and sustained release oral dosage forms are available to prevent attacks.
- Digoxin is used to treat heart failure to relieve symptoms although it does not improve survival. The heart more efficiently pumps blood due to the effect of digoxin, and consequently, blood flow to the kidney also increases. Digoxin has a low therapeutic index and thus must be monitored for toxicity; hypokalemia increases the effect of digoxin and can precipitate toxic symptoms.

THERAPY OVERVIEW

Besides drug therapy, an important part of the overall treatment plan for cardiovascular diseases are the nondrug measures that can have a significant impact on the symptoms, disease progression, and effectiveness of drug therapy. These include the life-style modifications mentioned in the Foundational Concepts section of this chapter. Another nondrug measure is to promote compliance with drug therapy. As is the case with the treatment of other chronic diseases, lack of compliance is a major impedance to achieving therapeutic outcomes, contributing to inadequate control in over two-thirds of hypertensive patients. Poor compliance is particularly a problem with hypertension therapy because it often requires a multiple drug regimen and the lack of immediate symptoms associated with hypertension diminishes the incentive to maintain therapy. Two means of improving compliance is to educate the patient regarding the potential effects of uncontrolled hypertension and to reduce the complexity of the drug regimen. Regarding the latter issue, the therapy for patients with a multiple drug regimen should be reviewed to determine whether a switch from multiple dosing per day to once-a-day or twice-a-day dosing is appropriate. Another option is to replace therapy with the corresponding fixed-dose combina-

Table 12-10. Selected Fixed-Dose Combination Products to Treat Hypertension

Category	Drug Components	Trade Name[1]
Diuretic + Diuretic	hydrochlorothiazide + triamterene	Dyazide
	hydrochlorothiazide + spironolactone	Aldactazide
	hydrochlorothiazide + amiloride	Moduretic
Diuretic + β-blocker	chlorthalidone + atenolol	Tenoretic
	hydrochlorothiazide + metoprolol	Lopressor HCT
	hydrochlorothiazide + propranolol	Inderide
	hydrochlorothiazide + timolol	Timolide
Diuretic + ACE Inhibitor	hydrochlorothiazide +benazepril	Lotensin HCT
	hydrochlorothiazide + enalapril	Vaseretic
	hydrochlorothiazide + lisinopril	Zestoretic
	hydrochlorothiazide + moexipril	Uniretic
Diuretic + Angiotensin II Receptor Blocker	hydrochlorothiazide + losartan	Hyzaar
	hydrochlorothiazide + valsartan	Diovan
Calcium Channel Blocker + ACE Inhibitor	amlodipine + benazepril	Lotrel
	diltiazem + enalapril	Teczem
	verapamil + trandolapril	Tarka
	felodipine +enalapril	Lexxel

[1]Most trade name products are available in multiple dosage combinations of the respective pair.

tions (ie, more than one drug in the same dosage form) that are available (Table 12-10). Using combinations like these reduces the number of tablets or capsules that the patients must remember to take each day.

Another aspect of treating hypertension and heart disease is the use of drugs that can have an indirect impact on the disease. Because elevated blood lipids are risk factors contributing to cardiovascular disease, patients with hypertension or heart disease may also be taking drugs to reduce blood triglyceride and *LDL cholesterol* or increase the *HDL cholesterol*. Use of antiplatelet therapy (eg, aspirin) or anticoagulant therapy (eg, warfarin) may also be a part of the patient's drug regimen to prevent thrombus formation, which is a potential ramification of heart disease. The use of drugs to reduce LDL cholesterol or to prevent thrombosis adds to the complexity of the dosage regimen and contributes to the compliance issues and introduces an additional layer of potential adverse effects and drug interactions. Typically, therefore, there is necessity for the patient's drug therapy to be monitored by the physician and/or pharmacist.

Because some pharmacological categories of drugs are used to treat more than one cardiovascular disease, and because multiple drug therapy is often necessary to treat hypertension and heart disease, a few aspects regarding drug therapy are provided below.

Hypertension

- The JNC 7 recommended first step for drug treatment of uncomplicated stage 1 hypertension (ie, no coexisting condition) in most patients is the use of a thiazide-type diuretic. For stage 2 hypertension, two drugs should be a part of the initial therapy: a thiazide-type diuretic plus ACE inhibitor or ARB or β-blocker or CCB. If the initial therapy is well-tolerated but the hypertension is not controlled, another drug should be added from a different category (ie, different mechanism of action). A third drug from another category can be added if the two-drug combination does not control the hypertension. Most patients will require two or more drugs to adequately control the hypertension.

- If adverse effects are not well-tolerated, a drug from another category should be substituted rather than added to the therapy.
- Initial doses of antihypertensive therapy should be low and doses increased gradually as needed. Because chronic hypertension generally does not place the patient in immediate danger, it is better to place the patient at lower risk of adverse effects as the dose is gradually increased. Also, baroreceptor responses are less dramatic when blood pressure is gradually decreased.
- Use of specific antihypertensive drug categories may be preferred for patients with certain coexisting conditions because the antihypertensive drugs in those categories may also have favorable results on the coexisting condition. In other situations, certain antihypertensive drugs should be avoided because they may exacerbate the coexisting condition. Examples are:
  1. If angina exists, consider β-blockers or CCBs.
  2. If history of MI, consider β-blockers, ACE inhibitors, or possibly CCBs.
  3. If heart failure exists, consider ACE inhibitors, diuretics, or possibly ARBs.
  4. If renal insufficiency, ACE inhibitors or ARBs are recommended.
  5. If diabetes, β-blockers and high-dose diuretics are less desirable.
  6. If heart failure, avoid β-blockers and CCBs that affect the heart.
  7. If asthma or COPD, β-blockers are contraindicated.
  8. If pregnant, ACE inhibitors and ARBs are contraindicated.
- In general, African Americans respond better to diuretics and CCBs than to β-blockers and ACE inhibitors. Nonetheless, β-blockers and ACE inhibitors should be used if there is a therapeutic benefit (eg, coexisting conditions); however, higher doses may be necessary.
- After hypertension has been controlled for at least 1 year, consideration should be given to a step-down in dosage and number of antihypertensive drugs being used, especially if the patient has also made lifestyle changes.

Angina

- A goal of chronic stable angina therapy is to reduce the oxygen demand with β-blockers or increase oxygen supply with CCBs and organic nitrates. Treatment of variant angina is aimed at increasing cardiac oxygen supply with CCBs and organic nitrates; β-blockers are not useful because oxygen demand is not increased in variant angina. Organic nitrates and CCBs decrease the frequency and severity of angina but do not decrease the mortality risk (from MI).
- Other therapy (not discussed) is used to decrease the risk of mortality in patients with angina. This includes antiplatelet therapy (eg, low-dose aspirin), cholesterol-lowering drugs, and antihypertensive therapy.
- Short-acting nitroglycerin tablets or spray are standard therapy for relief of an acute angina attack.

- β-blockers or CCBs that affect the heart (diltiazem, verapamil) are often used in combination with long-acting organic nitrates to offset the reflex tachycardia.

Myocardial Infarction, Prevention

- Long-term treatment to prevent subsequent MI includes treatment of underlying conditions of hypertension, angina, and hyperlipidemia.
- Antiplatelet therapy with low-dose aspirin (75 to 81 mg/day), unless contraindicated, is effective in preventing recurrent MI. Larger doses have not been shown to provide an additional advantage. Specific pharmacology related to aspirin is covered in Chapters 6 and 7.
- Long-term therapy with β-blockers is standard therapy following MI except in low-risk patients and if β-blockers are otherwise contraindicated.
- Angiotensin-converting enzyme inhibitors are useful after MI to prevent recurrent MI and heart failure. Depending on the symptoms and clinical evidence, patients may benefit from therapy for several weeks to indefinitely.

Heart Failure

- Angiotensin-converting enzyme inhibitors, β-blockers, and spironolactone improve survival and symptoms of heart failure. Digoxin and diuretics improve symptoms but do not affect survival.
- Angiotensin-converting enzyme inhibitors are the cornerstone of therapy for patients with heart failure and should be a part of the drug therapy for all patients with heart failure unless a specific contraindication exists.
- Diuretics are also a standard component of therapy for patients to relieve peripheral or pulmonary edema. Diuretics are used in combination with ACE inhibitors and β-blockers. Thiazide diuretics are preferred; loop diuretics are used if renal function is impaired.
- Long-term use of β-blockers is standard therapy for patients with class II or III heart failure. Previously thought to be a contraindication for β-blocker use, heart failure patients benefit from the decrease in sympathetic tone. Patients who also have hypertension, angina, and elevated heart rate are more likely to benefit from β-blockers, whereas patients who also have asthma, bradycardia, or hypotension are not good candidates.
- Use of ARBs is an alternative in patients who cannot tolerate adverse effects of ACE inhibitors.
- Spironolactone (Aldactone) is a potassium-sparing diuretic but is used in lower doses as an *aldosterone antagonist* to treat heart failure. It is recommended for patients with class III and IV heart failure, spironolactone may be used in combination with the patient's standard care but particular care should be taken to avoid hyperkalemia in patients also receiving ACE inhibitors.
- Digoxin (Lanoxin) does not improve survival but can be used to improve symptoms of heart failure. It can be added to standard therapy of β-blockers, ACE inhibitor, and diuretics.

Summary

Treatment of hypertension and heart disease very often require multiple drug therapy to obtain adequate control of symptoms and prevent progression of the disease. Combination of drugs sometimes proves useful beyond the therapeutic effect of the individual drug on the disease. For example, use of ACE inhibitors along with diuretics not only provides two drugs with antihypertensive activity but the ACE inhibitors help prevent the *hypokalemia* that often arises from diuretic therapy. Similarly, the use of β-blockers is useful with selective CCBs to prevent reflex tachycardia.

Although drugs of first choice have been established as part of treatment protocol (eg, diuretics and β-blockers for hypertension, ACE inhibitors and diuretics for heart failure), selection of the drug regimen must also include a consideration for other aspects of the patient's clinical history. For example, use of β-blockers in patients with coexisting asthma or diabetes presents the potential for additional risks. If the patient is pregnant, use of ACE inhibitors and ARBs must be avoided. Thiazide diuretics would not be a choice to treat hypertension in a patient with history of allergic reactions to sulfonamide antibiotics. Consequently, coexisting diseases, other physiological conditions, history of previous drug use, potential drug interactions, race, and age become more important considerations when multiple drug therapy is necessary.

ROLE OF THE ATHLETIC TRAINER

As evidenced by the array of categories of drugs available for the treatment of hypertension and heart disease, the issue of therapeutic effectiveness, adverse effects, and drug interactions are considerably complex. Consequently, the role of the athletic trainer in assisting athletes directly regarding drug therapy may be somewhat limited. Nonetheless there are some points worth emphasizing, especially regarding recurrent themes that may be useful for the athletic trainer.

- If the athlete is experiencing new symptoms (or adverse effects) or a change in severity of symptoms, the drug therapy should be considered as a cause. The recent addition of another drug to therapy, the occurrence of a drug interaction, or a change in compliance are possible reasons for new symptoms to appear.
- The athletic trainer should encourage the athlete to comply with the prescribed therapeutic regimen. Poor compliance is a major cause of treatment failures. If the regimen seems too difficult for the athlete to reasonably comply with therapy, a review of the medications by a physician or pharmacist may be useful to determine if dosage regimens can be simplified by the use of combination products or by using drugs that require fewer doses per day.
- The athletic trainer can help the athlete understand the necessity for the drug therapy and the important role of nondrug measures. Educating the athlete about the disease and the potential impact the therapy can have on symptoms and/or progression of the disease may improve compliance with therapy. For example, although an athlete may be asymptomatic for chronic essential hypertension, treatment is necessary to reduce the long-term consequences such as heart disease or stroke.
- An athlete who is beginning an exercise regimen after being diagnosed with hypertension or heart disease is likely to require a gradual increase in exercise. The starting point for this exercise, as well as the target level of exercise, must be planned carefully to accommodate the individual's needs and abilities.
- Exercise intolerance is an anticipated effect when β-blockers are used. Not only do these drugs limit the heart's ability to properly respond to the increased demand during exercise, but β-blockers decrease the liver's ability to provide glucose to the blood. Therefore, the ability for vigorous and sustained exercise may be compromised, and therefore, the athletic trainer should be sure that the athlete understands these limitations.
- Nonsteroidal anti-inflammatory drugs can diminish the effectiveness of diuretics, β-blockers, and ACE inhibitors. Athletes should be aware that self-medicating with OTC analgesic and anti-inflammatory drugs have the potential to cause this drug interaction.

BIBLIOGRAPHY

AHA Medical Scientific Statement. 1994 revisions to classification of functional capacity and objective assessment of patients with diseases of the heart. *Circulation.* 1994;90:644-645.

Bottorff M. Recent advances in the treatment of congestive heart failure. *Annals of Long-Term Care.* 2001;9:47-56.

Chintanadilok J, Lowenthal DT. Exercise in treating hypertension. *The Physician and Sportsmedicine.* 2002;30:11.

Dina R, Jafari M. Angiotensin II-receptor antagonists: an overview. *Am J Health Syst Pharm.* 2000;57:1231-1241.

Drugs for hypertension. *The Medical Letter.* 2001;43:17-22.

Hilleman DE. Role of angiotensin-converting-enzyme inhibitors in the treatment of hypertension. *Am J Health Syst Pharm.* 2000;57(Suppl 1):S8-S11.

National Heart, Lung, and Blood Institute, NIH. Data Fact Sheet. Congestive heart failure in the United States: a new epidemic. www.nhlbi.nih.gov/health/public/heart/other/chf.pdf. Accessed March 3, 2003.

National High Blood Pressure Education Program. *The Seventh Report of the Joint National Committee on Prevention, Detection, Evaluation, and Treatment of High Blood Pressure.* Bethesda, Md: National Heart, Lung, and Blood Institute; 2003. NIH publication No. 03-5233.

National High Blood Pressure Education Program. *The Sixth Report of the Joint National Committee on Prevention, Detection, Evaluation, and Treatment of High Blood Pressure.* Bethesda, Md: National Heart, Lung, and Blood Institute; 1997. NIH publication No. 98-4080.

Parker JD, Parker JO. Nitrate therapy for stable angina pectoris. *N Engl J Med.* 1998;338:520-531.

Sutton PR, Fihn SD. Chronic stable angina: treatment and follow-up. *J Clin Outcomes Manage.* 2001;8:52-67.

Waugh WJ. Factors to consider in selecting an angiotensin-converting-enzyme inhibitor. *Am J Health Syst Pharm.* 2000;57(Suppl 1):S26-S30.

Which beta-blocker? *The Medical Letter.* 2001;43:9-11.

White CM. Angiotensin-converting-enzyme inhibition in heart failure or after myocardial infarction. *Am J Health Syst Pharm.* 2000;57(Suppl 1):S18-S25.

Wing LMH, Reid CM, Ryan P, et al. A comparison of outcomes with angiotensin-converting-enzyme inhibitors and diuretics for hypertension in the elderly. *N Engl J Med.* 2003;348:583-592.

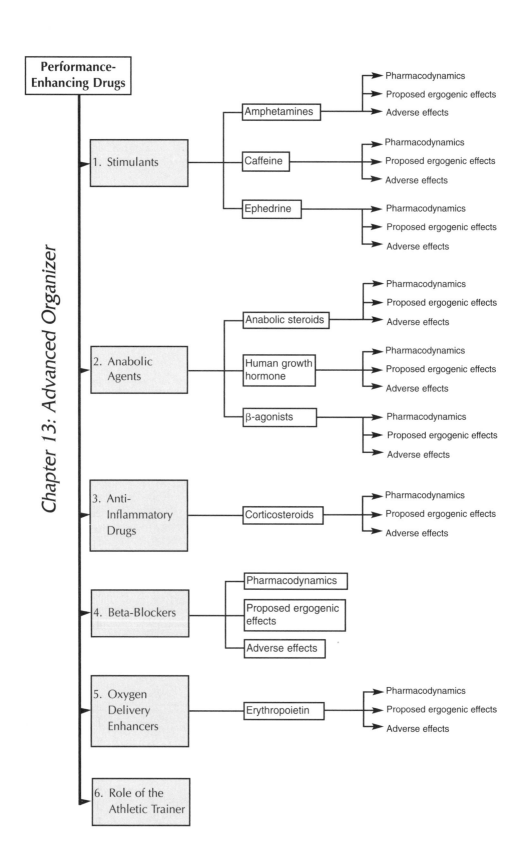

Chapter 13: Advanced Organizer

Performance-Enhancing Drugs

1. Stimulants
- Amphetamines
  - Pharmacodynamics
  - Proposed ergogenic effects
  - Adverse effects
- Caffeine
  - Pharmacodynamics
  - Proposed ergogenic effects
  - Adverse effects
- Ephedrine
  - Pharmacodynamics
  - Proposed ergogenic effects
  - Adverse effects

2. Anabolic Agents
- Anabolic steroids
  - Pharmacodynamics
  - Proposed ergogenic effects
  - Adverse effects
- Human growth hormone
  - Pharmacodynamics
  - Proposed ergogenic effects
  - Adverse effects
- β-agonists
  - Pharmacodynamics
  - Proposed ergogenic effects
  - Adverse effects

3. Anti-Inflammatory Drugs
- Corticosteroids
  - Pharmacodynamics
  - Proposed ergogenic effects
  - Adverse effects

4. Beta-Blockers
- Pharmacodynamics
- Proposed ergogenic effects
- Adverse effects

5. Oxygen Delivery Enhancers
- Erythropoietin
  - Pharmacodynamics
  - Proposed ergogenic effects
  - Adverse effects

6. Role of the Athletic Trainer

PERFORMANCE-ENHANCING DRUGS

Michael Powers, PhD, ATC, CSCS

CHAPTER OBJECTIVES

At the end of this chapter, the reader will be able to:
- Identify the classifications of ergogenic drugs and the drugs within each classification.
- Explain the pharmacodynamics of each drug and specific physiological and psychological effects each has on the human body.
- Discuss the efficacy of each drug as it relates to athletic performance.
- Identify the adverse effects associated with each drug.
- Identify the drugs that are available over-the-counter (OTC) and those available by prescription only.
- Discuss the ethical and legal issues associated with ergogenic drug use.

Ergogenic drug use or doping, as it is often referred to, is defined by the International Olympic Committee (IOC) as the administration of or use by a competing athlete of any substance foreign to the body or of any physiological substance taken in abnormal quantity or taken by an abnormal route of entry into the body with the sole intention of increasing in an artificial manner his or her performance in competition. The modern day competitiveness of both professional and amateur athletics has resulted in ergogenic drug use by many athletes in hopes of achieving an edge over the competition. However, this type of drug use is not new. Ancient Greek Olympic athletes consumed herbs and mushrooms to improve performance, whereas the use of drugs by American athletes dates back to the 1800s. The use of stimulants, anabolic steroids, and other drugs was popularized in the 1950s and 1960s forcing the IOC to begin drug testing at the 1968 Olympic Games in Mexico City. It was during these Games that the first drug disqualification occurred, as a Swedish entrant in the modern pentathlon tested positive for excessive alcohol.

Today, numerous drugs are ingested or otherwise administered for a performance-enhancing effect. Many drugs can be purchased OTC, whereas others require a prescription from a licensed physician. When the United States Food and Drug Administration (FDA) passed the Dietary Supplements Health and Education Act of 1994, it allowed numerous compounds to be classified as nutritional supplements instead of drugs. Although many athletes turned to these products because of their availability and implied safety, drug use in professional and amateur athletics is still widespread. In 1998, a large number of prohibited drugs were found by police in a raid during the Tour de France. The scandal led to a major reappraisal of the role of public authorities in antidoping affairs. It also highlighted the need for an independent international agency, which would set unified standards for drug testing and coordinate the efforts of sports organizations. The IOC took the initiative and convened the World Conference on Doping in Sport in February 1999. Following the proposal of the Conference, the World Anti-Doping Agency (WADA) was established in November 1999. Four years later, at the 2003 World Conference on Doping in Sport, all major sports federations and nearly 80 governments gave their approval to the WADA by backing a resolution that accepts the WADA Code as the basis for the fight against doping in sports. The World Code was put into effect prior to the 2004 Olympic Games in Athens, Greece, with the mission of promoting, coordinating, and monitoring on an international basis, the fight against doping in sport. Some of the primary classifications of drugs used in the athletic setting and targeted by WADA include stimulants, anabolic agents, anti-inflammatory agents, beta-blockers, and oxygen delivery enhancers (Table 13-1).

STIMULANTS

Stimulant is a name given to several groups of drugs that tend to increase arousal and alertness via central nervous system (CNS) stimulation. These groups include pharmaceuticals such as the street drugs commonly called "uppers" or "speed." This class of drugs has also found its way into the athletic arena and, in one form or another, they have been used to enhance performance for almost two centuries. In fact, stimulants were some of the first drugs used and studied as ergogenic aids and were the first class of drugs to be banned by the IOC (Tables 13-1 and 13-2). Those more commonly found in the athletic setting include amphetamines, ephedrine, and caffeine.

Amphetamines

Amphetamine was first synthesized in 1887 by a German chemist named Edeleano and was originally named phenylisopropylamine, which is marketed as a mixture of the d and l isomers under the brand name Benzedrine. In the 1930s, ephedrine was the only effective drug being used in the treatment of asthma, and at that time, it was obtained naturally from the ephedra plant. Fear that the demand for the ephedrine could not be met by its natural supply led to numerous attempts at producing synthetic ephedrine. In an attempt to do this, a University of California Los Angeles graduate student, named Gordon Alles, produced the d isomer of phenylisopropylamine, later named dextroamphetamine (Dexedrine). Before that time, a Japanese chemist accidentally produced methamphetamine while also attempting to produce synthetic ephedrine. This was later marketed under the brand name Methedrine. These three drugs became collectively referred to as amphetamines and in the late 1930s became available by prescription (in tablet form) for the treatment of narcolepsy and attention deficit hyperactivity disorder. It was not long after the medical use that their psychomotor stimulant effects were realized, and during World War II amphetamines were widely distributed to soldiers from both sides to help them keep fighting. Although it is unclear when amphetamine use by athletes began, the American Medical Association (AMA) and the National Collegiate Athletic Association (NCAA) alleged in 1957 that there was widespread use in athletics to improve performance. Concern for safety began when a Danish cyclist collapsed and died during the 1960 Olympic Games in Rome, Italy. Originally diagnosed as excessive heat, the cyclist's death was later revealed as a result of amphetamine overdose. However, amphetamine use became more than a question of ethics and safety with the passage of the Controlled Substance Act (Title II of the United States Comprehensive Drug Abuse Prevention and Control Act of 1970). Under this act, ampheta-

Table 13-1. The World Anti-Doping Code Prohibited Substance List (effective March 26, 2004)

Substances Prohibited in Competition

S1. STIMULANTS
The following stimulants are prohibited, including both their optical (D- and L-) isomers where relevant:

- adrafinil
- amfepramone
- amiphenazole
- amphetamine
- amphetaminil
- benzphetamine
- bromantan
- carphedon
- cathine[†]
- clobenzorex
- cocaine
- dimethylamphetamine
- ephedrine[††]
- etilamphetamine
- etilefrine
- fencamfamine
- fenetylline
- fenfluramine
- fenproporex
- fenfenorex
- mefenorex
- mephentermine
- mesocarb
- methamphetamine
- methylamphetamine
- methylenedioxyamphetamine
- methylene-dioxymethamphetamine
- methylephedrine[††]
- methylphenidate
- modafinil
- nikethamide
- norfenfluramine
- parahydroxyamphetamine
- pemoline phendimetrazine
- phenmetrazine
- phentermine
- prolintane
- selegiline
- strychnine
- and other substances with similar chemical structure or pharmacological effect(s)

[†] *Cathine is prohibited when its concentration in the urine exceeds 5 µg/mL*

[††] *Ephedrine and methylephedrine are prohibited when the concentration in the urine exceeds 10 µg/mL*

S2. NARCOTICS
The following narcotics are prohibited:

- buprenorphine
- dextromoramide
- diamorphine (heroin)
- hydromorphone
- methadone
- morphine
- oxycodone
- oxymorphone
- pentazocine
- pethidine

S3. CANNABINOIDS
Cannabinoids (eg, hashish and marijuana) are prohibited.

S4. ANABOLIC AGENTS
Anabolic agents are prohibited.
1. Anabolic Androgenic Steroids (AAS)
a. Exogenous AAS including but not limited to:

- androstanedione
- bolasterone
- boldenone
- boldione
- clostebol
- 4-hydroxytestosterone
- 4-hydroxy-19-nortestosterone
- mestanolone
- mesterolone
- methandienone
- norethandrolone
- oxabolone
- oxandrolone
- oxymesterone
- oxymetholone

continued

Table 13-1. The World Anti-Doping Code Prohibited Substance List (effective March 26, 2004) (continued)

- danazol
- dehydrochlormethyl -testosterone
- delta1-androstene-3,17-dione
- drostanediol
- fluoxymesterone
- formebolone
- gestrinone

- metenolone
- methandriol
- methyltestosterone
- mibolerone
- nandrolone
- 19-norandrostenediol
- 19-norandrostenedione
- norbolethone

- quinbolone
- stanozolol
- stenbolone
- 1-testosterone
- trenbolone
- and other substances with similar chemical structure or pharmacological effect(s)

b. Endogenous AAS including but not limited to:
- androstenediol
- androstenedione
- dehydroepiandrosterone
- dihydrotestosterone testosterone
- and other substances with similar chemical structure or pharmacological effect(s)

A sample will be deemed to contain a prohibited substance if the concentration of the prohibited substance or its metabolites or markers and/or any other relevant ratio(s) in the sample so deviates from the range of values normally found in humans so as not to be consistent with normal endogenous production.

If the laboratory reports that the ratio of the total concentration of testosterone to that of epitestosterone in the urine is greater than 6:1, further investigation is necessary to determine whether the ratio is due to a physiological or pathological condition.

2. Other Anabolic Agents
- clenbuterol
- zeranol

S5. PEPTIDE HORMONES
The following substances and their releasing factors are prohibited:
- erythropoietin (EPO)
- growth hormone (hGH) and insulin-like growth factor (IGF-1)
- chorionic gonadotrophin (hCG) prohibited in males only
- pituitary and synthetic gonadotrophins (LH) prohibited in males only
- insulin
- corticotrophins

A sample will be deemed to contain a prohibited substance if the concentration of the prohibited substance or its metabolites or markers and/or any other relevant ratio(s) in the sample so deviates from the range of values normally found in humans so as not to be consistent with normal endogenous production.

continued

Table 13-1. The World Anti-Doping Code Prohibited Substance List (effective March 26, 2004) (continued)

S6. BETA-2 AGONISTS
All beta-2 agonists including their D- and L- isomers are prohibited except that formoterol, salbutamol, salmeterol, and terbutaline are permitted by inhalation only to prevent and/or treat asthma and exercise-induced asthma/bronchoconstriction.

S7. AGENTS WITH ANTI-OESTROGENIC ACTIVITY
Aromatase inhibitors, clomiphene, cyclofenil, and tamoxifen are prohibited only in males.

S8. MASKING AGENTS
These are products that have the potential to impair the excretion of prohibited substances, to conceal their presence in urine or other samples used in doping control, or to change the hematological parameters. Masking agents include, but are not limited to, diuretics, epitestosterone, probenecid, and plasma expanders (eg dextran, hydroxyethyl starch).
Diuretics include:

- acetazolamide
- amiloride
- bumetanide
- canrenone
- chlorthalidone
- ethacrynic acid
- furosemide
- indapamide
- mersalyl
- spironolactone
- thiazides
- and related compounds

S9. GLUCOCORTICOSTEROIDS
Glucocorticosteroids are prohibited when administered orally, rectally, or by intravenous or intramuscular injection.

Substances Prohibited In and Out of Competition
S4. ANABOLIC AGENTS
S5. PEPTIDE HORMONES
S6. BETA-2 AGONISTS
S7. AGENTS WITH ANTI-OESTROGENIC ACTIVITY
S8. MASKING AGENTS

Substances Prohibited in Particular Sports
P.1 ALCOHOL
Alcohol is prohibited in-competition only in the following sports:

- Aeronautic
- Archery
- Automobile
- Billiards
- Boules
- Gymnastics
- Karate
- Modern pentathlon
- Motorcycling
- Roller sports
- Skiing
- Triathlon
- Wrestling

continued

Table 13-1. The World Anti-Doping Code Prohibited Substance List (Effective March 26, 2004) (continued)

P.2 BETA-BLOCKERS

Unless otherwise noted, beta-blockers are prohibited in competition only in the following sports:

- Aeronautic
- Archery (also prohibited out-of-competition)
- Automobile
- Billiards
- Bobsled
- Boules
- Bridge
- Chess
- Curling
- Gymnastics
- Modern pentathlon
- Motorcycling
- Nine-pin bowling
- Sailing
- Shooting (also prohibited out-of-competition)
- Skiing (ski jumping and freestyle snow board)
- Swimming (in diving and synchronized swimming)
- Wrestling

Beta-blockers include, but are not limited to, the following:

- acebutolol
- alprenolol
- atenolol
- betaxolol
- bisoprolol
- bunolol
- carteolol
- carvedilol
- celiprolol
- esmolol
- labetalol
- levobunolol
- metipranolol
- metoprolol
- nadolol
- oxprenolol
- pindolol
- propranolol
- sotalol
- timolol

For a current list of banned substances, visit the WADA Web site at http://www.wada-ama.org.

mines are classified as controlled substances, making it a felony to possess them without a prescription from a licensed physician.

Pharmacodynamics

Amphetamines are stimulants of both the CNS and the sympathetic division of the peripheral nervous system. These *sympathomimetic* amines basically affect the body in two ways—by interfering with the body's normal metabolism of neurotransmitters and by acting directly on some of the same receptors as *norepinephrine*. They are structurally related to *epinephrine*, the body's "fight or flight" hormone and bind to α- *and* β-*adrenergic receptors*, thus acting as α- *and* β-*agonists*. As discussed in Chapter 12, α- and β-*sympathetic* receptors are cell membrane receptors sensitive to the *catecholamines* epinephrine and norepinephrine and are found on most cells throughout the body, including the cells of the heart, lungs, and surrounding blood vessels. Consequently, the amphetamines exert effects such as increased blood pressure, respiratory rate, heart rate, metabolic rate, and increased plasma free fatty acid levels. Amphetamines also cause a release of the excitatory neurotransmitters dopamine and norepinephrine from storage vesicles in the CNS and, at the same time, prevent their reuptake. This results in greater amounts of these neurotransmitters in the synaptic cleft where they can act on receptors. Dopamine is a neurotransmitter that, in certain parts of the brain, activates the pleasure center. Unlike true catecholamines, amphetamines are able to readily cross the blood-brain barrier, which allows them to act as CNS stimulants.

Table 13-2. The National Collegiate Athletic Association List of Banned Drug Classes

(a) Stimulants

- amiphenazole
- amphetamine
- bemigride
- benzphetamine
- bromantan
- caffeine†
- chlorphentermine
- cocaine
- cropropamide
- crothetamide
- diethylpropion
- dimethylamphetamine
- doxapram
- ephedrine
- ethamivan
- ethylamphetamine
- fencamfamine
- meclofenoxate
- methamphetamine
- methylene-dioxymethamphetamine
- methylphenidate
- nikethamide
- pemoline
- pentetrazol
- phendimetrazine
- phenmetrazine
- phentermine
- phenylpropanolamine
- picrotoxine
- pipradol
- prolintane
- strychnine
- synephrine
- and related compounds*

(b) Anabolic Agents

- anabolic steroids
- androstenediol
- androstenedione
- boldenone
- clostebol
- dehydrochlormethyl-testosterone
- dehydroepiandrosterone
- dihydrotestosterone
- dromostanolone
- fluoxymesterone
- mesterolone
- methandienone
- methyltestosterone
- nandrolone
- norandrostenediol
- Other anabolic agents: clenbuterol methenolone
- norandrostenedione
- norethandrolone
- oxandrolone
- oxymesterone
- oxymetholone
- stanozolol
- testosterone††
- and related compounds*

(c) Substances Banned for Specific Sports

Rifle:
- alcohol
- atenolol
- metoprololv
- nadolol
- pindolol
- propranolol
- timolol
- and related compounds*

(d) Diuretics

- acetazolamide
- bendroflumethiazide
- benzthiazide
- bumetanide
- chlorothiazide
- chlorthalidone
- ethacrynic acid
- flumethiazide
- furosemide
- hydrochlorothiazide
- hydroflumethiazide
- methyclothiazide
- metolazone
- polythiazide
- quinethazone
- spironolactone
- triamterene
- trichlormethiazide
- and related compounds*

continued

Table 13-2. The National Collegiate Athletic Association List of Banned Drug Classes (continued)

(e) Street Drugs

- heroin
- marijuana[†††]
- THC (tetrahydrocannabinol)[†††]

(f) Peptide Hormones and Analogues

- chorionic gonadotrophin (HCG—human chorionic gonadotrophin)
- corticotrophin (ACTH)
- growth hormone (HGH, somatotrophin)

All the respective releasing factors of the above-mentioned substances also are banned.

- erythropoietin (EPO)
- sermorelin

(g) Definitions of Positive Depends on the Following:

*The term "related compounds" comprises substances that are included in the class by their pharmacological action and/or chemical structure.

[†]For caffeine—if the concentration in the urine exceeds 15 μg/mL.

[††]For testosterone—if the administration of testosterone or the use of any other manipulation has the result of increasing the ratio of the total concentration of testosterone to that of epitestosterone in the urine to greater than 6:1, unless there is evidence that this ratio is due to a physiological or pathological condition.

[†††] For marijuana and THC— if the concentration in the urine of THC metabolites exceeds 15 ng/mL.

For a current list of banned substances, visit the NCAA web site at http://www.ncaa.org.

Possible Ergogenic Effects

Amphetamines increase respiratory rate, heart rate, blood pressure, and metabolic rate. Increased levels of *catecholamines* also lead to increased arousal and alertness. They induce exhilarating feelings of power, strength, energy, self-assertion, focus, and enhanced motivation and diminish the need to sleep or eat. The release of dopamine typically induces a sense of aroused euphoria, which may last several hours.

Reports have been mixed regarding the effects of amphetamines on athletic performance. Some studies conducted over 40 years ago on trained runners, swimmers, and track and field athletes showed positive results, whereas other studies on untrained athletes failed to demonstrate a performance benefit following amphetamine use. Many of the earlier studies came under a great deal of criticism, mainly due to small subject number, methodological flaws, and lack of appropriate statistical analyses. Studies conducted 10 to 20 years later demonstrated improvement in anaerobic endurance when amphetamines were administered. However, because there was no increase in oxygen consumption (VO_2) and lactic acid levels increased, it was concluded that amphetamines did not provide any true physiological improvement, but only provided a masking of the fatigue due to their CNS stimulant effects. Overall, the amount of change induced by the amphetamines appears to be small, on the order of a few percent. However, in many events, a percent improvement can make the difference between winning and losing. Thus, many athletes still feel that the margin of improvement provided by these drugs is beneficial.

Table 13-3. Signs of Amphetamine Use

- Dilated pupils
- Dry mouth
- Frequent lip licking
- Restlessness, difficulty sitting still
- Reduced appetite
- Abdominal cramps
- Weight loss
- Irritable, moody
- Tremors
- Argumentative
- Talkative, rapid speech
- Anxiety
- Hallucinations

Adverse Effects

Some of the possible signs of amphetamine use can be found in Table 13-3. The minor adverse effects associated with amphetamine use include decreased appetite, fever, sweating, headache, restlessness, anxiety, blurred vision, sleeplessness, and dizziness. The serious adverse effects associated with amphetamine abuse are essentially the same as for cocaine and include arrhythmias, sudden cardiac death, stroke, and psychosis.

All amphetamines can cause *catecholamine-mediated* cardiotoxicity. Other cardiovascular adverse effects include hypertension, myocardial hypertrophy, aneurysm, and coronary artery disease. Amphetamine use is also associated with both hemorrhagic and ischemic stroke. Although the mechanism for this is unclear, hypertension has been suggested as the cause. Users of large amount of amphetamines over a long period of time can develop an amphetamine psychosis, a mental disorder similar to paranoid schizophrenia. Although amphetamine users may feel a temporary boost in self-confidence and power, abuse of the drug can lead to delusions, hallucinations, and a feeling of paranoia. Auditory, tactile, and visual hallucinations are also common. These feelings can cause a person to act in a bizarre, and even violent, fashion. In most people, these effects disappear when they stop using the drug.

Amphetamines cause psychological dependence due to the euphoria they produce. Users also become dependent on the drug to avoid the "down" feeling they often experience when the drug's effect wears off. Amphetamines also cause physical dependence. People who abruptly stop using amphetamines often experience withdrawal symptoms, such as fatigue, long periods of sleep, irritability, and depression. The length and severity of the depression is related to the dose and frequency of amphetamine use. Amphetamines also have the potential to produce *tolerance* (see Chapter 3), which means that when the drug is used on a regular basis, an increased amount of the drug is needed to achieve the desired effects.

Caffeine

Caffeine, known chemically as trimethylxanthine, is a methylxanthine derivative related to theophylline and theobromine. It is probably the most popular drug in the world, as it is found

Table 13-4. Caffeine Content of Some Common Foods and Over-the-Counter Drugs

Item	Size (oz)	Caffeine Content (mg)
Coffee	8	60 to 150
Coffee, decaf	8	2 to 5
Tea	8	15 to 80
Hot cocoa	8	1 to 8
Jolt Cola	12	71
Josta	12	58
Mountain Dew	12	55
Surge	12	52
Diet Coca Cola	12	46
Dr. Pepper	12	42
Sunkist Orange Soda	12	42
Mr. Pibb	12	40
Pepsi Cola	12	38
Coca Cola	12	35
Barq's Root Beer	12	22
RC Cola	12	18
7-Up or Diet 7-Up	12	0
Mug Root Beer	12	0
Sprite	12	0
Anacin	tablet	32
Excedrin	tablet	65
No-Doz	tablet	100
Vivarin and Dexatrim	tablet	200

in coffee, tea, cocoa, chocolate, some soft drinks, and numerous medications (Table 13-4). It is also widely used by athletes in their daily lives and during training and competition. However, caffeine is banned by the NCAA (see Table 13-2). A test is considered positive if the concentration in the urine exceeds 15 µg/mL. This would be the equivalent of ingesting about six cups of coffee before testing. Although the IOC had also banned caffeine at one time, the WADA did not include it on its list of banned substances that took effect in January 2004 (see Table 13-1). Thus, it is no longer banned by the IOC. However, the WADA will continue to monitor the use of caffeine during competition and, if trends are observed, it is possible that it will once again be banned.

Pharmacodynamics

Caffeine, like amphetamines and cocaine, stimulate the brain; however, the effects are milder than those of amphetamines and cocaine. It crosses the membranes of all tissues in the body, including the blood-brain barrier. Because of this, it can exert its effects on both the CNS and the peripheral tissues, resulting in a number of physiological effects. Caffeine interferes with adenosine at multiple sites in the brain. Adenosine is another xanthine that occurs naturally in the human body and acts as a neurotransmitter. As adenosine is created in the brain, it binds to adenosine receptors, causing drowsiness by depressing nerve cell activity. In the brain, adenosine

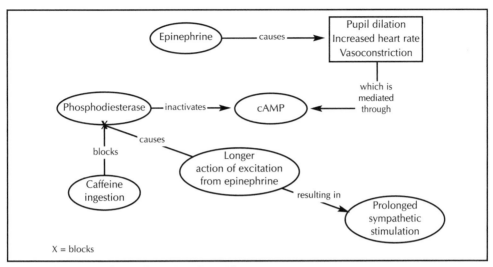

Figure 13-1. How caffeine affects physiological function.

binding also causes vasodilation (presumably to let more oxygen in during sleep). Caffeine is an adenosine receptor antagonist and thus has the opposite effect as adenosine. Therefore, instead of slowing down nerve cell activity, caffeine increases the cell's activity. Because it also blocks adenosine's ability to cause vasodilation, caffeine causes cerebral vasoconstriction. This effect is one reason for the use of caffeine in some headache medicines like Anacin, as caffeine will constrict the blood vessels to help relieve some types of headaches. As discussed in Chapter 7, caffeine may enhance the general analgesic effect when used in combination with other pain relievers, although the mechanism is unclear and caffeine has no analgesic properties when used alone. As mentioned previously, epinephrine is the "fight or flight" hormone and it has a number of effects on the body such as pupil dilation, increased heart rate, and vasoconstriction. Some of this activity of epinephrine is mediated through the *second messenger* cyclic adenosine monophosphate (cAMP). Caffeine blocks phosphodiesterase, an enzyme that inactivates cAMP, so the excitatory signals from epinephrine, through cAMP, persist longer. Thus, the effect of caffeine is to disable braking systems in the brain (adenosine) and the body (phosphodiesterase), resulting in a prolonged sense of wakefulness and alertness (Figure 13-1).

Possible Ergogenic Effects

There appear to be three primary mechanisms by which caffeine might provide an ergogenic effect. First, the metabolic theory suggests that caffeine will provide improved endurance due to an increase in fat availability and muscle lipid oxidation with a consequent glycogen sparing effect. The binding of caffeine to adenosine receptors might also block muscle glucose uptake and further reduce carbohydrate use. Second, caffeine may also provide a performance effect via changes in skeletal muscle ion handling. It has been proposed that caffeine can stimulate Na^+-K^+ ATPase activity and Ca^{2+} kinetics. An increase skeletal muscle Ca^{2+} presumably could enhance the strength of muscle contraction. Finally, caffeine has direct effects on the CNS as a stimulant, which can alter the perception of fatigue, increase alertness, and increase motor unit recruitment. The first mechanism would make this a drug of choice for the endurance athlete whereas the latter two would play a greater role in strength and power competitions and events requiring arousal and alertness.

In the 1970s, a number of studies provided support for the ergogenic use of caffeine, as improvements in time to exhaustion, work rate, and other measures of endurance were observed. Increased free fatty acids levels and decreased respiratory exchange ratios (indicating increased fat oxidation) were commonly observed, providing support for the metabolic theory. However, during the 1980s there was a great amount of variability in published findings and conclusions. One factor making caffeine research difficult is the fact that individuals ingest varying levels of caffeine in their habitual diet. Thus, it is difficult to establish groups of subjects with similar tolerance levels to the drug. Several well-controlled studies were published in the 1990s reexamining the performance effects of caffeine. Overall, varying doses of caffeine (ranging from 3 to 13 mg/kg) were shown to improve endurance performance by approximately 20% to 50%. The improvements in performance were associated with increases in plasma epinephrine and free fatty acids and an associated glycogen sparing effect. However, improvements did not always occur at lower doses. Furthermore, not all studies have reported hormonal and metabolic changes along with improvements in performance. These observations support the central fatigue theory and the ergogenic role of caffeine as a CNS stimulant. Thus, it appears unlikely that increased fat oxidation and glycogen sparing is the prime ergogenic mechanism. It is interesting to note that performance improved following ingestion of 6 and 9 mg/kg body mass, whereas urinary levels remained within acceptable limits for NCAA drug testing.[1] Only a 13 mg/kg dose or higher would have produced a positive urine test. However, in a separate study, ingesting 9 and 13 mg/kg body mass would have resulted in a positive urine test.[2]

When higher intensity, shorter duration aerobic exercise is investigated, improvements similar to the above mentioned studies have been observed. However, not all studies have shown improvements. Table 13-5 provides a summary of selected studies investigating performance effects. Overall, caffeine appears to provide a performance improvement during intense aerobic exercise. If this type of exercise is preceded by long-term submaximal exercise, performance does not improve.[3] When high intensity anaerobic exercise has been investigated, the results are not as positive as the aerobic studies. For example, in one study, caffeine improved performance when subjects exercised below anaerobic threshold, however, it had no effect when they exercised above their anaerobic threshold.[4] Likewise, caffeine also failed to improve performance during Wingate anaerobic cycle tests.[5] Although some evidence supports improvements in muscle strength and power, the majority of the studies do not.

Adverse Effects

The adverse effects associated with caffeine ingestion have been well established. The more minor ones include anxiety, jitters, dizziness, headache, inability to focus, irritability, insomnia, diuresis, and gastrointestinal distress. In the performance studies mentioned previously, these adverse effects were rare at dosages at or below 6 mg/kg, but were prevalent at higher doses. One of the more common problems is the effect that caffeine has on sleep. Adenosine receptor activity is important to sleep, and especially to deep sleep. Under the influence of caffeine, one might still be able to fall asleep, but the benefits of deep sleep would probably be missed.

Caffeine is also classified as a diuretic. This is of concern for the athlete as dehydration could not only impair performance, but can lead to heat illness. However, the majority of the research suggests that core temperature, sweat loss, plasma volume, and urine volume are normal when exercising following caffeine ingestion. As with most drugs, ingesting higher doses worsens the adverse effects. Adverse effects associated with higher doses also include cardiac arrhythmias and hallucinations. In massive doses, caffeine is lethal. A fatal dose of caffeine can range from 3 to 10 g (about 170 mg/kg body mass) resulting in seizures, tachycardia, or ventricular dysrhythmias. Like the performance effects, the adverse effects associated with caffeine ingestion vary considerably across individuals.

Table 13-5. The Effects of Caffeine Supplementation on Performance

Reference	Research Protocol	Results
Bell et al[6]	Caffeine users vs nonusers 5 mg/kg caffeine Time to exhaustion at 80% VO_{2max}	Nonusers experienced greater increases in time to exhaustion than users and the effect lasted longer in the nonusers.
Berry et al[7]	Aerobically trained subjects 7 mg/kg caffeine Incremental treadmill test	No change in VO_2, VCO_2, or RER.
Bond et al[8]	Intercollegiate sprinters 5 mg/kg caffeine Muscle strength	No change in knee extension strength. No change in knee flexion strength. No change in muscle power.
Casal & Leon[9]	Endurance trained subjects 400 mg caffeine 45-min run at 75% VO_{2max}	Serum free fatty acids increased. No change in VO_2, VCO_2, or RER.
Collump et al[10]	Recreationally active subjects 5 mg/kg caffeine Wingate anaerobic test	No change in anaerobic power or capacity. No change in power decrease. Increased catecholamines and blood lactate.
Collump et al[11]	Trained and untrained swimmers 250 mg caffeine 2 x 100-m swim sprints	Trained subjects increased swim velocity. Blood lactate increased in both groups.
Dodd et al[12]	Moderately trained subjects 3 mg/kg caffeine 5 mg/kg caffeine Graded VO_2 test to exhaustion	Increased resting heart rate. Increased resting and exercise FFAs. No change in VO_2 or anaerobic threshold.
Falk et al[13]	Endurance trained subjects 5 mg/kg caffeine Time to exhaustion at 90% VO_{2max}	No change in time to exhaustion. No change in free fatty acid levels.
Fisher et al[14]	Habitual caffeine users 5 mg/kg caffeine 60-min run at 75% VO_{2max}	Increased exercise VO_2. RER decreased. Free fatty acid levels increased.
Graham & Spriet[15]	Endurance trained subjects 9 mg/kg caffeine Time to exhaustion at 85% VO_{2max} (running/cycling)	44% increase in running time to exhaustion. 51% increase in cycling time to exhaustion. Increased plasma epinephrine. No change in free fatty acids or RER.
Graham & Spriet[1]	Endurance trained subjects 3, 6, or 9 mg/kg caffeine Time to exhaustion at 85% VO_{2max}	3 mg/kg: 22% increase in time to exhaustion. 6 mg/kg: 22% increase in time to exhaustion. 9 mg/kg: No change in endurance. Increased plasma epinephrine, glycerol, and FFAs.
Hunter et al[16]	Trained cyclists 6 mg/kg caffeine 100-km time trials	No change in performance. Mean heart rate higher with caffeine. No change in peripheral fatigue.

continued

Table 13-5. The Effects of Caffeine Supplementation on Performance (continued)

Reference	Research Protocol	Results
Ivy et al[17]	Endurance trained subjects 2 x 250 mg caffeine 120 min cycling at 80 rpm	Increased work production and VO_2. Increased fat oxidation.
Jackman et al[18]	Endurance trained subjects Time to exhaustion at 100% VO_{2max}	20% increase in time to exhaustion. Increased plasma epinephrine. No change in glycogen at fatigue.
Jacobson & Edwards[19]	Recreationally active subjects 300 mg caffeine 600 mg caffeine Muscle strength and endurance	No change in maximal strength. No change in muscle endurance.
Jacobson et al[20]	Trained athletes 7 mg/kg caffeine Muscle strength and power	Improvements were observed in some strength, work, and power parameters.

Pasman et al[2]	Endurance trained subjects
	5, 9, or 13 mg/kg caffeine
	Time to exhaustion at 80%
	  maximal power output
		5, 9, and 13 mg/kg increased time to
		  exhaustion 24% to 25%.
		Serum free fatty acids and glycerol
		  increased.

Spriet et al[3]	Recreational cyclists 9 mg/kg caffeine Cycling time to exhaustion at 80% VO_{2max}	27% increase in time to exhaustion. 55% decrease in muscle glycogenolysis.
Williams et al[21]	Physically active subjects 7 mg/kg caffeine Muscle strength and endurance	No change in hand grip strength. No change in endurance. No change in EMG characteristics.

There is also concern that ingesting caffeine on a regular basis (habitual use) might predispose an athlete to increased risk for a number of diseases, such as cardiovascular disease and cancer. However, the majority of studies examining cardiovascular health have concluded that caffeine consumption does not increase the risk of coronary heart disease and stroke. Habitual caffeine use can lead to a number of disorders, including anxiety, sleep disorders, dependence, and withdrawal (hence, a degree of physical dependence). Typical withdrawal symptoms associated with caffeine are headache, fatigue, and muscle pain. These symptoms can occur within 24 hours after the last dose of caffeine. Although caffeine is a mild CNS stimulant and may increase dopamine in the CNS, it is generally not considered addicting. This is because most caffeine users, unlike amphetamine users, do not lose control of their caffeine intake.

Ephedrine

The plant species *ephedra sinica, ephedra equisetina,* and *ephedra intermedia,* collectively known by their Chinese name ma-huang, are indigenous to northwestern India, Pakistan, and China. For centuries, the dried stem of these plants has been used as a remedy for numerous medical conditions. In 1923, scientists discovered that the ma-huang plant has two primary active ingredients, ephedrine and pseudoephedrine, and in the 1930s, ephedrine was the only effective drug being used in the treatment of asthma. At that time, ephedrine was sold OTC and

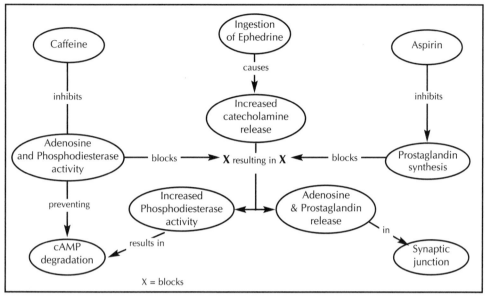

Figure 13-2. How caffeine and aspirin can potentiate the effects of ephedrine.

was available without a prescription until 1954. Like amphetamine, ephedrine and certain ephedrine alkaloids are banned by both the NCAA and the WADA (see Tables 13-1 and 13-2). Pseudoephedrine was also originally listed as a banned substance, but both organizations have since removed it from their lists. The National Football League (NFL) decided to ban ephedrine before the start of the 2002 season, during which time a number of players tested positive and were suspended.

Pharmacodynamics

Like amphetamine, ephedrine and pseudoephedrine are classified as *sympathomimetic* alkaloids because they directly stimulate the sympathetic or "fight or flight" nervous system. They are structurally similar to amphetamine and have direct α- and β-agonistic properties, as well as catecholamine releasing actions. Thus, they augment the availability and action of the natural neurotransmitter norepinephrine in the brain and in the heart. Ephedrine is easily absorbed following oral administration, with peak plasma levels occurring within 1 hour of ingestion. Its plasma half-life is approximately 3 to 6 hours and varies depending on urine pH. Unlike pseudoephedrine, ephedrine also mediates its effects by causing the release of circulating epinephrine.

The increased catecholamine release following ephedrine ingestion is subjected to negative feedback systems, which then tend to inhibit catecholamine release and actions (Figure 13-2). These negative feedback systems include adenosine and prostaglandin release in the synaptic junction and elevated phosphodiesterase enzyme activity, which results in degradation of cAMP. Caffeine interferes with this negative feedback mechanism by inhibiting both adenosine and phosphodiesterase activity and preventing degradation of cAMP. Aspirin also interferes with the negative feedback mechanism via its inhibition of *prostaglandin* synthesis. Thus, it is conceivable that either of these mechanisms would potentiate the effects of ephedrine. Because of this, it is common to find athletes ingesting the combination of ephedrine, caffeine, and aspirin.

Possible Ergogenic Effects

Because ephedrine is a *sympathomimetic* and a CNS stimulant, it is commonly used as an energy enhancer. *Thermogenic* and *lypolytic* effects have also led to the claim that ephedrine can improve endurance via increased fat utilization and glycogen sparing during exercise, similar to caffeine. It has been suggested that the thermogenic effects of combining ephedrine and caffeine are *synergistic*. Like ephedrine, caffeine has a stimulating effects on the CNS and energy metabolism. However, the primary reason for combining the two drugs is to potentiate the effects of the ephedrine (see previous paragraph). Many of the ergogenic claims associated with ephedrine originated from earlier studies investigating its antiobesity and anorectic effects. For some time now, ephedrine and the combination of ephedrine and caffeine have been considered effective weight loss agents, although not all studies support this. Originally, the observed weight loss was attributed solely to the appetite suppressing effects of ephedrine. More recently, increases in metabolism and, more specifically, fat metabolism have been suggested as the mechanism. For example, increases in resting VO_2, fat oxidation, and fat loss were commonly observed during clinical trials investigating the effects of ephedrine and the combination of ephedrine and caffeine. However, it must be noted that only clinically obese individuals were used as subjects in these investigations. Thus, it is likely that the subjects may have been deficient in metabolic rate and/or fat metabolism.

Although the research concerning ephedrine and performance in an athletic population is limited, most of the investigations do not support ergogenic claims. Although ephedrine ingestion has been observed to increase resting VO_2 and fat oxidation in healthy individuals, these changes have not been observed during exercise. Similar observations have been made following pseudoephedrine ingestion. Like VO_2 and fat oxidation, a number of other performance measures have also been unaffected by supplementation. Sidney and Lefcoe[22] administered 24 mg of ephedrine and found no improvements in muscle strength, endurance, power, lung function, reaction time, hand-eye coordination, anaerobic capacity, speed, cardiorespiratory endurance, ratings of perceived exertion, or recovery. Similarly, a single 120-mg dose of pseudoephedrine had no effect on 40-km cycling time, maximal muscle force, or muscle endurance during repeated isometric contractions.[23] More recently, Swain et al[24] administered pseudoephedrine (1 and 2 mg/kg) to trained cyclists and found no changes in ratings of perceived exertion or time to exhaustion.

Performance improvements have been observed when higher doses of ephedrine and caffeine have been combined. Bell et al[25] observed that the combination of caffeine and ephedrine significantly increased cycling time to exhaustion by 38% over a placebo condition, whereas caffeine and ephedrine on their own failed to provide such an effect. In a separate study, the combination of caffeine and ephedrine improved cycling time to exhaustion by 64% over a placebo condition.[26] In both of these studies, ratings of perceived exertion were significantly lower following supplementation, but heart rate was significantly elevated as well. The authors attributed the improvement to CNS stimulation as no changes were observed for VO_2, carbon dioxide production, or fat oxidation. More recently, Bell and Jacobs[27] administered 75 mg of ephedrine with 375 mg of caffeine and observed a slight (5%) but significant improvement running time during a Canadian Forces Warrior Test (3.2-km run while wearing field gear).

Adverse Effects

The spectrum of adverse health events associated with the use of ephedrine cannot be overlooked. Adverse effects were commonly observed in many performance studies. Although it is likely that the occurrence of adverse effects in many cases was the result of misuse, they have also been regularly observed in subjects involved in clinical trials with controlled doses. Some of the minor adverse effects associated with ephedrine include tremors, palpitations, headache, restlessness, anxiety, and insomnia. Because of its direct *sympathomimetic* effects, ephedrine can cause increases in heart rate, contractility, cardiac output, and peripheral resistance. Thus, increases in both heart rate and blood pressure are common observations following ephedrine ingestion. Although these effects are not serious in most users, the consequences can be severe in those with underlying heart disease, hypertension, diabetes, and those sensitive to ephedrine. The more serious adverse effects include seizures, severe hypertension, arrhythmias, psychosis, hepatitis, stroke, myocardial injury, and intracranial hemorrhage. It is important to note that the adverse effects do not always depend on the dose consumed, as serious problems can occur in susceptible persons with use of low dosages. Furthermore, the toxicity of *sympathomimetic* agents is exacerbated by physical exercise, dehydration, and increases in body temperature, which are all commonly experienced by athletes during training and competition. Although they are not common, cases of fatal intoxication following ephedrine ingestion have been reported. In instances of ephedrine overdose, cardiovascular and CNS stimulant effects predominate, with myocardial infarction and cerebrovascular accident causing death most often.

Summary

Although their efficacy as ergogenic aids can be debated, stimulants continue to be some of the most popular drugs used to enhance performance. The performance gains achieved through amphetamine use appear to be minimal and primarily via CNS stimulation and a masking of fatigue. Greater improvements have been observed from caffeine and the combination of caffeine and ephedrine. Although CNS stimulation is most likely the cause of this, physiological effects such as enhanced fat utilization and glycogen sparing may contribute as well. All stimulants are associated with adverse effects, which worsen with increasing dosages. At this time only caffeine and pseudoephedrine can be sold OTC. Caffeine is found in coffee, tea, cocoa, chocolate, some soft drinks, and numerous nutritional supplements marketed as energy boosters and fat burners, whereas pseudoephedrine is an active ingredient in many sinus and allergy medications. Ephedrine and amphetamines are only available with a prescription from a licensed physician for the treatment of medical conditions, thus their use as performance enhancers would be considered illegal. With the exception of pseudoephedrine, all of the stimulants discussed in this chapter are banned by various sport organizations.

ANABOLIC AGENTS

Anabolic agents are those substances that promote tissue growth. This can occur through a number of pathways; however, the most notable is through protein synthesis. Many athletes turn to drugs developed to enhance tissue growth in the hopes of increasing muscle size and strength. The most common drugs used for this purpose include anabolic-androgenic steroids, human growth hormone, and *β-agonists*.

Anabolic Steroids

Testosterone is the natural steroid hormone primarily produced by the testes that is responsible for the *androgenic* and *anabolic* effects observed during male adolescence and adulthood. The natural and synthetic derivatives of this hormone are known as anabolic-androgenic steroids (AAS). These steroids were first developed as treatments for medical conditions including delayed puberty, micropenis, aplastic anemia, and hypogonadism in children and for reproductive dysfunction, anemia, hereditary angioedema, metastatic breast cancer, and protein deficiency in adults. They are also commonly used in the management of infection, surgery, burns, acquired immunodeficiency syndrome (AIDS), and trauma. It was not long after the medical use began that their possible influence on performance was recognized, dating as far back as World War II when they were used to improve performance and increase aggressiveness in German troops. In the 1960s, the apparent use of these drugs by Olympic athletes was severe enough to warrant testing for them. However, it was not until the 1976 Olympic Games in Montreal, Canada that suitable methods were available to enforce a ban. A list of banned anabolic agents can be found in Tables 13-1 and 13-2. Probably the most notorious violation of the IOC's drug policy came in 1988, when Canadian sprinter Ben Johnson was stripped of his gold medal in the 100 meter after testing positive for the use of AAS. In the 1980s, widespread use was also reported in professional football, while use at the collegiate level was realized following the first drug test administered by the NCAA in 1986. Since that time, a number of studies have reported use at the collegiate level. Even more alarming is the fact that a number of studies also report use of AAS by high school students, many of them not even involved in athletics. Once considered drugs for strength and power sports only, AAS use has spread into many other areas, including swimming, boxing, track and field, and winter sports such as snowboarding and bobsledding. More recently, claims of widespread use in baseball have created a great deal of concern. It is important to note that the controversy surrounding AAS use is more than a question of ethics and moral judgment. The Anabolic Steroid Control Act of 1992 classified AAS as schedule III controlled substances. Because of this, it is a felony to possess AAS without a prescription from a licensed physician. Likewise, the illicit distribution of these drugs is also a felony.

Pharmacodynamics

Steroid hormones are lipid soluble and passively diffuse across the cell membrane. Once inside the cell, they bind to receptors and interact with the cell's genetic material (*DNA*). The stimulation of messenger ribonucleic acid (*RNA*) results in the production of new proteins that mediate the hormone's function. Virtually every cell in the body has receptors for AAS. However, physiologically, the anabolic and androgenic effects of AAS are inseparable. When the steroid molecule binds with receptor molecules in various tissues, the same type of receptor produces the anabolic and the androgenic effects. Thus, the effect the steroid has on the cell depends on the following:

- The location of the cell
- The type of cell
- The type of steroid-metabolizing enzymes contained within the cell

Some of the anabolic effects from the endogenous hormone include increased muscle mass, accelerated bone growth; increased bone density; increased heart, liver, and kidney size; enhanced erythropoiesis; and an enlarged larynx. These are seen in both men and women. The androgenic effects include spermatogenesis; changes in genital size and function; and axillary, facial, and pubic hair growth. Many attempts have been made in the production of synthetic steroids to reduce the androgenic effects and enhance the anabolic effects. However, this is most likely physiologically impossible.

Anabolic steroids can be administered orally or *parenterally* (by intramuscular injection). Those taken orally usually have short half-lives, generally on the order of several hours, whereas those injected tend to have longer half-lives, usually around 1 to 3 days. Orally ingested compounds are absorbed from the gastrointestinal tract and must first pass through the liver before entering the blood to be distributed throughout the body. To prevent rapid breakdown by the liver, many oral AAS are chemically modified by the manufacturer by a process called *alkylation* (C-17 alkylated steroids). Injected steroids are slowly absorbed into the bloodstream without a first pass through the liver (see Chapter 2). Consequently, the liver experiences a much lower concentration than with orally administered AAS. Most injected steroid compounds are not *alkylated* but they are chemically modified to form *esters*. Esters increase the half-lives of injectable AAS because they have a slower rate of breakdown. The ester also makes the steroid compound less water soluble and more fat soluble. This makes it more difficult for the blood to pick it up and carry it into circulation, and likewise slows the rate the drug can leave the injection site. When a steroid has an ester attached, the steroid is rendered inactive because the ester prevents it from binding to a receptor. As a result, an inactive deposit of steroid can sit at the site of injection, releasing slowly for days into the bloodstream. Once free in the blood, the ester is removed by enzymes, and the steroid is rendered active.

Proposed Ergogenic Effects

Regardless of administration, AAS are believed to increase muscle mass and strength by three mechanisms. First, AAS increase protein synthesis. As mentioned above, the binding of the steroid hormone to specific steroid receptors located in cells of target tissues stimulates an increased production of messenger and ribosomal *RNA*.[28] The increased amount of RNA is then used by the muscle cells to produce more protein, leading to increases in muscle mass and strength. Second, AAS inhibit protein degradation. Glucocorticoids are hormones that have a *catabolic* effect on the body via protein degradation. They are released during times of stress, which would include intense exercise or training. Anabolic steroids compete with glucocorticoids for receptor sites, thus inhibiting protein degradation. It has been suggested that it is through this mechanism that AAS provide the greatest increases in muscle size and strength. Through an improved use of protein, AAS can convert a negative nitrogen balance to a positive one, increasing nitrogen retention. Finally, it has been suggested that the use of AAS provides a psychological effect. Individuals taking AAS frequently exhibit aggressive behavior, a state of euphoria, and a diminished sense of fatigue allowing them to train at higher intensities and longer durations. The possibility of a placebo effect associated with this psychological result cannot be ruled out.

A number of studies have shown that increased levels of testosterone can increase protein synthesis, muscle strength, and lean body mass. However, other studies investigating the efficacy of AAS use for enhanced strength provide inconsistent results. This is primarily due to numerous methodological differences. For example, in an analysis of studies investigating AAS and muscle strength, Haupt and Rovere[29] concluded that an athlete must have been intensively trained in resistance training prior to AAS use and that the intense training must continue during this use. They also concluded that improvements in muscle strength can only occur if the athlete maintains a high-protein, high-caloric diet when using AAS. Likewise, Elashoff et al[30] attempted to analyze 30 studies investigating the effects of AAS on muscle strength. Twenty-one of those studies were eliminated from the analysis, primarily due to methodological flaws. From the remaining nine studies, they concluded that AAS may slightly enhance muscle strength in previously trained athletes. However, no firm conclusion could be made regarding the effects of AAS on overall athletic performance. They also pointed out that the studies they reviewed used low dosages and that it is difficult to generalize the results of clinical investigations to the actual athletic setting. Individuals who use AAS often use 10 to 100 times the therapeutic dose and often stack (taking more than one AAS simultaneously) a number of different steroids. In one study of weight-training athletes taking AAS, the lowest dosage reported was equivalent to 350% of the usual therapeutic dose.[31]

The majority of strength-training studies in which body weight was assessed report greater increases in weight under steroid treatment than under placebo treatment. Although it has been suggested that the increase is due to greater lean body mass, the extent to which increased water and electrolyte retention accounts for body mass changes remains to be resolved. However, the American College of Sports Medicine acknowledges that AAS, in the presence of adequate diet, can contribute to increases in body weight, often in the lean mass compartment and the gains in muscular strength achieved through high-intensity exercise and proper diet can be increased by the use of AAS in some individuals. It is generally accepted that adequate protein intake and high-intensity training in previously trained individuals are required for these gains to occur.

Adverse Effects

The immediate and long-term adverse effects associated with AAS use are well established and typically involve the hepatic, reproductive, cardiovascular, musculoskeletal, immune, and psychological systems. Hepatic abnormalities are probably the most serious adverse effects of AAS use currently documented. Changes in liver enzyme levels are generally used to monitor liver function. Elevations in these enzymes have been reported during AAS use, but return to normal when use is discontinued. Cholestatic jaundice and peliosis hepatis (blood-filled cysts of unknown etiology) are relatively common and typically occur when *alkylated* agents, such as methyltestosterone, methandrostenolone, oxymethalone, oxandrolone, and stanozolol, are used. As mentioned previously, the alkylated agents are those primarily administered orally. However, a few alkylated steroids that are usually administered orally are also available as injectable compounds (methandrostenolone and stanozolol), and these have similar effects on the liver as the oral AAS. Nonalkylated agents, such as testosterone and nortestosterone, are less likely to produce liver damage.

Hypogonadism has also been associated with AAS use. This results in a decline in sperm count, abnormal sperm morphology, and testicular atrophy. The mechanism for this involves a negative loop of the pituitary and gonads, causing a dose-dependent depression of luteinizing hormone (LH) and follicle stimulating hormone (FSH). This is also associated with significant decreases in plasma testosterone. *Androgenic* hormones can also be converted to the female sex hormones estradiol and estrone in the extragonadal tissues. This results in feminizing effects such as increased voice pitch and gynecomastia in males.

The use of AAS can lead to detrimental changes in serum lipid profiles. These changes, which include decreases in high-density lipoprotein (*HDL*) cholesterol and increases in low-density lipoprotein (*LDL*) cholesterol, have been associated with the development of cardiovascular disease. The more serious cardiovascular effects include hypertension, myocardial ischemia, and sudden cardiac death. As an example, electrocardiographic changes reflecting altered myocardium in the hypertrophied heart were observed in power athletes taking large doses of AAS. However, the true relationship between AAS use and serious cardiovascular effects is not fully understood at this time.

Aggressive behavior, mood changes, and psychiatric events including acute paranoia, delirium, mania or hypomania, and homicidal rage have been reported with AAS use. Episodes of depression, anxiety, and hostility have also been reported. Anabolic steroid users have reported higher rates of aggressive feelings, verbal aggression, and aggression toward objects while on the agents as compared to while off of them. The general conclusion is that these episodes are not frequent when lower dosages are used, but are more prevalent at higher dosages. It has also been suggested that AAS are addictive and that body type dissatisfaction and an obsession with increases in size and strength obtained with AAS contribute to patterns of dependent use and abuse.[32,33]

Table 13-6. Signs of Anabolic Steroid Use

- A dramatic increase in body bulk.
- Wide and erratic mood swings.
- Increased aggressiveness ("steroid rage") and irritability.
- Irrational behavior and depression.
- Increased presence of acne (oily skin and hair).
- Jaundice, usually only with the use of oral anabolic steroids.
- Hypertension, increased low density lipoprotein cholesterol, and decreased high density lipoprotein cholesterol.
- In males, premature balding, gynecomastia (increased breast size), testicular atrophy, and decreased sperm production.
- In females, male pattern balding, enlarged clitoris, growth of coarse facial hair, deepened voice, reduction in breast size, and change in or cessation of menstruation.

Although the effects of AAS use by females are not as well documented as those of males, adverse effects include hirsutism (changes in hair growth patterns, including facial hair), acne, deepening of the voice, clitoral hypertrophy, kidney and liver dysfunction, decreased breast mass, increased abdominal fat accumulation, male pattern baldness, and general virilization. The non-medical use of AAS can also have serious consequences for adolescents, such as severe facial and body acne, premature skeletal maturation (premature closing of the growth plates), and decreased spermatogenesis.

Although clinical testing is the most reliable method of detecting illicit AAS use, there are numerous physical signs that may cause suspicion (Table 13-6). These include muscular hypertrophy, oily skin and acne, jaundice in the skin or eyes, gynecomastia, hepatomegaly, testicular atrophy and edema, and mood changes or aggression.

Human Growth Hormone

Human growth hormone (hGH), otherwise known as somatotropin, is a *polypeptide* hormone that mediates numerous metabolic and growth processes in the human body. Although a number of growth hormone peptides exist in the body, the most common is a single strand polypeptide composed of 191 *amino acids* (about 21% of all circulating hGH). This hormone is used clinically to treat children's growth disorders and adult growth hormone deficiency. In recent years, replacement therapies with hGH have become extremely popular in the battle against aging. Touted as the "fountain of youth," reported effects of hGH therapy include decreased body fat, increased lean mass, increased bone density, increased energy levels, improved skin tone and texture, improved immune system function, and an enhanced sense of well-being. However, the research involving hGH has not been limited to the aging, as its role as an anabolic agent in a young, healthy population has also been investigated. At this time, hGH is still considered to be a very complex hormone and many of its functions are still unknown.

It has been used by competitors in a variety of sports since the 1970s. Although hGH has been banned by the NCAA and IOC for quite some time (see Tables 13-1 and 13-2), traditional urine analyses were not able to distinguish between its natural and synthetic forms. Thus, the ban could not be enforced. However, in the early 2000s, blood tests were developed that could detect doping with hGH. Because of this, the WADA collected approximately 3000 blood samples at the 2004 Olympic Games in Athens, Greece, with hGH being the primary target.

Pharmacodynamics

Human growth hormone is synthesized in and secreted from the anterior pituitary gland in a pulsatile manner throughout the day. Under basal conditions, hGH levels in a normal adult are relatively low. Surges of secretion occur at 3- to 5-hour intervals, with the greatest surge occurring 60 to 90 minutes after the onset of deep sleep. The secretion of hGH is regulated by two hypothalamic hormones: GH-releasing hormone (GHRH), which stimulates its release, and somatostatin, which inhibits it. A number of factors are known to affect these hormones and hGH secretion, such as age, gender, diet, exercise, stress, and other hormones. Secretion can be suppressed by a negative feedback on the hypothalamus and pituitary. This occurs when blood levels of hGH increase.

The effects of hGH on tissues are exerted directly and through the mediation of insulin-like growth factors. Because *polypeptide* hormones are not fat soluble, they cannot penetrate the *sarcolemma*. Thus, hGH exerts its effects directly by binding to receptors on target cells, such as muscle and fat cells. The binding to a receptor activates a *secondary messenger*, which then directs its actions to specific areas in the cell. Through this mechanism, hGH is a potent anabolic agent, as it promotes muscle, bone, and cartilage growth via enhanced cellular *amino acid* uptake and protein synthesis. However, hGH also exerts its anabolic effect indirectly via another potent anabolic hormone, insulin-like growth factor-1 (IGF-1).

Human growth hormone also mediates numerous metabolic processes, such as promotion of glucose and amino acid transport into muscle and fat, diversion of amino acids from oxidation to protein synthesis, retention of intracellular electrolytes, and stimulation of *lipolysis* in fat and muscle. Thus, it has the ability to alter the source of fuel from carbohydrate to fat.[34] However, because more than one form of it exists in the human body, the overall physiological effects of hGH are not completely understood at this time.

Proposed Ergogenic Effects

Exogenous hGH administration requires intramuscular or subcutaneous injection of *recombinant* hGH. Recombinant hGH is primarily used to increase muscle size and strength. However, the possible anabolic effects combined with the *lipolytic* effects make it an appealing drug for bodybuilders and those concerned with cosmetic appearance. Increases in lean body mass have been observed in hGH- or IGF-1-deficient adult patients and in an elderly population (who have typically low hGH concentrations) after receiving hGH treatment. In addition to increases in muscle mass, improvements in muscle strength and exercise capacity have also been observed in the hGH-deficient population. When groups of young healthy subjects are administered hGH, the results are not as consistent. In an examination of power-trained athletes, Deyssig et al[35] observed significant increases in serum hGH, IGF-1, and IGF-1 binding protein following 6 weeks of hGH treatment. However, these increases were not associated with any changes in lean body mass or strength. Likewise, in two separate studies, hGH administration failed to increase muscle protein synthesis and muscle strength in both trained[36] and untrained[37] young men. Whole body protein synthesis rates increased, but were attributed to decreased amino acid oxidation. They concluded that the increases in fat-free mass commonly observed during hGH treatment were probably from lean tissue other than skeletal muscle. In contrast, Crist et al[38] observed a significant increase in fat-free weight, a significant decrease in percent body fat, and an improved ratio of fat-free weight to fat weight in highly conditioned subjects following 6 weeks of hGH treatment. The primary cause of these changes appeared to be *lipolysis*. Elevations in circulating levels of IGF-1 were also observed in that study. It is important to note that when exogenous hGH is administered, it is only in one form. As mentioned previously, numerous forms of hGH are found in the body and these may be the true source of the anabolic potential.

Adverse Effects

Although the use of exogenous hGH is fairly common among athletes and bodybuilders, the data from this population are limited. Thus, the majority of what is known regarding the adverse effects of excess hGH has been obtained through the clinical evaluation of acromegaly (Table 13-7). Acromegaly is the clinical condition in which the pituitary gland naturally oversecretes hGH. It is characterized by bony overgrowth, which is particularly noticeable in the mandible, the supra-orbital ridges, and the enlargement of the hands and feet. Other clinical symptoms can include facial and aural soft tissue swelling; profuse sweating; deepening of the voice; gigantism; accelerated osteoarthritis; and visceral growth of cardiac, hepatic, renal, pulmonary, and thyroidal tissue. Growth hormone administration may have profound adverse effects on other hormonal systems and metabolic processes. Prolonged exposure to excessive amounts of hGH can also cause a suppression of endogenous hGH release and insulin resistance. In one of the few studies involving an athletic population, diminished hGH response to natural stimuli was observed following 6 weeks of exogenous hGH treatment.[38] However, a complete understanding of the adverse effects experienced by a healthy athletic population injecting hGH is not possible at this time.

β-Agonists

As discussed in Chapter 12, a β-*agonist* is defined as any compound that stimulates β-*adrenergic receptors*. Although β-agonists have traditionally been used for the treatment of bronchial ailments, it has become apparent that they have the ability to improve performance. This has become more apparent over the past decade, as their popularity as performance enhancers has grown. Common β-agonists include albuterol, bambuterol, clenbuterol, salmeterol, and terbutaline. At this time, clenbuterol, which is probably the most popular β-agonist used to enhance performance, is not approved by the FDA for human use and has been banned by the NCAA and the WADA (it was banned by the IOC in 1992 as a stimulant, but is now classified as an anabolic agent). In fact, during the 1992 Olympic Games in Barcelona, Italy, two American athletes tested positive for clenbuterol and were disqualified from competition. However, because many medications used for the treatment of asthma contain β_2-agonists (see Table 9-6), the NCAA and the WADA allows for the use of some in aerosol or inhalant form, but only with prior written notification (Table 13-8).

Pharmacodynamics

As mentioned previously, β-adrenergic receptors are characterized by their interaction with epinephrine and norepinephrine. The β-receptors can be classified as either β_1 or β_2 based on their affinity for certain compounds (see Chapter 12). Stimulation of β_1 *receptors* is associated with increased heart rate and cardiac contractility. Simulation of β_2 receptors is generally associated with bronchial and vascular smooth muscle relaxation and a stabilizing effect on mast cells, thus preventing the release of histamine and other inflammatory mediators. In general, β_2-agonists can be classified as *sympathomimetic* amines (eg, amphetamine and ephedrine). Thus, they mimic the β_2 actions of epinephrine.

Interest in β_2-agonists as performance enhancers began with studies involving veterinary applications. In animal models, β_2-agonists have been shown to prevent protein breakdown,

Table 13-7. Adverse Effects Associated With Excessive Growth Hormone

Metabolic Changes

- Diabetes mellitus
- Hypercalciuria
- Impaired glucose tolerance
- Insulin resistance

Neuromuscular Manifestations

- Headache
- Hypertrophic neuropathy
- Myopathy
- Nerve impingement (carpal tunnel syndrome)
- Sleep apnea
- Visual field loss

Skin and Connective Tissue Growth

- Excessive sweating
- Facial and acral (fingers, feet, etc) soft tissue swelling
- Hirsutism
- Laryngeal thickening (causing deep voice)
- Skeletal and articular changes
- Articular cartilage growth (accelerated osteoarthritis)
- Cranial growth
- Costal growth (barrel chest)
- Gigantism
- Mandibular growth (lantern jaw)
- Nasal cartilage growth
- Phalangeal bony overgrowth
- Vertebral bony overgrowth

Visceral Growth

- Cardiac (ventricular and septal thickening)
- Hepatic
- Pulmonary
- Renal
- Thyroid

Table 13-8. β-Agonists Permitted by WADA in Aerosol or Inhalant Form With Written Notification

Generic Name	Trade Name
Salbutamol*	Proventil
	Ventolin
Salmeterol	Serevent
Terbutaline	Brethaire
Salbutamol/Ipratropium	Combivent

Below 1000 ng/mL, a therapeutic justification and/or an examination by a medical panel is necessary, whereas above 1000 ng/mL is considered as having an anabolic effect and is considered a doping violation.

For a current list of banned substances, visit the WADA web site at http://www.wada-ama.org.

increase skeletal muscle hypertrophy, and decrease fat deposition. The primary mechanism behind the anabolic effects appears to be a reduction of protein degradation. At this time, however, the majority of the research remains limited to animal studies. In those studies, the dosages used to achieve the anabolic and lipolytic effects were much greater than those used for bronchodilation (up to 100 times).

Proposed Ergogenic Effects

The proposed ergogenic mechanism is primarily based on anabolic effects observed in animals. At this time, there are no studies relating the effects of oral β_2-agonists on muscle mass or strength in athletes. Maltin et al[39] administered clenbuterol to patients following knee surgery and observed a faster recovery of extensor strength in the injured leg. No change was noted in the healthy leg and neither leg experienced an increase in muscle cross-sectional area. Likewise, Martineau et al[40] administered oral, extended-release albuterol to untrained men and observed significant increases in muscle strength compared to a placebo group. Again, no changes in lean body mass were noted. Caruso et al[41] also observed improvements in isokinetic strength following 6 weeks of albuterol treatment. Like the studies above, these changes were not associated with any changes in muscle size. Also, the changes in isokinetic strength mainly occurred eccentrically. It would be expected that true changes in physiological strength would present concentrically as well. Eccentric testing is difficult for untrained individuals, so part of the increase might be explained by a learning or training effect. Thus, caution should be used when generalizing their results. Despite the lack of solid evidence from human trials, these drugs have become very popular at all levels of competition. Like hGH, the lipolytic potential of β_2-agonists makes them desirable for bodybuilders as well as strength and power athletes.

A lack of evidence supporting β_2-agonist use also exists when other types of performance are investigated. McKenzie et al[42] administered therapeutic doses of albuterol in aerosol form to healthy track and field athletes and found no change in pulmonary function, VO_{2max}, heart rate, and anaerobic threshold. In a separate study, Signorile et al[43] administered an acute therapeutic dose of aerosolized albuterol to nonasthmatic subjects who were recreationally active and observed an increase in anaerobic power and decreased fatigue. However, no changes were observed in respiratory function and cardiac response. In contrast, Meeuwisse et al[44] and Lemmer et al[45] failed to observe improvements in anaerobic power following administration of

Table 13-9. Potential Adverse Effects Associated with β-Agonists

System	Effect/Adverse Effect
Cardiovascular	Tachycardia
	Vasodilation
	Electrocardiogram changes
	Cardiac arrhythmia
	Myocardial ischemia
	Myocardial necrosis
	Potential inotropy
Skeletal muscle	Tremor
	Spasms/cramps
Other metabolic parameters	Glycogenolysis
	Gluconeogenesis
	Insulin production
	Hypokalemia
	Decreased magnesium
	Lipolysis
	Increased lactate production
Central nervous system	Nervousness
	Insomnia
	Migraine
	Paresthesia
	Psychosis

Adapted from Lynch GS. Beta-2 agonists. In: Bahrke MS, Yesalis CE, eds. *Performance Enhancing Supplements in Sport and Exercise.* Champaign, Ill: Human Kinetics; 2002:47-64.

albuterol. Unlike the previous study, both used highly trained athletes, which might account for the conflicting results. Furthermore, Lemmer et al[45] administered twice the normal dosage (360 μg) of albuterol and still found no improvement.

At this time, the efficacy of β-agonist use for performance enhancement remains unclear. There is minimal support for increases in strength in nonathletic populations; however, these were not associated with an anabolic effect (the proposed ergogenic mechanism). Thus, the majority of the research does not support ergogenic claims.

Adverse Effects

The majority of what is known regarding adverse effects associated with β_2-agonists has been obtained from patients being treated with these drugs and from people who have eaten meat from animals treated with the drugs. Common adverse effects can be found in Table 13-9. Adverse effects of β_2-agonists are considered minimal if they are inhaled using recommended doses. These include skeletal muscle tremor, nervousness, and palpitations. Some of the other adverse effects include headaches and insomnia. However, the fact that little is known about β_2-agonists, particularly at dosages used for the anabolic effects, make it a very dangerous drug. At higher doses, more serious adverse effects could include cardiac arrhythmias. Myocardial hypertrophy has been reported as an adverse effect of clenbuterol treatment in animal studies. This is a known factor in sudden cardiac death in athletes. Reports of adverse effects by illegal users of clenbuterol in the United States are understandably minimal. However, it has been anecdotally reported that the deaths of two professional bodybuilders from Europe were the result of clenbuterol use.

Summary

Increased protein synthesis, decreased protein degradation, or a combination of the two is the primary mechanism by which anabolic agents promote muscle growth. There are conflicting reports regarding the efficacy of these drugs for increasing muscle size and strength. A number of studies report increases in strength and lean body mass when AAS are administered. However, not all studies are in agreement with this. Human growth hormone appears to be effective when treating hGH- or IGF-1-deficient patients, whereas its effects on a healthy population remain unclear and, at this time, the scientific literature is lacking in any evidence to support the ergogenic use of β_2-agonists. All of the anabolic agents discussed in this chapter have been associated with negative adverse effects, some serious in nature. These drugs are not available OTC, and each one has been banned by various sport organizations.

ANTI-INFLAMMATORY DRUGS

Musculoskeletal breakdown is almost inevitable during athletic competition and intense training. This type of breakdown is generally accompanied by pain and inflammation. Because of this, the use of nonprescription and prescription anti-inflammatory drugs is one of the most common pharmaceutical interventions in athletics. Anti-inflammatory drugs are generally separated into two classifications, nonsteroidal anti-inflammatory drugs (NSAIDs) and corticosteroids (see also Chapter 6).

Corticosteroids

Corticosteroids are drugs with a sterol structure similar to that of cortisol, which is the primary circulating glucocorticoid found in the human body. Levels of these hormones are elevated in stressful situations, such as intense training, and are thought to be the primary endocrine response to starvation, as amino acids are converted to carbohydrate to maintain essential glucose levels in the brain. The therapeutic effects of glucocorticoids were first realized when it was unexpectedly reported that cortisone had powerful anti-inflammatory activity that dramatically improved the condition of patients with rheumatoid arthritis. Thus, these hormones are mainly used as anti-inflammatory drugs, which also provide an analgesic effect as inflammation is relieved. Some examples used in the treatment of musculoskeletal injury include dexamethasone, cortisone, prednisolone, and prednisone. At this time, the systemic use of glucocorticoids is prohibited by the WADA when administered orally, rectally, or by intravenous or intramuscular injection. The use of adrenocorticotropic hormone (ACTH), which stimulates the secretion of glucocorticoids, is also prohibited (see Tables 13-1 and 13-2). However, local and intra-articular injections of glucocorticoids are permitted if the governing body receives medical notification.

Pharmacodynamics

Glucocorticoids are produced in the adrenal gland and are generally regarded as protein *catabolic* hormones. As mentioned above, the secretion of these hormones is stimulated by ACTH. Glucocorticoids stimulate gluconeogenesis from amino acids derived from protein catabolism, decrease glucose use, and can cause insulin resistance. The direct effect on skeletal muscle is known from the marked muscle wasting and weakness in Cushing's syndrome (increased glucocorticoid production). Likewise, loss of muscle protein due to increased protein breakdown and decreased protein synthesis has been observed in response to glucocorticoid treatment. Like many other hormones, glucocorticoids exert their effect by binding to specific receptors.

As endogenous anti-inflammatory compounds, glucocorticoids protect tissue from damage caused by its own defense reactions and the products of these reactions during stress. They inhibit the synthesis of almost all known *cytokines* and other molecules required for immune function. Thus, they inhibit the function of key cells that comprise the inflammatory response. They also prevent the breakdown of phospholipids and their conversion to inflammatory mediators. One of the most important anti-inflammatory effects is their ability to inhibit the recruitment of leukocytes to the inflammatory site and to modify the capillary and membrane permeability that occurs during the tissue injury response. By doing so, glucocorticoids inhibit a critical step in the initiation of the inflammatory process.

Proposed Ergogenic Effects

Theoretically, the reduced glucose use and increased use of fatty acids associated with corticosteroids would provide a glycogen-sparing effect and improve performance. However, the research involving corticosteroid use and performance is limited, and the studies that do exist do not support the claims of enhanced performance. The *catabolic* properties of these drugs would suggest that their use would only impair performance. Thus, their use in athletics appears to be restricted to the treatment of chronic and painful musculoskeletal injury. Local injection is the method of choice in this situation. However, it is possible that a reduction in pain could allow an athlete to continue training and competing at a more intense level, providing an ergogenic effect. Once again, clinical studies supporting the ergogenic benefits of corticosteroids do not exist.

Adverse Effects

There are numerous ways in which corticosteroids can be administered. When taken orally, these drugs act systemically and can have profound effects on the body. *Cushing's syndrome* provides a primary example of adverse effects associated with elevated glucocorticoid levels. Some of these adverse effects include hypertension, acne, glaucoma, avascular necrosis, obesity, psychiatric problems, and poor wound healing. The development of diabetes mellitus is possible with long-term corticosteroid use and existing diabetes can be worsened.

Although local injection reduces the risks of systemic effects, there are still complications. The anti-inflammatory and *catabolic* properties can adversely affect the healing process. Because the pain feedback mechanism is lost, the potential for further injury exists. The possibility of tendon and ligament weakening justifies concern for joint injury and tendon rupture. It is actually recommended that athletes be kept out of training for several weeks following corticosteroid injection. One of the primary concerns in an athletic population would be the long-term complication of corticosteroid-induced osteoporosis.

Summary

At this time, evidence supporting the ergogenic use of corticosteroids in healthy individuals does not exist. When used by an injured athlete, the decreased inflammation and resultant reduction in pain may allow training and competition to continue. However, this may also increase the risk of reinjury. Although the adverse effects appear to be minor, continued use and increasing doses can increase the risk of more serious adverse effects. Although the use of glucocorticoids is prohibited by a number of organizations when administered orally, rectally, or by intravenous or intramuscular injection, local and intra-articular injections are generally permitted.

BETA-BLOCKERS

Beta-adrenergic antagonists, also known as *beta-blockers* (β-blockers), are drugs primarily used for conditions that affect the cardiovascular system (see Chapter 12). In an athletic population, these drugs are more commonly prescribed to control hypertension. As performance enhancers, β-blockers are used to counteract the effects of anxiety associated with athletic competition, which include increases in heart rate, nervousness, and skeletal muscle tremor. Although the physiological response to beta blockade may not be desirable for many types of sports or athletic events, it may provide benefit for activities requiring precision and accuracy. Thus, the IOC banned β-blockers in 1985. This ban was subsequently altered and now affects only precision sports such as archery, shooting, fencing, equestrian events, biathlon and modern pentathlon, bobsled, diving, synchronized swimming, and ski jumping (see Table 13-1). Likewise, the NCAA has banned the use of β-blockers during rifle competition (see Table 13-2). However, the extent of β-blocker use in athletic competition is not fully understood. There have even been anecdotal reports of use during golf competition, including the Professional Golfers' Association (PGA) tour. Whether this actually occurs is unknown, as neither the PGA nor the NCAA test for β-blockers during golf competitions.

Pharmacodynamics

β-blockers are drugs that were developed to bind to *sympathetic* cell membrane receptors sensitive to the *catecholamines, epinephrine* and *norepinephrine*. As mentioned previously (see amphetamines), these receptors are found on most cells throughout the body, including the cells of the heart, lungs, and surrounding blood vessels. They work by decreasing heart rate, stroke volume (overall cardiac output), and mean arterial blood pressure. They are used to lower blood pressure and decrease the work of the heart in ischemic heart conditions and congestive heart failure. β-blockers are commonly used to treat hypertension, angina, arrhythmias, migraine headache, and anxiety and are frequently given after myocardial infarction. Their central *anxiolytic* effect occurs in direct proportion to their *lipophilic* binding and their ability to cross the blood-brain barrier.

Proposed Ergogenic Effects

β-blockers are commonly used to reduce performance anxiety in musicians, teachers, and business executives. Although reports are mostly anecdotal, short-acting, low-dose preparations, such as propranolol, are generally recommended. Improvements have been observed in these populations; however, it is difficult to generalize these improvements to sport competition. Sport competition creates anxiety, which is associated with an increase in *sympathetic* nervous system activity and increased levels of *catecholamines*. Even before competition begins, an athlete will experience anxiety symptoms such as elevations in heart rate and blood pressure and skeletal muscle tremor. β-blockers are used to decrease this type of anxiety during athletic competition. Although decreases in cardiac output would not be beneficial for an endurance athlete, β-blocker use could improve performance in sports requiring precision and accuracy. For example, experienced shooters fire during diastole. Thus, a slower heart rate would increase time during diastole and possibly improve shooting performance. At this time, investigation into the efficacy of β-blocker use during sport competition is very limited. Metoprolol use has been associated with a 13% improvement in pistol shooting, with the greatest effect being observed in the more skilled shooters.[46] It was suggested that the improvement was more due to the drug's effect on hand tremor rather than on heart rate. Similar observations have been made when oxprenolol is administered. However, not all studies have shown improvement. For example, although cardio-vascular changes have been observed, β-blockade has not been shown to improve bowling performance. It appears that their effects on performance and physiological changes, such as lipid and lactic acid levels, depend on the intensity of the activity and whether a cardioselective or nonselective drug is used. β-blockers have no effect on strength or power, and their negative *inotropic* and *chronotropic* effects are undesirable for endurance athletes.

Adverse Effects

The most common adverse effects associated with beta blockade are bradycardia and hypotension. Other adverse effects include bronchospasm, heart failure, arrhythmias, fatigue, impaired glucose control in diabetes, and aggravation of peripheral vascular disease. It is important to note that these reactions can be accentuated with alcohol. Endurance athletes should avoid using β-blockers because of their negative effect on cardiac output, oxygen consumption, and overall exercise capacity. Other possible adverse effects during exercise include increased perceived exertion levels, earlier lactate threshold and fatigue, and possible exacerbation of exercise-induced bronchospasm or asthma. Because these drugs can inhibit *lipolysis* and *glycogenolysis*, hypoglycemia may occur after intense exercise. β-blocker use should also be avoided by athletes with first- or second-degree heart block and by those with asthma.

Summary

Although the benefit of beta blockade in the treatment of various medical conditions is well accepted, their use as performance enhancers is not. Any possible benefit would only apply to sports requiring precision such as shooting and archery. However, at this time support for their ability to improve this type of performance is very limited. Furthermore, any sport requiring strength, power, speed, or endurance would only be impaired by β-blockade. There are also numerous adverse effects associated with these drugs. Thus, caution is warranted with their use.

OXYGEN DELIVERY ENHANCERS

In endurance sports such as running, cycling, and cross-country skiing, the ability to deliver oxygen to the working muscles over long periods of time is a critical component to performance. This is evident as VO_2 during exercise and maximal VO_2 are generally higher in trained athletes compared to untrained. Oxygen consumption by the working muscles is dependent on the cardiovascular system's ability to deliver the oxygen from the lungs. Erythrocytes, or red blood cells (RBCs), are responsible for this delivery. Red blood cells contain hemoglobin, which binds to oxygen to form an unstable compound called oxyhemoglobin. In tissues where the oxygen concentration is low, hemoglobin releases its oxygen. Thus, changes in the hemoglobin concentration (Hb) or its oxygen saturation can have an impact on physical performance. Because of this, numerous attempts have been made to alter these variables. In blood doping, units of whole blood are collected from an athlete. The RBCs are then separated from the plasma, frozen, and stored in glycerol. This is usually done 2 to 3 months before competition to allow for erythropoiesis (the production of RBCs) and restoration of normal Hb. Three to five days before competition, the RBCs are infused resulting in an increased Hb. It is well accepted that this procedure can improve oxygen delivery and endurance performance. However, this is an invasive procedure and is associated with certain risks. Because of this, attempts have been made to find alternative pharmaceutical methods for increasing Hb and oxygen delivery. One of the more popular drugs used for this purpose is erythropoietin.

Erythropoietin

Erythropoietin (EPO) is a glycoprotein hormone that plays a primary role in erythropoiesis. It is secreted by the kidneys and liver in response to low oxygen levels in the blood, resulting in an increased bone marrow production of RBCs. The gene encoding EPO was cloned in 1985, which led to its synthetic production. *Recombinant* EPO (r-EPO) is produced by inserting the gene into a cell and stimulating the cell to produce it. It was originally developed for treating patients suffering from bone marrow failure and those with certain types of anemia, such as anemia due to chronic renal failure, anemia associated with cancer and chemotherapy, and anemia secondary to zidovudine treatment of AIDS. The r-EPO assists these patients in raising their hematocrit (index of RBC level) and oxygen-carrying capacity, relieving the symptoms of their chronic disease. However, it was not long after its development that the ergogenic potential of r-EPO was also realized. Although the prevalence of r-EPO use in sport is unknown, anecdotal reports suggest that it is widespread among endurance athletes. Because r-EPO potentially gives an unfair advantage in competition, it has been banned by various sport governing bodies (see Tables 13-1 and 13-2). Probably the greatest controversy surrounding the use of r-EPO has occurred during the Tour de France. Before the start of the 1998 Tour, a team masseur named Willy Voet was stopped at the Franco-Belgium border where his car was found to contain >400 doping products, including r-EPO. This led to an investigation of teams and individual riders by authorities, resulting in numerous disqualifications. Since that time, a number of high-profile athletes have tested positive for r-EPO and have been penalized. However, despite improvements in doping control, penalties, and possible risks, r-EPO continues to be a very popular drug among athletes.

Pharmacodynamics

Normal levels of EPO are approximately 0 to 19 mU/mL; however, large individual and interindividual variations exist during the day and in response to different physiological situations. The kidney cells that make EPO are specialized and are sensitive to low oxygen levels in the blood. Thus, oxygen availability in the kidneys is the primary regulator of EPO production. Hypoxia due to anemia or low plasma oxygen pressure leads to an increase in EPO secretion. Following secretion, EPO binds to receptors in the bone marrow, which stimulate the differentiation and proliferation of erythroid precursors. This also stimulates the release of reticulocytes into the circulation and the synthesis of cellular hemoglobin. The end result of this process is an increased RBC production and Hb. *Exogenous* r-EPO is administered intravenously or subcutaneously and has a plasma half-life ($t\frac{1}{2}$) of approximately 6 to 8 hours (the half-life is longer following subcutaneous injection). It binds to the same receptors and has the same physiological effect as *endogenous* EPO. Early clinical trials showed that r-EPO was capable of increasing the hematocrit by 3% to 4% in as little as 3 to 4 weeks. This treatment has also resulted in a restoration of Hb and physical performance levels and an overall improvement in quality of life in patients with certain diseases. In patients with chronic heart failure, r-EPO has been shown to increase oxygen delivery and Hb and enhance exercise capacity. It is important to note that these patients can be considered a deficient population. The question is whether the same changes would occur in healthy individuals.

Proposed Ergogenic Effects

Like a diseased population, improved physical performance in healthy individuals would depend on an increased Hb and enhanced maximal VO_2. Although large variations have been observed across subjects, the general conclusion is that r-EPO will increase the Hb and hematocrit in trained subjects. Other variables such as blood volume, resting heart rate, and VO$_2$ during submaximal exercise do not appear to change. However, the increases in Hb and hematocrit have been associated with increases in maximal VO$_2$. These observations have been consistent across most individuals. In fact, the increases observed are similar to those observed following blood doping. Even in well-trained athletes, it appears that r-EPO will increase erythropoiesis and enhance physical performance. Increases in maximal VO$_2$ following r-EPO administration have been associated with improvements in time to exhaustion, which is a standard measure of endurance performance. Thus, it has become well-accepted that the use of r-EPO can provide an ergogenic effect. However, many have suggested that the use of r-EPO as a performance-enhancing agent is a dangerous practice.

Adverse Effects

The use of r-EPO can cause a reduction in *endogenous* EPO production. Although the effects of long-term use are not fully understood, endogenous levels return to normal when short-term use is discontinued. The use of r-EPO also has the potential for increased blood viscosity and thrombosis with potentially fatal results. Exercise training can stimulate RBC production and increase Hb, but this is usually associated with an increase in plasma volume as well. In contrast, the increase in RBC mass during r-EPO therapy generally occurs without an increase in the total blood volume. When used to gradually elevate the hematocrit in anemic patients, r-EPO therapy usually is uneventful. The same cannot be said for healthy subjects. When r-EPO is administered to healthy individuals and the normal hematocrit level is exceeded, blood viscosity increases. Thus, the increased RBC density caused by r-EPO can increase the viscosity of the blood and increase the risk for thrombotic events. The increased viscosity can also overload the heart, increasing the chances of heart attack and stroke. Because of this, it has been suggested that r-EPO use contributed to the unexpected deaths of several well-trained endurance athletes during the 1990s. This may be of even greater concern with athletes during training or competition, as dehydration can further increase the viscosity of the blood.

Other adverse effects associated with r-EPO include headaches, hypertension, and seizures. Hypertension develops in 20% to 30% of renal patients treated with r-EPO, whereas elevations in systolic blood pressure have been observed in trained athletes during submaximal exercise. Those with a history of thrombosis, heart disease, or hypertension may have increased chances of adverse effects. The chance of seizures may be increased in those with history of seizures. Rare side effects include flu-like symptoms and bone and muscle pain. There are also rare reports of antibody formation toward r-EPO in humans.

Summary

Very few would debate the ergogenic value of r-EPO. However, very few would also debate the dangers associated with this prescription drug. For this reason, r-EPO has been banned by numerous sport governing organizations. In the absence of a valid procedure to detect r-EPO doping, in-competition health checks were introduced by organizations such as the International Ski Federation and the International Cycling Union. These health checks excluded athletes from competition when their Hb or hematocrit values exceeded an arbitrary limit. This limited the danger to athletes, but did nothing to eliminate the use of r-EPO. Through the past decade, both direct and indirect methods for detecting r-EPO were investigated. No single indirect marker was found that satisfactorily demonstrated r-EPO use. Because of this, a combination of blood and urine tests together formed the procedure and strategy approved by the IOC for detecting r-EPO use at the 2000 Olympic Games in Sydney, Australia, and the 2002 Salt Lake City Winter

Olympics. However, until a more definitive test is developed for detection of r-EPO, it will continue to be a part of athletic competition.

ROLE OF THE ATHLETIC TRAINER

Ergogenic drug use continues to create controversy at all levels of athletic competition. At this time, there is support in the scientific literature for the use of some drugs (eg, caffeine, AAS), whereas it does not exist for others (eg, β-agonists, glucocorticoids). The potential for adverse effects, sometimes serious in nature, exists with the use of any drug. Because of the health risks associated with ergogenic drug use, it is important that athletic trainers and other health care professionals provide intervention in the form of education, information, medical care, and referral when necessary. In addition, the athletic trainer's role in ergogenic drug use includes the following:

- It is imperative that athletic trainers and other health care professionals become educated themselves with regards to the efficacy, safety, and legalities of ergogenic drug use.
- Because many athletes may not be open about their drug use, it is also important that the athletic trainer recognizes the adverse effects and general signs and symptoms of this type of drug use.
- The athletic trainer must also accept the role of liaison and refer the athlete to counseling when it is believed that this type of intervention is necessary.

REFERENCES

1. Graham TE, Spriet LL. Metabolic, catecholamine and exercise performance responses to varying doses of caffeine. *J Appl Physiol.* 1995;78:867-874.
2. Pasman WJ, VanBaak MA, Jeukendrup AE, DeHaan A. The effect of different dosages of caffeine on endurance performance time. *Int J Sports Med.* 1995;16:225-230.
3. Spriet LL, MacLean DA, Dyck DJ, Hultman E, Cederblad G, Graham TE. Caffeine ingestion and muscle metabolism during prolonged exercise in humans. *Am J Physiol.* 1992;262:E891-E898.
4. Denadai BS, Denadai ML. Effects of caffeine on time to exhaustion in exercise performed below and above the anaerobic threshold. *Braz J Med Biol Res.* 1998;31:581-585.
5. Greer F, McLean C, Graham TE. Caffeine, performance, and metabolism during repeated Wingate exercise tests. *J Appl Physiol.* 1998;85:1502-1508.
6. Bell DG, McLellan TM. Exercise endurance 1, 3, and 6 h after caffeine ingestion in caffeine users and nonusers. *J Appl Physiol.* 2002;93:1227-1234.
7. Berry MJ, Stoneman JV, Weyrich AS, Burney B. Dissociation of the ventilatory and lactate thresholds following caffeine ingestion. *Med Sci Sports Exerc.* 1991;23:463-468.
8. Bond V, Gresham K, McRae J, Tearney RJ. Caffeine ingestion and isokinetic strength. *Br J Sports Med.* 1986;20:135-137.
9. Casal DC, Leon AS. Failure of caffeine to affect substrate utilization during prolonged running. *Med Sci Sports Exerc.* 1985;17:174-179.
10. Collomp K, Ahmaidi S, Audran M, Chanal JL, Prefaut Ch. Effect of caffeine ingestion on performance and anaerobic metabolism during the wingate test. *Int J Sports Med.* 1991;12:439-443.
11. Collomp K, Ahmaidi S, Chatard JC, Audran M, Prefaut Ch. Benefits of caffeine ingestions on sprint performance in trained and untrained swimmers. *Eur J Appl Physiol.* 1992;64:377-380.
12. Dodd SL, Brooks E, Powers SK, Tulley R. The effects of caffeine on graded exercise performance in caffeine naïve versus habituated subjects. *Eur J Appl Physiol.* 1991;62:424-429.

13. Falk B, Burstein R, Ashkenazi I, et al. The effect of caffeine ingestion on physical performance after prolonged exercise. *Eur J Appl Physiol.* 1989;59:168-173.

14. Fisher SM, McMurray RG, Berry M, Mar MH, Forsythe WA. Influence of caffeine on exercise performance in habitual caffeine users. *J Sports Med.* 1986;7:276-280.

15. Graham TE, Spriet LL. Performance and metabolic responses to high caffeine dose during prolonged exercise. *J Appl Physiol.* 1991;71:2292-2298.

16. Hunter AM, St Clair Gibson A, Collins M, Lambert M, Noakes TD. Caffeine ingestion does not alter performance during a 100-km cycling time-trial performance. *Int J Sport Nutr Exerc Metab.* 2002;12:438-452.

17. Ivy JL, Costill DL, Fink WJ, Lower RW. Influence of caffeine and carbohydrate feedings on endurance performance. *Med Sci Sports Exerc.* 1979;11:6-11.

18. Jackman M, Wendling P, Friars D, Graham TE. Metabolic, catecholamine, and endurance responses to caffeine during intense exercise. *J Appl Physiol.* 1996;81:1658-1663.

19. Jacobson BH, Edwards SW. Influence of two levels of caffeine on maximal torque at selected angular velocities. *J Sports Med Phys Fitness.* 1991;31:147-153.

20. Jacobson BH, Weber MD, Claypool L, Hunt LE. Effect of caffeine on maximal strength and power in elite male athletes. *Br J Sports Med.* 1992;26:276-280.

21. Williams JH, Barnes WS, Gadberry WL. Influence of caffeine on force and EMG in rested and fatigued muscle. *Am J Phys Med.* 1987;66:169-183.

22. Sidney KH, Lefcoe NM. The effects of ephedrine on the physiological and psychological responses to submaximal and maximal exercise in man. *Med Sci Sports Exerc.* 1977;9:95-99.

23. Gillies H, Derman W, Noakes T, Smith P, Evans A, Gabriels G. Pseudoephedrine is without ergogenic effects during exercise. *J Appl Physiol.* 1996;81:2611-2617.

24. Swain RA, Harsha DM, Baenziger J, Saywell RM. Do pseudoephedrine or phenylpropanolamine improve maximum oxygen uptake and time to exhaustion? *Clin J Sports Med.* 1997;7:168-173.

25. Bell DG, Jacobs I, McLellan TM, Zamecnik J. Reducing the dose of combined caffeine and ephedrine preserves the ergogenic effect. *Aviat Space Environ Med.* 2000;71:415-419.

26. Bell DG, Jacobs I, Zamecnik J. Effects of caffeine, ephedrine, and their combination on time to exhaustion during high intensity exercise. *Eur J Appl Physiol.* 1998;77:427-433.

27. Bell DG, Jacobs I. Combined caffeine and ephedrine ingestion improves run times of Canadian Forces Warrior Test. *Aviat Space Environ Med.* 1999;70:325-329.

28. Rogozkin V. Metabolic effects of anabolic steroid on skeletal muscle. *Med Sci Sports Exerc.* 1979;11:160-163.

29. Haupt HA, Rovere GD. Anabolic steroids: a review of the literature. *Am J Sports Med.* 1984;12:469-484.

30. Elashoff JD, Jacknow AD, Shain SG, Braunstein GD. Effects of anabolic androgenic steroids on muscular strength. *Ann Intern Med.* 1991;115:387-393.

31. Burkett LN, Falduto MT. Steroid use by athletes in a metropolitan area. *Phys Sports Med.* 1984;12:69-74.

32. Brower KJ, Blow FC, Young JP, et al. Symptoms and correlates of anabolic-androgenic steroid dependence. *Br J Addict.* 1991;86:759-768.

33. Copeland J, Peters R, Dillon P. Anabolic-androgenic steroid use disorder among a sample of Australian competitive and recreational users. *Drug Alcohol Depend.* 2000;60:91-96.

34. Goodman HM, Grichting G. Growth hormone and lipolysis: a reevaluation. *Endocrinology.* 1983;113:1697-1702.

35. Deyssig R, Frisch H, Blum WF, Waldhor T. Effect of growth hormone treatment hormonal parameters, body composition and strength in athletes. *Acta Endocrinol.* 1993;128:313-318.

36. Yarasheski KE, Campbell JA, Smith K, Rennie MJ, Holloszy JO, Bier DM. Effect of growth hormone and resistance exercise on muscle growth in young men. *Am J Physiol.* 1992;262:E261-E267.

37. Yarasheski KE, Zachwieja JJ, Angelopoulos TJ, Bier DM. Short-term growth hormone treatment does not increase muscle protein synthesis in experienced weight lifters. *J Appl Physiol.* 1993;74:3073-3076.

38. Crist DM, Peake GT, Egan PA, Waters DL. Body composition response to exogenous GH during training in highly conditioned adults. *J Appl Physiol.* 1988;65:579-584.

39. Maltin CA, Delday MI, Watson JS, et al. Clenbuterol, a beta-adrenoceptor agonist, increases relative muscle strength in orthopaedic patients. *Clin Sci* (Lond).1993;84:651-654.

40. Martineau L, Horan MA, Rothwell NJ, Little RA. Salbutamol, a beta 2-adrenoceptor agonist, increases skeletal muscle strength in young men. *Clin Sci* (Lond). 1992;83:615-621.

41. Caruso JF, Signorile JF, Perry AC, et al. The effects of albuterol and isokinetic exercise on the quadriceps muscle group. *Med Sci Sports Exerc.* 1995;27:1471-1476.

42. McKenzie DC, Rhodes EC, Stirling DR, et al. Salbutamol and treadmill performance in non-atopic athletes. *Med Sci Sports Exerc.* 1983;15:520-522.

43. Signorile JF, Kaplan TA, Applegate B, Perry AC. Effects of acute inhalation of the bronchodilator, albuterol, on power output. *Med Sci Sports Exerc.* 1992;24:638-642.

44. Meeuwisse WH, McKenzie DC, Hopkins SR, Road JD. The effect of salbutamol on performance in elite nonasthmatic athletes. *Med Sci Sports Exerc.* 1992;24:1161-1166.

45. Lemmer JT, Fleck SJ, Wallach JM, et al. The effects of albuterol on power output in non-asthmatic athletes. *Int J Sports Med.* 1995;16:243-249.

46. Kruse P, Ladefoged J, Nielsen U, Paulev P, Sorensen J. Beta-blockade used in precision sports: effect on pistol shooting performance. *J Appl Physiol.* 1986;61:417-420.

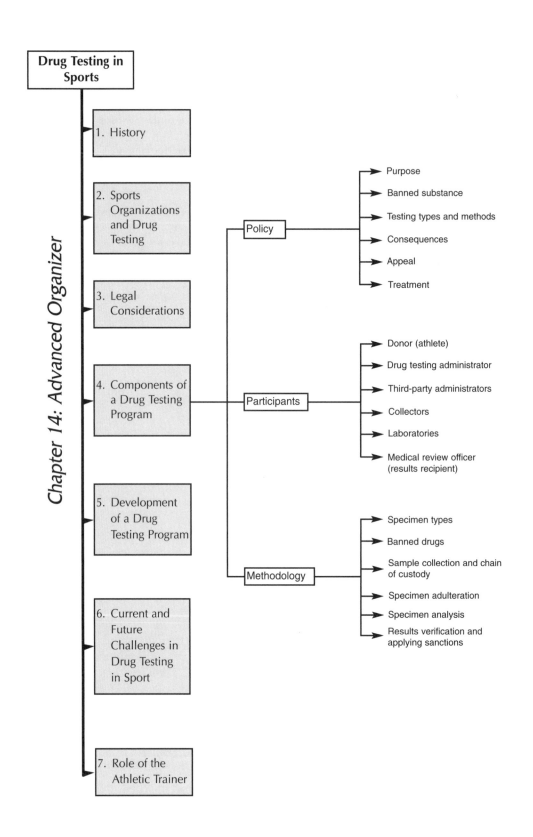

Chapter 14: Advanced Organizer

Drug Testing in Sports

1. History

2. Sports Organizations and Drug Testing

3. Legal Considerations

4. Components of a Drug Testing Program

5. Development of a Drug Testing Program

6. Current and Future Challenges in Drug Testing in Sport

7. Role of the Athletic Trainer

Policy
- Purpose
- Banned substance
- Testing types and methods
- Consequences
- Appeal
- Treatment

Participants
- Donor (athlete)
- Drug testing administrator
- Third-party administrators
- Collectors
- Laboratories
- Medical review officer (results recipient)

Methodology
- Specimen types
- Banned drugs
- Sample collection and chain of custody
- Specimen adulteration
- Specimen analysis
- Results verification and applying sanctions

DRUG TESTING IN SPORTS

Cindy Thomas, ATC

CHAPTER OBJECTIVES

After the end of this chapter, the reader will be able to:

- Discuss the historical progression of performance enhancing drug use in sport from the ancient Olympic Games to current day.
- Identify and compare the various sports organizations that administer drug testing programs.
- Explain relevant case law pertaining to drug testing in sport, including an understanding of the protections guaranteed by the Constitution of the United States.
- Identify and describe the necessary components of a sports drug testing policy.
- Explain the responsibilities of the drug testing administrator, collector, and laboratory.
- Compare the applicability, methodology, advantages, and disadvantages of the various types of biological specimens used in drug testing.
- Identify and locate sports organizations' banned drug lists and explain why specific drug classes are prohibited.
- Explain why the specimen collection process is an integral part of the drug testing process and include a discussion on specimen adulteration.
- Describe the difference between laboratory specimen screening and confirmation procedures and provide examples of each method.
- Identify the steps necessary in the development and implementation of a sports drug testing program.

Sport has a responsibility to maintain a level playing field. Competitors are expected to abide by the rules of fair play. Some athletes use chemical and pharmacological substances in pursuit of competitive superiority.[1] The sports world has responded to this unethical and risky behavior of manipulating performance to dominate the opponent by developing drug testing programs. Unfortunately, these programs are not accepted as the total solution to the doping woes tarnishing sport today. To the contrary, drug testing in sport is often considered a necessary evil. It is necessary to deter the use of performance-enhancing substances and other dangerous drugs by athletes, yet the very process has been challenged as an invasion of privacy and regarded as inconvenient, time consuming, humiliating, and ineffective. Heralded as the cure for athlete doping practices, drug testing has become commonplace in sport. As long as athletes choose an unethical path of improving performance and endangering their lives, drug testing programs will continue as an attempt to promote integrity in athletics.

The purpose of this chapter is to provide the athletic trainer with a detailed understanding of sports drug testing. A chronological history is presented demonstrating how performance-enhancing substances have been used since the earliest recorded competitive setting. Conversely, numerous sports organizations have developed antidoping initiatives in response to drug use in sport, and these programs are described along with the legal battles that have been fought in an effort to eliminate these unethical and risky behaviors. A breakdown of the various components necessary to implement drug testing is explained and provides details on policy content and methodology. Finally, a perspective of doping issues facing the future of sport is examined.

Drug use or doping in sport has become a complex, multidimensional problem. The term "doping" is believed to be derived from the Dutch word "doop," which is a viscous opium juice, the drug of choice of the ancient Greeks. "Doping control" has been adopted as a common international term for drug testing in sports.[2,3] The International Olympic Committee (IOC) defines doping as "the administration of or use by a competing athlete of any substance foreign to the body or any physiological substance taken in abnormal quantity or taken by an abnormal route of entry into the body with the sole intention of increasing in an artificial or unfair manner his or her performance in competition."[4] Although anabolic steroids and other performance-enhancing agents and processes are most widely used by athletes, many routinely use and abuse alcohol, tobacco, marijuana, cocaine, and a variety of other licit and illicit drugs. Like performance-enhancing substances, these drugs also pose serious health-related problems and their use must be addressed. It is well documented that athletes use a variety of drugs for a multitude of reasons.[5] It is important to recognize that abuse of drugs in sport is not just an individual problem limited to athletes; it is a burgeoning problem threatening our youth and public health.[6] Drug testing has been shown to be extremely effective at reducing drug use in schools and businesses nationwide.[7] The growth of drug testing has been fueled by the fact that it deters drug use, yielding an immeasurable benefit.[8] To fully understand today's antidoping initiatives in sport, a historical perspective of substances used to enhance performance or "doping" for a competitive advantage must be examined.

HISTORY

The practice of using performance-enhancing agents to gain a competitive advantage is not new to athletics. In ancient Olympic Games, athletes drank various alcohol concoctions and herbal infusions in the pursuit of victory.[4] The ancient Greeks ate sesame seeds attempting to enhance performance, and the gladiators were known to ingest plants containing stimulants to prevent the effects of fatigue.[9,10] The Berserkers, an ancient class of Nordic warriors, fought frenziedly, a "berserk" behavior attributed to a deliberate dish of wild mushrooms containing bufotein for its stimulating effects.[11]

The reasons for anabolic steroid and stimulant doping in sport today are the same as those described in the earliest recorded history of drugs and physical activity—to increase strength and overcome fatigue. Early competitors discovered the anabolic and androgenic properties of the testes through the observation of castrating domesticated animals. Many indulged in organotherapy, the practice of eating animal and human organs to cure disease and improve vitality. As early as 1400 BC, the Susruta of India advocated consumption of testis tissue to cure impotence. During the eighth century, testicular extract was prescribed as an aphrodisiac.[10]

Early use of stimulants to enhance performance was accomplished by ingesting plants. West Africans and Andean Indians chewed the leaves of the cola plant and drank tea to increase endurance. Mexican Indians used peyote plants along with strychnine for its stimulant effects during long runs, whereas Austrian lumberjacks ingested arsenic to increase endurance.[10]

The first drug-related death in sport was documented in 1886 when an English cyclist died from an overdose of trimethyl, probably a slang term for a form of ether. Prior to the 1940s, most drug use in sport consisted of ingesting a mixture of strychnine and alcohol. Strychnine taken in low doses has a stimulant effect, but higher doses are toxic.[4,10] During the late 19th and early 20th centuries, a variety of concoctions were tried including milk-punch, champagne and brandy, belladonna, strychnine, and "morphine in hot drops" in an effort to prolong performance efforts.[10] In the 1930s, amphetamines replaced the popular strychnine cocktail.[11] During the 1952 Winter Olympic Games, several speed skaters became ill from alleged amphetamine use.[4] The most significant amphetamine-related tragedy occurred in the 1960 Summer Olympic Games in Rome, Italy, when Danish cyclist Knud Jensen collapsed and died.[4,11] An autopsy revealed Jensen probably died of dehydration after taking amphetamines and cough medicine.[4]

In the mid-1930s, scientists began synthesizing the hormone testosterone. Following this discovery, oral and injectable testosterone preparations became available to the medical community.[10] It was rumored that some German athletes were given testosterone for the 1936 Berlin Olympic Games and that during World War II German soldiers were given steroids before battle to enhance aggressiveness. However, the first recorded case of an "athlete" using testosterone was documented in the early 1940s when an 18-year-old horse named Holloway was administered testosterone in an attempt to improve his slowing performance on the track. After hormone administration and training, Holloway went on to win a number of races, establishing a trotter record at age 19.[10]

During the 1950s, it was reported that the Soviets were experimenting with hormone manipulation. At the 1956 World Games in Moscow, Russia, American physician John Ziegler witnessed the use of testosterone in highly successful Soviet athletes. During this time period, CIBA Pharmaceutical Company was developing an oral anabolic steroid methandrostenolone (Dianabol). Although designed for legitimate medical uses, athletes obtained and began using Dianabol at 10 to 20 times the therapeutic doses.[4,10] There seemed to be no widespread problem with athletes using anabolic steroids during the 1960 Olympic Games, as only a few Soviet strength athletes and a few American weight lifters were suspected of using.

By the 1960s, the startling success of a number of strength athletes, known to be using anabolic steroids, created an epidemic of use. Weight lifters, track and field throwers, sprinters, and others were using steroids and breaking world records at a phenomenal pace. It was estimated that one-third of the US track and field team used steroids at the 1968 pre-Olympic training camp. This was at a time when steroid use was not banned and users were actually boasting of the enhanced performance effects from anabolic steroids.[10]

In response to Knud Jensen's untimely death in 1960, the sports world began exploring ways to control the use of drugs in athletics. Pharmacist Arnold Beckett introduced the first documented antidoping initiatives.[11] Beckett and some of his colleagues developed procedures capable of detecting several different stimulants and began drug testing cyclists participating in Tour of Britain races.[12] However, it was not until the death of British cyclist Tommy Simpson during the 1967 Tour de France that official antidoping programs were implemented banning amphetamines from sport internationally. Simpson died while under the influence of amphetamines.[11,12] In 1963, in response to the widespread use of potentially life-threatening drugs in sports, the Council of Europe (COE) established the following definition of doping:

> *The administering or use of substances in any form alien to the body or of physiological substances in abnormal amounts and with abnormal methods by healthy persons with the exclusive aim of attaining an artificial and unfair increase in performance in competition. Furthermore, various psychological measures to increase performance in sports must be regarded as doping. Where*

treatment with a medicine must be undergone, which as a result of its nature or dosage is capable of raising physiological capability beyond normal level, such treatment must be considered doping and shall rule out eligibility for competition.

The COE also published the first list of banned substances, which included narcotics, amine stimulants, alkaloids, analeptic agents, respiratory tonics, and certain hormones.[3]

Finally, the international sports world recognized that using performance-enhancing drugs was not only immoral but also posed significant health risks. By 1965, gas chromatography (GC) was introduced and implemented in laboratories for specimen analysis. In 1968, the IOC appointed a Medical Commission, adopted a Medical Code, and developed its first list of banned list of drugs. The IOC conducted preliminary testing during the Munich Summer Games in 1972. Comprehensive testing with anabolic steroid analysis did not begin until the Montreal Olympic Games in 1976.[4,11,12] Other sports-governing bodies quickly established rules against doping. During the 1980s, major athletic organizations in the United States, including the National Collegiate Athletic Association (NCAA), the National Football League (NFL), USA Track and Field (USATF), and the United States Olympic Committee (USOC) implemented comprehensive drug testing programs.[13]

In 1970, the NCAA Drug Education Committee was formed because of concern about increasing drug use and abuse among college student-athletes. Three years later, NCAA member institutions voted to establish legislation banning use of unauthorized drugs that could endanger athletes' health and safety or provide an unfair competitive advantage. More than a decade later the NCAA Committee on Drug Testing was formed and developed a drug testing plan including a list of banned drugs. On November 24, 1986, the NCAA implemented its first drug testing program during the Division I Women's Cross Country Championships in Tucson, Arizona. During the 1986 to 1987 academic year, >3000 student-athletes were drug tested at NCAA championships. Two years later, the NCAA implemented out-of-competition drug testing for anabolic steroids.[14] The NCAA drug testing program was not established without challenge, but the legal battles in the United States courts ultimately served to strengthen both the drug testing program and its ideals. The NCAA's current drug testing program includes both in-competition and out-of-competition drug testing of >10,000 student-athletes annually. In addition to the organization's drug testing programs, the NCAA encourages member schools and offers guidelines to develop and implement institutional drug testing programs.

Communities nationwide are adopting middle and high school drug testing programs out of concern for the welfare of young people. Recent national studies that monitor drug use by youth in the United States indicate significant increases in illicit drug use. The Supreme Court has continued to uphold the constitutionality of drug testing athletes and other student groups because of its effectiveness in preventing, deterring, and detecting drug use.[7]

Athletic performance-enhancing substances and their associated dangers are a matter of public concern today. The use of dietary supplements by athletes looking for any competitive edge is commonplace. A 2001 NCAA student-athlete, drug-use survey indicated an increased use of ephedrine.[15] Of the respondents who indicated ephedrine use, 50% indicated intent to improve performance as the reason for use. Anecdotal reports of athletes using large quantities of pseudoephedrine, phentermine, nicotine, and caffeine to enhance performance are supported by positive drug tests at the 1999 Pan American Games and by police actions involving prominent athletes.[13,15] Organizations worldwide are constantly being challenged to develop solutions for the doping epidemic in sport. Regardless of the substance chosen in attempting to gain the competitive edge, this historical perspective demonstrates the ongoing need to confront the very fabric of the unethical and dangerous practice of using drugs in sport today.

SPORTS ORGANIZATIONS AND DRUG TESTING

Antidoping initiatives in sport are as varied and diverse as the organizations governing them. From international federations and national governing bodies to local school boards and private schools, organizations are attempting to deter drug use in sport. Although the list of banned drugs may vary, the mission is generally the same—to deter the use of drugs by athletes. There are international efforts underway to harmonize antidoping programs in an attempt to increase the effectiveness of drug detection. The United States emphasizes those same goals through its international consortium of athletic organizations and through independent amateur and professional sports groups within this country. The policies differ depending on the organization, and sometimes athletes must comply with multiple antidoping programs as they compete in more than one sports organization. It is important to be aware of the multitude of athletic organizations and their respective antidoping policies.

The IOC is an international, nongovernmental, nonprofit organization and creator of the Olympic Movement. It is an umbrella organization with primary responsibility for supervising the summer and winter Olympic Games. Over time, the IOC has designated many commissions and associations to guide it in its daily activities. The IOC Medical Commission was established to address the increasing problem of doping in sport. The three fundamental principals of the IOC Medical Commission are to protect the health of athletes, promote respect for both medical and sport ethics, and encourage equality for all competing athletes. For >40 years, the IOC Medical Commission has worked in the antidoping field by establishing the Olympic Movement Anti-Doping Code, which is applicable to all constituents of the Olympic Movement. One of the Anti-Doping Code's fundamental objectives is to eliminate doping in sport. The Code applies to the Olympic Games, various championships, and all competitions to which the IOC grants its patronage or support and has provisions that enable appeals to be lodged with the Court of Arbitration for Sport (CAS).[16]

The role of the testing organization is critical and complicated. At Olympic competition, the IOC rules are clear, but they only apply at Olympic Games. Otherwise, each international federation or national governing body sets the rules.[17]

Under the umbrella of the IOC are the National Olympic Committees (NOCs). NOCs serve to disseminate the fundamental principles of Olympic sport at the national level. Representatives from NOCs meet at least once every 2 years to exchange information and experiences to consolidate their role within the Olympic Movement. Recommendations from these meetings are intended to foster Olympic solidarity, including antidoping initiatives.[18]

Also under the IOC umbrella are the International Athletic Federations (IAFs). These nongovernmental organizations serve to administer one or more sports at the world level and are responsible for the integrity of their sport. While maintaining their independence and autonomy in the administration of their sports, IAFs seeking IOC recognition must ensure that their statutes, practice, and activities conform to the Olympic Charter. The IAFs administer antidoping programs under the statutes of the IOC Medical Code.[19]

Individual sports governing bodies demonstrate great variation in their response to positive drug tests; some are very sophisticated with clear rules whereas others have minimal expertise and confusing rules.[17] IAFs are not democracies, but obtain authority from sovereign states that are members of the federations. International Athletic Federations base policies and structures on the perceived value to the sport, not on the interest of any of the nations that contribute to these federations. The IAFs and IOC act as virtual sovereigns within the area of athletics.[20]

The IOC also works with a variety of Olympic Movement Partners. The CAS is one such partner. It was developed to deal with legal problems faced by athletes. The purpose of the CAS is to resolve sports-related disputes submitted through ordinary arbitration or through appeal against the decisions of sports bodies or organizations, including appeals from athletes who test positive for an IOC-banned substance.[21,22]

Another recent partner to the Olympic Movement is the World Anti-Doping Agency (WADA). In response to the continued phenomenon of doping in sport, the IOC organized a World Conference on Doping in Sport in 1999, which resulted in the establishment of WADA.[21] The newly formed association is an independent body that coordinates antidoping enforcement for the Olympics and other international competitions.[23] The WADA's mission is the promotion and coordination of activities against doping in sport worldwide. The international sports world anticipates WADA to intensify efforts to banish drugs from sport. The purposes of WADA and the subsequent Anti-Doping Code are to protect athletes' fundamental rights to participate in doping-free sport, ensuring fairness and equality for athletes worldwide and to ensure harmonized and effective antidoping programs at the international and national level with regard to detection, deterrence, and prevention of doping. The WADA Foundation Board is composed of representatives of the Olympic Movement (IOC, NOCs, IFAs, and athletes).[24]

Antidoping efforts within the United States involve broader interests by including the national branches of the Olympic Movement. The USOC is one of 199 National Olympic Committees worldwide (www.usoc.org). The USOC was established by the Amateur Sports Act in 1978 and was the first sports organization to conduct drug testing in the United States beginning in 1984.[17] In 2000, the USOC outsourced its antidoping operations to the United States Antidoping Agency (USADA) giving it full authority for testing, education, research, and adjudication for United States, Olympic, Pan Am Games, and Paralympic Games. The USADA's responsibility is to develop a comprehensive national antidoping program for the Olympic Movement in the United States (www.usaantidoping.org).

The NFL and the National Football League Players Association (NFLPA) have maintained policies and programs regarding substance abuse for a number of years.[25] In the mid-1980s, the NFL began testing for illicit drugs and anabolic steroids with the primary purpose of assisting players who misuse substances of abuse. However, players who do not comply with the requirements of the drug testing policy are subject to discipline. The league performs random drug testing of its players year-round and bases its drug testing program on the premise that substance abuse can lead to on-the-field injuries, alienation of the fans, diminished job performance, and personal hardship. Both the NFL and NFLPA are committed to deterring and detecting substance abuse and to offering programs of intervention, rehabilitation, and support to players who have substance abuse problems. An important principle of this drug testing policy is that a player will be held responsible for whatever goes into his body.[25]

In addition to the organization's substances of abuse policy, the NFL prohibits players from using anabolic steroids (including exogenous testosterone), human or animal growth hormones, whether natural or synthetic, and related or similar substances. The NFL believes these substances have no legitimate place in professional football and threaten the fairness and integrity of competition. The NFL bans performance-enhancing agents because it is concerned about the adverse health effects of steroid use, and steroid use by players sends the wrong message to young people. High school and college students use steroids with alarming frequency, and NFL players should not by their own conduct suggest that such use is either acceptable or safe.[25]

Other professional sports organizations struggle to provide the quality of antidoping initiatives seen by the NFL. Professional sports organizations are often divided on drug testing issues because of the various subgroups involved (eg, players unions, owners). Following drug-use disclosures by former players, Major League Baseball and the Major League Baseball Players'

Association have negotiated plans to implement unannounced, reasonable cause drug testing; however, players and owners must agree on the exact process and upon implementation display a commitment to deterring drug use by players in the sport of baseball. Professional athletes, like it or not, are role models for young athletes today. Allowing or endorsing dangerous supplements and drugs sends the wrong message—"drug use is not only permissible, but desirable if an individual wants to perform at his or her best."[26]

The NCAA is a nonprofit athletic association comprised of approximately 1200 colleges and universities, athletic conferences, and sports organizations. Membership is voluntary. NCAA member schools strive to maintain intercollegiate athletics as an integral part of the educational program and its athletes as an integral part of the student body. Among the NCAA's goals is the protection of student-athletes through standards of fairness and integrity. The NCAA Committee on Competitive Safeguards and Medical Aspects of Sports (CSMAS) provides the NCAA with leadership and expertise on student-athlete health and safety issues. The CSMAS provides oversight for NCAA's drug education and drug testing programs, making recommendations on drug testing policies, procedures, and banned substances.[27] In addition, the Drug Education and Drug Testing Subcommittee of the CSMAS adjudicates appeals from institutions and student-athletes related to positive drug tests. The NCAA out-sources its drug testing program to The National Center for Drug Free Sport (Drug Free Sport). Drug Free Sport administers the NCAA in-competition and out-of-competition drug testing programs (www.drugfreesport.com).

The NCAA's drug testing programs were created to protect the health and safety of student-athletes and to ensure that no one participant might have an artificially induced advantage or be pressured to use chemical substances. The program involves urine collection on specific occasions and laboratory analysis of substances listed on the NCAA's banned drug classes list. The list, which was developed by the NCAA Executive Committee, consists of substances generally purported to be performance enhancing and/or potentially harmful to the health and safety of student-athletes. The drug classes specifically include stimulants and anabolic steroids, as well as street drugs. Under the direction of the CSMAS, the NCAA surveys student-athletes at all member institutions every 4 years regarding substance use and abuse habits. The committee uses this information and other scientifically researched data to maintain a sound drug testing program that accurately addresses drug use concerns among its student-athletes.

The NCAA encourages, but does not require, its member institutions to provide in-house drug testing programs independent of the NCAA's program. Of Division I-A institutions recently surveyed, 93% reported operating independent drug testing programs for their student-athletes.[28]

Since the early 1990s, high school administrators have been attempting to address the alarming increase in drug use by children and adolescents by implementing random drug testing programs. National drug use studies indicate substance abuse contributes to thousands of deaths annually, having an economic impact in the billions of dollars. Half of the nation's youth use illegal drugs before completing high school.[29] Due to Constitutional restraints, public schools cannot require the general student body to participate in random testing because it is an unreasonable invasion of one's privacy. However, landmark Supreme Court decisions now permit schools to randomly drug test participants in athletics and other extracurricular activities. Currently, about 5% of middle and high schools in the United States administer athlete drug testing programs; another 2% include testing for students involved in extracurricular activities.[30] With courts deciding that drug testing of athletes is constitutional, school boards nationwide are implementing drug testing programs because of legitimate concerns in preventing, deterring, and detecting drug use by high school students. The national problem of adolescent substance abuse is compelling enough to justify random drug testing of America's youth, at least for those participating in sport and extracurricular activities.

In the United States, many sports organizations' drug testing programs have been compared to workplace drug testing implemented during the 1980s by the Substance Abuse and Mental Health Services Administration (formally the National Institute on Drug Abuse) of the US government. Although the two programs have some similarities, the purpose and implementation of the programs are different. For example, the Substance Abuse and Mental Health Services Administration (SAMHSA) Five Drugs of Abuse drug testing panel has not changed in content since the inception of the program. Administrative cut-off concentrations or detection levels have been imposed for each of the five analytes for the purpose of identifying individuals who have a drug abuse problem that affects the work environment. In contrast, the number of compounds included on a full sports drug testing panel exceeds 125 with an average of five compounds added each year. Sports drug testing programs involve testing at both competitive events and during out-of-competition times to assess drug use at the time that the drug is most beneficial to performance. For example, anabolic steroids may be beneficial in off-season or pre-season training whereas a β-blocker would be more beneficial during competition.[13] In reality, workplace drug testing addresses concerns about safety and productivity in the workplace and must confront societal drug use trends. Sports organizations choose to address performance-enhancing substances, but also include testing for drugs athletes may use that are dangerous to their health although nonenhancing.

Regardless of the organization and its antidoping policies and procedures, due to their competitive nature, athletes will continue to search for substances or methods to enhance performance whether legal or not, whether safe or not. Although diverse and broad, organizations must continually focus on antidoping in sport. Former IOC President Juan Antonio Samaranch was quoted as he relinquished his position, "In doping, the war is never won."[23] A listing of sports drug testing organizations and appropriate contact information is found in Table 14-1.

LEGAL CONSIDERATIONS

Courts are frequently called upon to decide issues involving competing interests that are both fundamental and important to society. Drug testing is certainly an issue involving two competing fundamental interests and one that has been argued in the legal system numerous times.[31] In amateur sports, drug testing has raised many legal issues, including concerns about an athlete's constitutional right to due process, equal protection, and privacy, as well as protection against illegal search and seizure and self-incrimination.[32] Although the legal implications of sports drug testing vary from jurisdiction to jurisdiction, case law historically supports the reasonableness of drug testing athletes. It is important to understand the protections guaranteed by the Constitution of the United States when developing and implementing a sports drug testing program.[33] In addition, it is prudent for administrators of such programs to be familiar with case law relevant to drug testing in sport.

One of the first legal principles to consider is "state action." If an athlete is attempting to invoke constitutional law protection in a drug testing challenge, he or she must be able to prove the school, association, or other amateur governing body is a state actor. The organization administering drug testing must be shown to be part of the federal government, state government, or an agency of state government. As a general rule, public colleges and universities are state actors, as are public high schools. Private organizations, such as the NCAA, are not subject to constitutional challenges.[34] In Barbay v. NCAA (1987), a Louisiana State University football player tested positive for steroids as part of the NCAA drug testing program. He sought to pre-

Table 14-1. Organization Contact Information

Organization	Contact Information	Mission
World Anti-Doping Agency (WADA)	Stock Exchange Tower 800 Place Victoria (Suite 1700) PO Box 120 Montreal (Quebec) H4Z 1B7 Canada Phone: (514) 904-9232 info@wada-ama.org	To promote and coordinate the fight against doping in sport in all forms at an international level. Coordinates with IOC, International Sports Federations, National Olympic Committees, and athletes.
International Olympic Committee (IOC)	Château de Vindy 1007 Lausanne Switzerland Phone: (41.21) 621 61 11	Olympic Movement Anti-Doping Code: http://multimedia.olympic.org/pdf/en_report_21.pdf.
United States Antidoping Agency (USADA)	2550 Tenderfoot Hill St Suite 200 Colorado Springs, CO 809-7346 Phone: (719) 785-2000 Drug Reference: 800/233-0393 drugreference@usantidoping.org	Dedicated to eliminating the practice of doping in sport and to preserving the well being of sport and ensuring the health of athletes through research initiatives and educational programs. Administers research, education and testing for USOC, Pan Am, and Paralympic Games.
National Collegiate Athletic Association (NCAA)	PO Box 6222 Indianapolis, IN 46206-6222 Phone: (317) 917-6222 www.ncaa.org *Programs administered by:* The National Center for Drug Free Sport 810 Baltimore Kansas City, MO 64105 (816) 474-8655 www.drugfreesport.com	To protect the health and safety of student-athletes and to ensure that no one participant has an artificially induced advantage or pressured to use chemical substances.

continued

Table 14-1. Organization Contact Information (continued)

Organization	Contact Information	Mission
International Athletic Foundation (IAAF)	Stade Louis II Avenue Prince Hereditaire de Monaco MC 98000 Monaco Phone: (377) 92 05 70 68 www.iaaf.org	To charitably assist the world governing body for track and field athletics through affiliation with national governing bodies in perpetuating the development and promotion of athletics worldwide. IAAF Procedural Guidelines for Doping Control: http://www.iaaf.org/newsfiles/9600.pdf.
National Football League (NFL) & National Football League Players Association (NFLPA)	NFL 280 Park Ave New York, NY 10017 www.nfl.com Phone: (212) 450-2000 NFLPA 2021 L St NW, Suite 600 Washington, DC 20036 Phone: (202) 463-2200 www.nflpa.org	NFL Anabolic Steroid Drug Testing Policy: http://www.nflpa.org/agents/main.asp?subPage=Steroid+Policy. NFL/NFLPA Substance Abuse Drug Testing Policy:http://news.findlaw.com/legalnews/sports/drugs/policy/football/index.html or http://www.nflpa.org/agents/main.asp?subPage=Drug+Policy.
National Basketball Association (NBA) & National Basketball Players Association (NBPA)	NBA 645 5th Ave #10 New York, NY 10022 Phone: (212) 826-7000 www.nba.com NBPA 2 Penn Plaza #2430 New York, NY 10121 Phone (212) 655-0880 http://www.nbpa.com	National Basketball Association (NBA) and National Basketball Players Association (NBPA) Anti-Drug Program: http://news.findlaw.com/legalnews/sports/drugs/policy/basketball/index.html#NBA.
Major League Baseball (MLB)	245 Park Ave, 31st Floor New York, NY 10167 Phone: (212) 931-7800 www.mlb.com	Major League Baseball Drug Policy and Prevention Program: http://news.findlaw.com/legalnews/sports/drugs/policy/baseball/index.html.

vent the NCAA from enforcing a penalty based on a violation of his Fourteenth Amendment right to due process. The Federal District Court of Louisiana held that the NCAA was not a state actor; thus the athlete had no constitutional claim against the NCAA. The State of Florida trial court reached a similar decision in <u>Mira v. NCAA</u> (1988).[32]

Athletes opposed to drug testing often times bring "due process" claims against their institutions or athletic organizations. Due process arguments in drug testing have included objecting to the consent forms that athletes are asked to read and sign as a condition of athletic eligibility, not being afforded an adequate hearing following a positive drug test, or an unreasonable penalty based on an unreliable test. Under the due process clause of the Fourteenth Amendment, the athlete must show he or she was deprived of a significant liberty or property interest before due process requirements are applied. Case precedent generally finds that athletes have neither liberty nor property interest in athletics.[32] As a result, the general requirement of notice and a hearing need not be met. Due process was challenged in <u>Bally v. Northeastern University and NCAA</u> (1989). The Superior Court of Massachusetts ruled that the NCAA consent form did not infringe upon any due process rights. The case was dismissed.[32]

Athletes also have argued, albeit unsuccessfully, that they are being discriminated against and will use an equal protection argument as their legal defense. Institutions or organizations are precluded from discriminating against any one group, such as requiring athletes to submit to drug testing, unless the institution or organization establishes a rational basis justifying such.[32] Often, the rational basis for drug testing is stated in the very purpose of the program—to protect the health and safety of the participants from the increased risks associated with drug use, to uphold the integrity of sport, and to prevent or deter use.

The unreasonable invasion of privacy has been a concern in drug testing programs as well. Courts have heard several arguments related to excessive or unjustified intrusion that drug testing causes. Does a college or school infringe upon an athlete's constitutional right to privacy to obtain a biological specimen for drug analysis? In the area of invasion of privacy, many courts have held that athletes have a diminished expectation of privacy. Courts generally site physical examinations and athletes disrobing in front of one another in locker rooms as examples of the lower expectation of privacy.[32] One of the most prominent cases challenging drug testing as an unconstitutional invasion of privacy was <u>Hill v. NCAA</u> (1993). In 1987, a Stanford University diver challenged a requirement that she submit to drug testing to participate in NCAA diving championships. A California Superior Court granted an injunction barring the NCAA from testing her at the competition. The suit alleged an unreasonable invasion of privacy under the state constitution. A trial court found the NCAA program to be an unconstitutional invasion of privacy. The NCAA appealed, and in 1994, the California Supreme Court reversed the lower court decision reasoning that student-athletes had diminished expectations of privacy. Additionally, the court found the NCAA's performance-enhancing drug testing program was beneficial because it allowed them to concentrate on competition without worrying about losing a competitive edge.[33]

High school drug testing programs also have been challenged as an unreasonable search and seizure under the Fourteenth Amendment. The Fourth Amendment of the United States Constitution provides for people to be secure in their persons, houses, papers, and effects against unreasonable searches and seizures. Before requiring athletes to provide biological specimens for drug analysis, the drug test must be deemed "reasonable."[32] In <u>Schaill v. Tippecanoe</u> (1988), the Seventh Circuit Court of Appeals held that a drug testing program was not an unreasonable search and seizure if it did not require observation of the student-athlete during specimen collection. Monitored specimen collections are considered less intrusive than observed collections but are not as effective in deterring manipulation or substitution of donated specimens. In <u>O'Halloran v. University of Washington and NCAA</u> (1988), O'Halloran claimed the drug testing process was an unreasonable invasion of privacy and unreasonable search and seizure. The Ninth Circuit Court held that the interests of the university and the NCAA were compelling and outweighed the hardships placed on the student-athlete. The court ruled in favor of the university, upholding that the drug testing program was constitutional. However, in 1993, the Colorado Supreme Court ruled differently. In Derdeyn v. University of Colorado (1993), the Colorado Supreme Court found the university's drug

> *The Fourteenth Amendment of the US Constitution prevents any state from depriving any person of life, liberty, or property without due process of law, nor deny any person equal protection of the law. The Fourth Amendment of the US Constitution protects any person from unreasonable searches and seizures without warrant of probable cause.*

testing program to be unconstitutional because observed specimen collections were an unreasonable search and seizure and that the consent form signed by its student-athletes was not voluntary. The Colorado court found that although promoting fair competition had value, it did not rise to a level of compelling government interest as required by the Constitution.[35]

Acton v. Vernonia (1994) and Pottawatomie County v. Earls (2002) are two landmark United States Supreme Court cases supporting suspicionless random drug testing of high school student-athletes and other students involved in school-related extracurricular activities. Both Vernonia and Earls allege Fourth Amendment and due process violations.

In Acton v. Vernonia, a seventh grader intended to participate in grade school football. He was not allowed to participate because his parents refused to sign the district's drug testing consent form, which was a condition of his eligibility. The United States Supreme Court ruled in favor of Vernonia School District recognizing an exception to the Fourth Amendment's search and seizure requirement in cases where a special need exists. The Court balanced the students' privacy rights against the school's interest in providing a safe athletic environment for all participants and found the search for potential drug use through urine specimen collection was reasonable.[36]

In Pottawatomie County v. Earls, students involved in extracurricular activities including athletics, in the Tecumseh, Oklahoma School District were required to consent to urinalysis testing for drugs. Parents of the students brought suit against the school district citing violation of the Fourth Amendment. The Court held the school district's drug testing policy to be a reasonable means of preventing and deterring drug use among school children and did not violate the Fourth Amendment. The health and safety risks identified in the Vernonia case were found to apply with equal force to the Tecumseh school district.[37]

Although courts have upheld sports drug testing to be constitutional, any institution or athletic organization developing a drug testing program must involve its legal counsel throughout the development process to draft policy and advise on laws specific to the organization's jurisdiction.

The law as it applies to drug testing is still evolving. Courts are still struggling with how to balance the interests of society against the privacy rights of individuals.[38] Athletes have legally challenged drug testing procedures on various constitutional grounds. In response to those challenges, the courts have consistently upheld legally sound programs.[38]

COMPONENTS OF A DRUG TESTING PROGRAM

The primary components of a drug testing program include a detailed written policy, educational opportunities for athletes, drug testing procedures, and consequences for positive drug tests—including a consistent adjudication process and provisions for substance use and abuse treatment for athletes. The ultimate goal of any drug testing program is to influence change in human behavior. To create change in behavior, all of the above components must be carefully observed and practiced.[39]

Policy

Before any type of drug testing can occur, a specific written policy must be developed, distributed to all participants, and publicized. Sports drug testing policies must include:

- A clear explanation of the purposes for the drug testing program
- A description of who will be tested and by what methods
- The banned drug list
- A description of the types of testing athletes will be subjected to
- The consequences for positive drug tests
- A description of the appeal process

Organizations should also include a process for addressing substance abuse by providing a systematic approach for athlete treatment and rehabilitation. All athletes must be provided with these policies in advance of implementing a drug testing program. Athletes must provide written consent to the administering organization indicating that he or she has received, read, and agrees to the policy as it applies to participation within the organization.[40] The very foundation of any drug testing program is the document that states the program's goals, regulations, and procedures.[39] Written drug testing policies should be carefully developed, reviewed, and when necessary, edited on an annual basis.

Purpose

The purpose of drug testing must be clearly explained in the introduction of any adopted policy. These purposes are generally considered benefits, and the benefits of drug testing athletes are many and varied. Opponents of drug testing will argue vehemently against these benefits, thus any individual or group appointed to the task of developing a drug testing program should consider opponents' views when tackling this issue. Opposing arguments include the idea that drug testing sends mixed messages, violates a person's rights, is viewed as a punitive measure, can be divisive, and is costly.[41]

Drug testing in athletics is basically intended to check for substances that could either provide an unfair advantage over those not using them or contribute to problems in the individual's life, including impaired athletic performance.[41] The misuse of drugs and other substances in the world of sport has been recognized as a significant problem for >30 years, with the two major concerns being ethics and health. These concerns are not independent of one another. Misuse of performance-enhancing drugs in sport is a health risk given the types of drugs abused, the large doses usually taken, and the stress that is already present in the body under competitive conditions. The all-encompassing purpose of drug testing in sport is to promote fair and equitable competition while protecting the health and safety of athletes. By subjecting athletes to drug testing, no one participant will have an artificially induced advantage, will be pressured to use chemical substances in attempting to remain competitive, and will not be exposed to the health risks associated with using potentially dangerous drugs and other substances.[42] The goals of all drug testing programs should be to deter the use of banned substances, identify individuals who have substance abuse problems, and provide access to treatment for such problems.[39]

In addition to ethical and health reasons for drug testing, organizations may also include detecting drug use, enforcing banned drug lists, punishing those found to be using banned substances, and deterring drug dependency as additional purposes for drug testing. Other reasons include protecting athletes from injury, enhancing the role model perceptions of athletes, and minimizing criminality. Properly conceived and implemented, a drug testing program can also serve as an educational vehicle.[7]

Because athletes are usually healthy individuals, signs and symptoms of drug use may not be apparent upon observation, even to the trained eye. Drug testing provides a very definitive method of detecting use of controlled or illegal substances. In addition, the threat of a positive drug test and the resulting consequences may deter or prevent athletes from using these substances.[41,43] This deterrent effect has perhaps been the most important contribution of drug testing to societal well-being. Testing and fear of detection forces a person to make the affirmative decision not to use drugs in an uncontrolled or illegal manner.[44] Results from the 2001 NCAA student-athlete drug use survey indicated >50% of the participants agreed that drug testing has a strong deterrent effect.[15] Of course, the deterrent effect is only present if policies are consistently enforced. The only thing worse than not drug testing is having a drug testing program and not enforcing it.

Banned Substances

Any sports organization adopting a drug testing program must develop a list of drugs for which athletes will be tested. In sport, there are two areas of drug use that must be deterred, performance-enhancing substances and other illicit drugs found to be detrimental to the health and well being of athletes. Performance-enhancing substances (see Chapter 13) are banned because of their coercive nature and their potential adverse effects. Anabolic agents (eg, anabolic steroids, testosterone, and growth hormone), stimulants, oxygenation enhancers, and certain relaxants are considered to be types of performance-enhancing substances and/or procedures that should be banned by any sports drug testing program.[39] Timing and purpose of performance-enhancing substances should be considered to effectively deter use through drug testing. For example, drug testing during competition may not adequately identify users of anabolic agents. These substances are more likely to be used during out-of-competition training for their long-term performance-enhancing goals, whereas stimulants are more likely to be used during competition to enhance performance on the day of an event. For this reason, athletes must be subjected to drug testing year-round for the total deterrent effect.

In addition to performance-enhancing substances, most athletic programs include testing for other drugs found to be potentially dangerous to an athlete's health. With national drug use studies indicating >4.5 million people over the age of 12 needing drug treatment, organizational drug testing programs would be negligent in the prevention of unacceptable drug use and addiction if they did not include testing for "drugs of abuse."[32] These drug categories include stimulants (eg, cocaine, methamphetamines, and Ecstasy), depressants (eg, marijuana, alcohol, and barbiturates), hallucinogens (eg, LSD and psilocybin mushrooms), and opiates (eg, morphine, codeine, and heroin).[39] Most athletic organizations choose to adopt an all-inclusive banned drug list providing the ability to test for any drug deemed performance-enhancing and/or dangerous to the health of its athletes. Banned drug lists should be included in any drug testing policy, readily available to participants, and updated regularly to adequately address drug use issues in sport. Banned drug lists are available from respective athletic organizations.

Testing Types and Methods

Organizations implementing drug testing programs must consider a number of logistical and technical issues that will ultimately define the types of testing and the methods used. These types and methods must be described in the drug testing policy. There are several types of testing available for sports drug testing with distinct reasons for each (Box 14-1). Random drug testing is the

Box 14-1. Types of Drug Testing

- Random testing
- Reasonable suspicion testing
- Preparticipation testing to identify at-risk athletes
- Follow-up testing on athletes with previous positive drug tests
- Monitoring of athletes following drug use interventions
- Precompetition drug testing
- Event testing

most popular type of testing used and is applied year-round to deter drug use and identify users.

Random drug testing involves maintaining a complete and accurate list of athletes and randomly selecting athletes for periodic drug testing. Effective random drug testing should be frequent, unpredictable, and unannounced. The random selection process should be completely objective, assuring nondiscriminatory identification of participating athletes to be tested. Athletes should be notified and required to report for testing at the designated collection site within preset parameters. Random testing is effective in deterring and identifying performance-enhancing drugs for training such as anabolic agents and "social/designer" drugs such as marijuana or Ecstasy. The notification of the athlete should be as short as logistically possible. The maximum time should be 24 hours prior to test time and the ideal would be testing immediately after being notified. Testing athletes should not interfere with academic schedules or practices.[39]

Reasonable suspicion testing provides organizations with another option for drug testing athletes. Organizations can selectively test an athlete based on specific objective facts and reasonable inferences drawn from those facts in light of documented experiences related to drug use. Reasonable suspicion testing must be based on physical symptoms or manifestations of being under the influence such as behavior or appearance consistent with prohibited use (eg, odor of alcohol); direct observation of prohibited use; a report of prohibited use from a reliable source; or evidence of use possession, sale, etc of prohibited drugs. An athlete notified of reasonable suspicion testing must immediately submit to a drug test.

Other types of drug testing to consider including in a sports drug testing program include preparticipation testing to identify at-risk athletes, follow-up testing on athletes with previous positive drug tests, monitoring of athletes following drug use interventions, and precompetition drug testing on athletes who have qualified for events where he or she will be subject to drug testing by other sports organizations. Sports organizations often perform event testing to ensure a level playing field for drugs taken on competition day. The NCAA and IOC perform event drug testing in an effort to deter performance-enhancing drug use and to identify users of such. Stimulants, relaxants, and oxygenation enhancers are classes of drugs athletes are tempted to use in an effort to enhance performance during a specific competitive time period.

Testing methods and procedures should also be described in the written drug testing policy. Specifically the type(s) of specimens to be used for testing should be identified as well as the collection protocol that will be followed in collecting specimens from athletes. Chain of custody procedures, laboratory procedures, and methods of specimen analysis must also be described in the policy.

Consequences

The drug testing policy should specifically describe the procedures for reporting results, including who receives results, who notifies the athletes, who the athlete is referred to for evaluation, who is granted knowledge of a positive drug test, and what disciplinary action is imposed for a positive drug test. Confidentiality is of primary concern when communicating a positive drug test. Once positive drug test results are reported, these results must be reviewed to determine if there is an acceptable explanation for the test result. A medical review of these results is essential prior to labeling an athlete

> *Chain of custody refers to the ability to completely document the handling of a specimen from the moment the donor provides a sample until it is completely processed by the laboratory and a result is reported.*

as testing positive under the program's policies. Once the result is deemed positive under the definition of the program policy, administrators must implement procedures for handling a positive drug test. Generally, the program director will meet with the athlete to discuss the nature and extent of drug use and to apply sanctions for policy violations as described. Sanctions for a positive drug test often include immediate suspension from sport participation until the athlete can be evaluated by medical and substance abuse specialists to determine the risks associated with physical exercise and prohibited drug use and a treatment plan for the athlete is implemented. Consequences for any refusal to comply with procedures or repeated positive drug test results must also be described in the written policy.

Appeal

All drug testing programs must include an opportunity for the athlete to appeal the decision and subsequent consequences associated with a positive drug test or noncompliance to procedures. The appeal process should include a designated committee made up of representatives from various relevant professions (eg, medicine, athletics) who meet to hear the athlete's reasons for testing positive. Technical experts, third-party administrators, and collectors may also serve as consultants to the committee when such matters are involved in the nature of the appeal. Unlike criminal litigation, civil cases require only that the preponderance of evidence support the finding of doping activity.[3] Following a hearing, the committee's decision will ultimately be accepted and any subsequent sanctions applied. The goal of effectively modifying behavior can only occur when the consequences are widely believed to impose accurate and even-handed results.[20]

Treatment

Following a positive drug test and subsequent evaluation by medical professionals regarding the nature and extent of drug use, an appropriate treatment plan must be implemented. At the very least, treatment should provide accurate and current information on the health hazards of drug abuse; help users overcome drug dependence; be directed based on age, interests, and special problems of athletes; emphasize immediate negative effects from drug use; and hold the athlete accountable for his or her actions.[9] Most athletes' evaluations following a positive test show a drug use problem, not dependency. Drug use is a behavioral problem, not a disease. These individuals respond well to counseling on decision-making and instruction on the potential hazards of drug use. If dependency or repetitive drug use occurs, more intensive treatment is indicated.[39] Appropriate substance abuse professionals must supervise any treatment or rehabilitation program.

Before any type of drug testing can be implemented, a detailed written policy must be adopted and presented to all participants. This policy must include purpose, banned drug list, testing

Box 14-2. Summary of Entities Involved in a Complete Drug Testing Program

- Donor (athlete)
- Drug testing administrator
- Third-party administrators
- Collectors
- Laboratories
- Medical review officer (results recipient)

methods, consequences, due process, and recommended treatment opportunities. Once policies and procedures are reviewed, participants must consent to drug testing as described and a signed consent form should remain on file throughout the effective date of the policy.

Participants

Developing, implementing, and administering an effective drug testing program involves a number of people with a variety of responsibilities. Early in the process when examining the need for program development, legal counsel should be recruited to review local, state, and federal statutes that apply. The legal aspects involved with each organization should be clarified. The development process should also involve representatives from various relevant academic departments and disciplines (eg, pharmacology, chemistry, and psychology), athletic administrators, athletes, athletic trainers, and medical doctors.[28] Ultimately, the administration of a complete drug prevention program will involve a number of entities (Box 14-2).

Donor (Athlete)

A donor is any person who is designated in the organization's drug testing policies as subject to drug and/or alcohol testing. As applied to sports drug testing, the term includes any athlete who is currently listed as a participant in sport within the organization. The term "donor" is a drug testing industry standard identifying the individual subjected to drug testing who is required to provide a biological specimen for analysis of drugs.[45] The donors in an institutional athletic drug testing program may include student-athletes, cheerleaders, managers, and athletic training students. Drug testing may also include all participants of competitive extracurricular programs (eg, club sports, debate, band). The organization's drug testing policies must identify and define all donors subject to drug testing. All donors must be provided with the drug testing policies, and administrators of the program should describe drug testing in detail. Once all donors have been provided accurate information about the program, each donor must read and sign a drug testing consent form, and if underage, parents of the donor must also sign the consent form prior to specimen collection and testing. Once a donor has consented to participating in the drug testing program, he or she will be expected to follow policies and procedures accordingly. Failures to abide by the policies usually have consequences similar to that of a positive drug test. These consequences should also be included in the written policy.

Drug Testing Administrator

Each organization with a drug testing policy should have an individual responsible for administering the program. Often, many people are involved in program administration, but one individual is identified as the program administrator. It is the drug testing administrator's responsibility to financially manage and oversee compliance with the entire program. Often this individual coordinates annual review and dissemination of policies to all participants, collects signed consent forms from donors, schedules required drug education programs and testing events for participants, and coordinates other individuals or entities with responsibilities related to drug testing. The drug testing administrator may have additional duties associated with actual drug testing and results handling. Athletic trainers are often responsible for administering sports drug testing programs, but sometimes find these responsibilities place them in conflict with athlete relationships, especially if duties include specimen collection and results handling. The program administrator can effectively oversee the entire drug testing program and maintain strong, trustworthy relationships with athletes by delegating or outsourcing specific components of program administration, including collections, results reporting, and applying sanctions.

Third-Party Administrators

Sports organizations have the option of contracting with outside agencies to provide or coordinate a variety of drug testing services. Third-party administrators offer organizations industry expertise and objectivity in administering drug testing programs and allow athletic organization personnel the ability to focus on day-to-day responsibilities associated with athletics management. Third-party administrators provide trained specimen collectors, laboratory discounts through consortium efforts, independently administered random selection services, and Medical Review Officer (MRO) expertise. When determining cost factors for considering outside agencies, organizations must include the value of time expended by the internal staff to perform these duties. In addition, using experts with extensive and detailed training further supports the effectiveness and ultimately the success of a drug testing program.

Collectors

The collection of biological specimens from selected donors (athletes) is crucial to the effectiveness of any drug testing program. The collector must be trusted to perform his or her job professionally and provide for privacy while ensuring integrity and security of the specimen throughout the entire collection process. Collectors must be knowledgeable in sports drug testing issues and maintain the skills necessary to perform specimen collections in a consistent manner. Collectors should be adequately trained and required to maintain proficiency in collection services according to industry standards and organizational diversity. Trained collectors eliminate costly and legally challenging chain of custody errors with regard to specimen handling and transfer to appropriate laboratories. In addition, collectors deter specimen *adulteration*, substitution, and manipulation attempts by donors at the collection site. Specimen adulteration is any attempt to change the outcome of an anticipated positive drug test by altering the biological specimen prior to analysis. Adulterated specimens significantly compromise drug testing programs by causing false negative results. If a drug testing program does not adequately deter specimen adulteration through on-site collection procedures, athletes will attempt to and successfully beat a drug test, ultimately creating a mockery of an organization's drug testing program.

Care should be taken when determining who will be responsible for the collection process if an organization elects to perform its own collections. For example, athletic trainers may be compromising their relationship with athletes by performing collections or other judicial processes in a drug testing program. Athletes often approach the athletic trainer in confidence when concerned about health issues, including drug use and may no longer trust or feel comfortable disclosing such issues if the athletic trainer performs these drug testing duties. In addition, if an organization chooses to use its own personnel because of budgetary constraints, it is important to consider the time costs this task imposes on already taxed employees.

Pharmacists are excellent candidates for drug testing collectors because they can develop and conduct drug testing protocols; educate athletes, coaches, and athletic trainers about drug use and abuse; and help ensure the safe and effective use of medications.[2] Other medical professionals such as nurses or medical technologists are also strong candidates. Third-party administrators and collection companies can also provide specimen collections. There are also unacceptable candidates for specimen collections. An athlete cannot serve as a collector for his or her own specimen; neither is it appropriate for athletic training students to perform collections. Employees of any participating laboratory should not perform specimen collections, and collectors of the opposite gender should not perform direct observation collections due to the sensitivity of the process and the increased risk of litigation based on an unreasonable invasion of privacy. If a same-sex validator cannot be provided, the test should either not be performed or a monitored collection should be used, depending on the organization's policy and procedures.

Laboratories

Credentialed laboratories are vital to the ultimate success of a drug deterrence program. Organizations must be confident that results generated by the laboratory are accurate and scientifically measured. There are a variety of credentialing entities responsible for certifying laboratories. Laboratory accreditation is an important criterion to consider when selecting a lab for specimen analysis. Accreditation and certification demonstrate reliability and quality assurance.[35] Before using a laboratory, the organization should request verification of the laboratory's standards of accreditation.

In 2004, the World Anti-Doping Agency (WADA) replaced the International Olympic Committee (IOC) as the official accrediting body for laboratories performing specimen analysis in sport. The World Anti-Doping Code International Standard for Laboratories outlines the specific requirements for WADA's accreditation process. Requirements include providing an official letter of support from the relevant national public authority responsible for the national anti-doping program, signing and complying with WADA's Code of Ethics, proficiency testing of samples, sharing of knowledge with other accredited laboratories and a strong commitment to research. Goals of the WADA accreditation program include promoting scientific excellence, harmonization of methodology, reliable scientific information and fostering good will and cooperation. WADA's Code of Ethics forbids testing samples unless they are from a bona fide sports program. Thus, WADA accredited laboratories are prohibited from testing to aid or abet athletes attempting to learn how to evade detection of drug use.[46]

Laboratories engaged in urine drug testing for federal agencies must be SAMHSA certified. This certification sets strict standards that laboratories must meet to conduct urine drug testing for federal agencies. To become certified, an applicant laboratory must undergo three rounds of performance testing plus on-site inspection. To maintain certification, a laboratory must participate in a quarterly performance testing program and periodic on-site inspections.[47]

Medical Review Officer (Results Recipient)

In workplace drug testing programs, a Medical Review Officer (MRO) is used to review positive drug test results to determine if there is a legitimate reason for the positive result. The MRO is defined in federal regulations as a licensed physician with a working knowledge of substance abuse disorders who has appropriate medical training to interpret and evaluate positive drug test results.[44] In sports drug testing programs, the team physician is often designated to receive positive drug test results to review for possible legitimate medical reasons contributing to the confirmed positive result. Results should be handled as part of an athlete's medical record and protected from disclosure by the laws protecting confidentiality of medical documents. Regardless

Box 14-3. Available Specimen Types for Drug Testing

- Urine
- Blood
- Oral fluid
- Hair
- Sweat

of the individual designated to receive results, the process must be administered with the utmost confidentiality. It is important for the laboratory to be "blind" with respect to the donor's identity, thus laboratory personnel cannot serve as review officers for their own work.[13] Laboratories are capable of providing results to the designated individual via a number of secure methods, such as certified mail, secure facsimile, or secure Internet access. The recipient of the results must maintain these confidential records, assure adequate medical review of positive results, and present the verified positive results to the individual responsible for meeting with the athlete and other designated parties to disclose the result, apply consequences, facilitate the appeal process if requested, and/or refer for necessary counseling and/or treatment.

There are a number of responsibilities involved in administering a sound sports drug testing program. A team of individuals generally completes these tasks, but the program administrator should play a leadership role in coordinating all aspects of drug testing.

Methodology

Before administering a sports drug testing program, an organization should review industry-adopted procedures and scientific methodologies currently being practiced. Often there are options available and the organization should select those options that best meet its needs in addressing drug use in sport. From the specimen type that will be analyzed to the actual method of analysis, these decisions must be made based on current and accurate information.

Specimen Types

Because of many advances in analytical technology, drugs and their metabolites can be detected in a variety of tissues and biological fluids. Chemical testing of biological fluids is the most objective means of diagnosis of drug use.[48,49] A wide variety of specimens are available today, each providing valuable information concerning prior and current drug use[50] (Box 14-3). The standard for drug testing in toxicology is the immunoassay screen, a quick method of determining the presence or absence of a drug or metabolite in a urine specimen. A positive screen is followed by confirmation using gas chromatography with mass spectrometric detection (GC/MS), a very specialized procedure that specifically identifies the metabolite qualitatively. Although initial research in alternative specimen testing used radioimmunoassay, newer nonisotopic commercial immunoassays are now widely available for screening of drugs and drug metabolites. *Enzyme-linked immunosorbent assay* (ELISA), a specific type of immunoassay screening, has been adapted for detection of analytes in extracts/digests of hair, oral fluid, and sweat patches. ELISAs are semiquantitative, cost-effective, highly sensitive, and especially applicable to alternative specimens because of their increased specificity to parent drugs such as cocaine, rather than drug metabolites such as benzoylecgonine, a major metabolite of cocaine. The selection of a specific biological specimen for drug analysis is influenced by a variety of factors, principally ease of spec-

Box 14-4. Identified Problems With Urine Testing

- A limited window of detection due to drug excretion in urine.
- The inability to correlate the concentration of drug in the urine with the effects on performance.
- The adulteration of specimen by donors.
- The occurrence of privacy issues.

imen collection, analytical and testing considerations, and interpretation of results. Interest has shifted from urine toward other specimens that can provide distinct advantages. The introduction of several laboratory-based drug test systems and on-site devices has expanded drug testing capabilities.[50] Today there are a number of specimens other than urine, such as saliva, sweat, meconium, or hair, demonstrating viable biological options for drug detection.[48-50]

Urine

Since the 1970s, urine has been the most common biological specimen used in detecting drugs of abuse. Although other biological matrices are now available for drug testing, urine continues to be the specimen of choice. The collection of urine in noninvasive and large volumes can be collected easily. Drugs and their metabolites are generally present in higher concentrations in urine than in other matrices because of the concentrating function of the kidneys. Urine is easier to analyze than other biological specimens because of less protein, and cellular constituents and drugs (and their metabolites) are usually stable in frozen urine, which allows for long-term storage of positive samples.[9] Although widely used, problems with urine testing have been identified (Box 14-4). Regardless of its limitations or the complications it imposes, urine remains the specimen standard in sports drug testing. Laboratories have extensive scientific basis for the testing methodology and scientists have developed extremely sophisticated instruments and procedures using urine specimens to effectively detect many of the more common substances currently being abused by athletes.

Blood

Compared to urine, the use of blood or plasma provides better correlations between the concentrations of the drug and its effects on performance. However, the use of blood as a specimen for analysis of drugs presents several limitations, including religious beliefs. It is an invasive technique requiring technical proficiency in collecting from the donor, analyses are expensive and more complex, specimens are smaller and drugs (and their metabolites) are found at significantly lower concentrations than in urine.[9] Because of the invasiveness of collecting a blood sample and the inherent risks associated with such, athletic organizations are not likely to use blood as a matrix for sports drug testing except on rare occasions.

Oral Fluid

Saliva, or the preferred term, oral fluid, was originally introduced to monitor therapeutic drugs and for insurance testing; however, it has been increasingly used as an analytic tool in the detection of environmental chemicals, illicit drugs, and many *endogenous* substances.[49,50] Saliva is the fluid secretion of the salivary glands, whereas oral fluid contains saliva, mucosal transudate, and crevicular fluid.[49] Advantages of oral fluid over other traditional fluids are the collection is almost noninvasive, is relatively easy to perform, and, in forensic situations, can be achieved under close supervision to prevent *adulteration* or substitution of samples.[49] It seems the concentrations of many drugs in oral fluid correlate well with blood concentrations, which suggest that quantitative measurements in oral fluid may be a valuable technique to determine the current degree of exposure to a definite drug at the time of sampling.[48] Caution must be taken when collecting oral fluid samples. Substances containing citric acid (eg, citrus fruits, fruit juices, and certain candies) cause an over stimulation of saliva and can skew concentration levels of certain substances. In addition, certain oral fluid collecting devices produce significantly different concentrations of marijuana after recent use. Devices placed between the gum and cheek for oral fluid collection demonstrated much higher concentrations of tetrahydrocannabinol (THC) than those with collecting procedures requiring the donor to spit oral fluid into a collection device.[48]

Perhaps the most effective use of oral fluid screening is the measurement of ethanol in saliva. Ethanol is a small molecule, is highly water-soluble, and is not bound to plasma protein. Because of these characteristics, plus the rich blood flow to the oral cavity, the concentration of alcohol in the saliva should reflect the concentration in arterial blood.

Currently on-site or point-of-collection oral fluid testing devices are not considered reliable, and screening sensitivity inconsistencies exist. Laboratory-based oral fluid testing services provide a potentially viable alternative to urine testing on certain drugs. Screening is performed with an instrumental laboratory enzyme immunoassay providing less interference from *endogenous* compounds than when using blood or urine samples. This technique allows for the detection of cocaine, methamphetamine, morphine, cannabinoids, and PCP. Because of the smaller sample volume of oral fluid, confirmed quantitative analytic procedures using MS in the chemical ionization mode, liquid chromatography (LC)-MS, and tandem MS–MS confirmation are being developed.[49] Overall, oral fluid testing demonstrates promise in detecting drugs of abuse, but science does not currently exist to support using oral fluid specimens for analyzing many of the drugs and substances listed as banned by many sports organizations.

Hair

Hair testing was originally used for metal detection and nutritional evaluation.[7] More recently, there are reported applications in forensic toxicology, clinical toxicology, occupational medicine, and doping control. The major practical advantage of hair for testing drugs, compared with urine and blood, is its larger detection window. The detection window is weeks to months, depending on the length of hair shaft analyzed. The average length of the hair sample to be tested should be 3.9 cm or 1.5 in, and because hair grows about 0.5 inch a month, the time period represents approximately 90 days. It is interesting to note that hair and urine testing are complementary of one another. Urine analysis provides short-term information on drug use, whereas long-term histories are accessible through hair analysis. The greatest use of hair testing may be in identifying a false-negative result from other biological specimen analysis. Urine does not indicate the frequency of drug use in subjects who might deliberately abstain for several days before screening. Hair analysis is a potentially fail-safe procedure in contrast to urine testing because an identical urine specimen cannot be obtained at a later date. However, there are still concerns about the qualitative results from hair due to the influences of external contamination or cosmetic treatment and results may vary due to race.[48,51]

To date, the scientific knowledge of hair biology in attempting to detect performance-enhancing substances in sport is not available. Analytical methods do not exist for several doping compounds, such as diuretics. Peptide hormones are not extractable. Hair washing, discoloring, tinting, and hair color (resulting in potential ethnic differences) appear to influence drug concentrations in hair.[48,49] Scientists have been able to detect *endogenous* steroids in hair using GC/MS, and physiologic concentrations of both testosterone and dehydroepiandrosterone (DHEA) are distinguishable in hair between male and female subjects. Hair analysis can be used to identify the exact nature of the parent compound (eg, nandrolone, norandrostenediol, or norandrostenedione, in the case of a urine sample positive for norandrosterone), allowing discrimination between nandrolone abuse from OTC preparations containing 19-norsteroids. Although hair is not yet a valid specimen option for the IOC, courts in Europe, Japan, and the United States have accepted drug test results from hair analysis. Recently, some conflicting results have occurred in athletes who tested positive in urine samples submitted to accredited IOC laboratories, but negative in hair samples sent to certified forensic laboratories. Since 2001, hair analysis has been allowed in France to document doping practices.[48,49] Certainly the question to be asked in considering whether to use hair testing is whether the drug testing program's purpose is to detect or to deter.

Sweat

Using the sweat patch as a detection vehicle is fairly simple. The patch contains an absorbent pad sandwiched between the skin and an outer protective membrane. A tamper-evident adhesive backing on the membrane of the patch allows easy adherence to the donor's skin. The outer membrane allows vapors from the sweat to pass through it. Thus, the donor's sweat moistens the pad, the water in the sweat eventually evaporates through the membrane, and any drugs or metabolites found in the sweat remain in the absorbent pad. Once the sweat patch is removed, it is returned to the laboratory for analysis. The sweat patch has been successful in the criminal justice system due to its reliability. It is a rugged and tamper-evident device; however, questions exist regarding possible external environmental contamination through the sweat patch membrane.[52] Profuse sweating can contribute to the susceptibility of environmental contamination by allowing external influences, such as cocaine powder, to penetrate the membrane of the patch and contributes to the ineffectiveness of its use in sports drug testing.

The value of alternative specimen analysis for the identification of drug users appears to be steadily gaining recognition.[49] Adding state-of-the-art techniques such as LC–MS and MS–MS technology will enable forensic toxicologists to facilitate the use of these additional matrices. In the future, testing of alternative specimens will expand the ability to understand the patterns of drug use and will become routine in forensic toxicology.[50] Alternative specimens, such as hair, appear to provide potential in the analysis of anabolic agents. At the very least, alternative specimens may complement traditional urine testing to further document results (Table 14-2).

Banned Drugs

In sport, substances are prohibited or banned because of performance-enhancing properties and/or the potential health risks associated with their use. The most significant difference between workplace drug testing and sports drug testing is the list of prohibited drugs and levels of detection or "cut-offs" used for analysis. Workplace drug testing is designed to identify prospective or current workers who have a drug problem, particularly with any of the five illegal substances: amphetamines, cocaine, heroin, marijuana, and PCP.[3] The cut-off levels are the values chosen for the determination of a positive or negative in a drug screen and adopted in workplace testing to identify individuals with substance abuse problems. The SAMHSA levels are recommended as the most appropriate established and legally defensible standards for workplace drug testing and have been set to avoid false positives.[38,45] It is often argued that these cut-offs are too high to effectively identify many substance abusers. In contrast, the purpose of sports drug testing is to detect the presence of substances identified as banned by testing organizations. Most high schools, college, and universities that drug test athletes continue to include testing for illegal substances because of the potential health risks and legal implications associated with their use, but tend to use detection levels lower than the workplace model. The IOC, NFL, and NCAA have similar banned drug lists and most substances on these lists have no administrative

Table 14-2. Specimen Comparison Chart

Matrix: Comparable Factors	Lab Urinalysis (Industry Standard)	On Site Urinalysis	Oral Fluid	Hair	Sweat	Blood
Applicability	Used to detect all types of drug use.	Up to 9 drug panel.	Up to 9 drug panel, including alcohol typical 5 panel most common.	Wide variety of drugs detected.	Wide variety of drugs detected, including alcohol.	Drugs detectable, but not applicable.
Collection procedure	Procedurally strong and legally defensible. May be embarrassing or uncomfortable.	Similar to lab urinalysis. Do not need scientific personnel to determine result.	Foam absorption pad inserted in mouth for 2 minutes. Pad then pressed into reagent device for on-site result with package to send positive screen specimen to lab for confirm.	Cut 1.5" sample of hair from back of head along scalp, package, and send to lab for testing.	Use a sweat patch that is adhesively applied to skin and worn over days to weeks and then sent to lab for testing.	Collecting sample is invasive and high risk, use of needles requires highly-trained medical personnel.
Performance criteria	Extensive research. Controlled and accurate. Extensive quality control testing. Accurate cut-off levels.	Lacks quality control. Variation in cut-off concentrations. No performance testing done.	Limited proficiency testing has been done. Not widely used. Fair amount of scientific acceptability.	No proficiency testing programs exist. Scientifically acceptable, but controversy exists (interpretation does, time relationships).	No performance testing has been done.	Accepted and widely used in the scientific community for therapeutic drug monitoring and for postmortem assessments.
Government approval	Yes, considered standard and operating.	Some kits are FDA approved.	Not yet approved by FDA.	Some devices approved by FDA.	Patch is approved by FDA.	Yes, primarily for medical use.
Adulteration testing	Lab screening and on-site screening available	Not available unless sample is sent to lab for confirmation.	Not available.	Not available.	Not available.	Available at laboratory.
Sample adulteration or manipulation probability	Dilution is factor. Observed collection controls.	Dilution is factor. Observed collection controls.	None if collection procedure followed correctly.	Products sold that claim to "cleanse" hair of drugs.	Patch removal or contamination.	None.

cut-off concentrations or have cut-offs much lower than the SAMHSA levels in attempting to identify the presence of such drugs. Banned substances are determined by athletic organizations, published, and updated regularly. In general, the IOC, NCAA, and NFL prohibit classes of compounds rather than publishing a list of individual compounds. The lists include examples within each class to act as a guide and also to ensure that new drugs and designer substances are covered, and include the words "and related substances," to describe drugs that are related to the class by their pharmacologic actions and/or chemical structure.[53] Complete and current banned drug lists are available by contacting individual athletic organizations. (See Table 14-1 for organization contact information.)

The typical testing menu in sports drug testing encompasses five classes of prohibited compounds: stimulants, narcotic analgesics, diuretics, anabolic agents, and peptide hormones. There are restrictions in selected circumstances on a number of other substances including alcohol, marijuana, local anesthetics, corticosteroids, and β-blockers. Blood doping procedures and agents that could mask drug detection or manipulate urinary excretion are also prohibited.[3] A short description of the classes of drugs banned by most sports organizations follows.

Stimulants

Stimulants (see Chapter 13) have been used in sport for their performance-enhancing properties for over two centuries. The earliest performance-enhancing compounds were stimulants such as amphetamine, caffeine, cocaine, ephedrine, and strychnine. These compounds have been used to improve concentration, increase aggressiveness, and to relieve the perception of fatigue during competition.[3] As examples of *sympathomimetic* amines, amphetamines are believed to improve physical and mental performance while masking pain and fatigue. Physiological effects include increased respiratory rate, heart rate, blood pressure, and metabolism. Caffeine is a socially acceptable drug, but probably the most widely abused drug in the world. Caffeine is also widely used by athletes as a performance enhancer in training and competitions. It is considered restricted by many athletic organizations, and urinary levels >12 µg/mL constitute a positive drug test in sport.[54] Ephedrine is another stimulant classified as a *sympathomimetic* drug. It has been found to be an effective bronchodilator due to its stimulation of β_2-*receptors* in the lungs, but because ephedrine is nonselective for β_1- and β_2-*receptors* it caused unwanted adverse effects such as increased heart rate and blood pressure. There are documented cases of ephedrine-related deaths in sport and efforts are underway to restrict sales of this potentially dangerous compound, especially in OTC dietary supplements.[55]

Narcotic Analgesics

Narcotic analgesics (opioids) are included on banned drug lists because they potentially increase performance and because of the vulnerability of the athletes to serious injury as a result of the analgesia.[3] Prohibiting opioids is based more on their reputation and dangers when used as illegal drugs than their performance-enhancing potential. Narcotics are more likely to reduce performance than improve it.

Diuretics

Diuretics (see Chapter 12) are used to mask the presence of other substances by diluting or altering the pH of the urine. They are also used to achieve rapid weight loss through water excretion for sports such as wrestling or bodybuilding.

Anabolic Agents

Anabolic agents are used to achieve increases in muscle mass, strength, and speed; improve recovery from training; and increase mental aggressiveness.[3] Athletes choose to use both *endogenous* (testosterone, DHEA) or *exogenous* (eg, nandrolone, stanozolol, mesterolone) anabolic steroids because of claims that they increase lean body mass, increase strength, increase aggressiveness, and lead to a shorter recovery time between workouts.[48] Nandrolone, a very popular anabolic agent, is metabolized to norandrosterone and noretiocholanolone. Other 19-norsteroids, such as norandrostenedione or norandrostenediol, classified as anabolic androgenic steroids by the IOC, NFS, and NCAA, are available OTC or through the Internet. β_2-*agonists* are also banned by the IOC because of their *sympathomimetic* properties (stimulant effects) and their activity as anabolic agents in higher dosages.[49] There is a high risk of adverse effects associated with continuous use of anabolic agents especially in women and adolescents. Highly toxic effects on the liver, growth disorders in youth, and female fertility disorders are common adverse effects.

Peptide Hormones

Peptide hormones (see Chapter 13) are typically large polypeptides (eg, human growth hormone [hGH], insulin, insulin-like growth factor-1 [IGF-1]), but may also be glycosylated (human chorionic gonadotropin, erythropoietin [EPO]). Many of these are now readily available as pharmaceutical products produced through genetic manipulation. This class of compounds is relatively easy to detect in *immunoassay*, but the metabolism of the substances is rapid and the detection window of the parent molecules in blood is very short. The natural levels are often low, but in some cases, they are released in a manner that causes enormous variations in blood levels. These factors make it difficult to confirm presence of the substances.[3,53]

β-Blockers

The use of β-*blockers* (see Chapter 12) was first reported in the sport of rifle where the twitch caused by blood pumping from the heart was thought to be sufficient to adversely affect aim. Studies found a 13% improvement in shooting related to decreased hand tremor when β-blockers were used. Testing for β-blockers is limited to sports requiring fine motor skill, such as diving, shooting, or archery.[3] Golfers also may experience performance benefits through the use of β-blockers.

Other Prohibited Substances and Manipulators

Substances used for performance enhancement are generally divided into two types of compounds: those that function during competition and those that are used during training for enhancement or have a delayed effect on performance during competition. An example of a delayed onset performance enhancer would be the use of EPO during training to achieve better oxygen-carrying capacity after EPO has disappeared from the system[3] (see Chapter 13). In addition to banning performance-enhancing drugs, athletic organizations also prohibit pharmaceutical, chemical, and physical means of urine manipulation designed to avoid detection.

> *A T/E ratio is the comparison of the quantity of testosterone to the quantity of epitestosterone during specimen analysis in an attempt to determine whether testosterone has been administered exogenously. A T/E ratio >6:1 is considered positive by most sports organizations.*

Probenecid, for example, has been shown to effectively block the urinary excretion of steroid glucuronates. Additionally, because of attempted manipulation of epitestosterone in an effort to alter T/E ratios, epitestosterone levels >200 µg/L are considered an attempt to manipulate urine. Bromantan is another recent addition to banned drug lists. Although listed in the stimulant category, bromantan metabolites excreted in the urine can also interfere with detection of steroids.

Recent interest in dietary supplements containing DHEA, androstenedione, androstenediol, and norandrostenedione indicate a continued interest in performance enhancement with *endogenous* steroids. Androstenedione is the immediate metabolic precursor of testosterone and DHEA enters the steroid metabolic pathway before testosterone, increasing the concentrations of all steroids downstream. Either can result in an elevated T/E ratio. Norandrostenedione metabolizes into nandrolone, a banned anabolic agent.[3]

Organizations will amend banned drug lists as needed to address the use of new compounds and methods introduced in sport to artificially enhance performance. The term "related compounds" will be consistently found throughout these lists because it would be extremely difficult, if not impossible, to maintain a complete and accurate listing of substances in each of the banned categories. Related compounds include any substances similar to a drug class by pharmacological action or chemical structure. In addition, because dietary supplements are not strictly regulated, most athletic organizations warn athletes of the risk involved from using any product and encourage abstinence.

Sample Collection and Chain of Custody

Collecting biological specimens for sports drug testing is an important and integral part of a total drug testing program, yet poses a significant legal risk. Specimen collections carry a great deal of responsibility for the collector and he or she is not immune from legal liability. There is undue risk of having a poorly managed process. Negligent collection processes by employers who choose to perform collections in-house instead of outsourcing to a third-party have been challenged in the courts. In <u>Mission Petroleum Carriers v. Roy Solomon</u>, the Court of Appeals of Texas found Mission created a danger when it chose to use its own employees to collect urine specimens rather than use an outside industry source. Furthermore, the court found Mission did not properly train its employees in urine collections and the process was routinely mishandled.[55] By following industry-adopted standard operating procedures, specimen collection protocols specific to the client, and using trained collectors, liability can be almost completely managed, reduced, or eliminated. An organization's drug testing policies should specifically describe the specimen collection process or reference any adopted protocol from another drug testing entity. Often colleges or universities adopt the NCAA's specimen collection protocol as standard operating procedure. By implementing a procedure, many athletes are already familiar with the consistency of the process; this familiarity facilitates compliance. Other essentials for minimizing risk include assuring collector proficiency and good collection site management.

The collection site may be a temporary or permanent facility. Any facility may require special attention to ensure that it meets requirements. The term "collection site" refers to the entire facility used to collect the urine specimen (ie, the rest room or toilet stall and the work area used by the collector). In all cases, the collection site must allow for an adequate amount of privacy and respect for the athlete while providing the urine specimen. It is appropriate for the collection site to have a source of water for washing hands prior to and following a specimen collection. The source of water should be separate from the immediate area where urination occurs. The use of personal hygiene is acceptable after the specimen has been provided. The collection site must have a suitable clean surface for writing so that the collector and the athlete can complete the required paperwork. The collection site must prevent unauthorized access that could compromise the integrity of the collection process or the specimen. Unauthorized access includes not only unauthorized personnel but also any unauthorized access to collection materials or supplies. The collection site must not allow the athlete access to any items that could be used to dilute or adulterate the specimen. A representative from the sports organization should ensure the security of the room(s) during the actual time of specimen collection.

The specimen collection area should be fully equipped with male and/or female restrooms adjacent to the quiet waiting area. Access to a shower is helpful.

The specimen should remain under the direct control of the athlete and observed by the collector until it is enclosed in the sample vials. Once it is sealed for shipment, it should be immediately shipped, maintained in secure storage, or remain under the personal control of the collector until shipped. Although most athletes provide a specimen in <20 minutes, adequate time should be given for reservation of the facility in the event that testing takes longer than expected.

When athletes arrive for testing, the collector must positively identify the athlete. If the athlete cannot be positively identified, the collection should be discontinued. Acceptable methods of identification include photo identification issued to the athlete from the institution, his/her driver's license, or a positive identification by the client representative/site coordinator. Athletes should arrive at the collection site by the predesignated time. If the athlete is delayed, the collector must inform the client representative/site coordinator to determine the appropriate measures for locating the athlete or when to consider the athlete as a "no show" based on the client's policies and procedures.

All urine specimens collected are accompanied by a Custody and Control Form (CCF). "Custody" refers to a chain of custody, which is the term used to describe the process of documenting the handling of a specimen from the time an athlete provides a specimen and the collector processes the specimen, through shipping to the laboratory, during the testing at the laboratory, and until the results are reported by the laboratory. The CCF documents all information pertinent to the collection and testing of the specimen. It is important to note that the CCF must be filled out completely, and that any unusual occurrences in the collection process should be noted in the collector's final report. Any error on the CCF is considered a "fatal flaw" and if caught during the information gathering process, the collector must have the athlete select another CCF for the collector to complete correctly. This documentation becomes an official statement of evidence that documents the possession of the specimen at all times. The collector must maintain the integrity and security of the specimen. Perhaps the most important aspect of this responsibility is maintaining absolute control of the specimen from the moment the collector receives the specimen until the specimen is transferred to the shipping agent. After the specimen is prepared for shipment, there is no requirement for couriers, express carriers, or postal service personnel to sign any custody documentation because they do not have access to the specimen or any CCF.

Other considerations for urine specimen collection include whether to perform observed or monitored collections and the decision to package single or split specimens. Direct observed urine collections involve having an observer accompany the athlete into the toilet area to observe the act of urination. Monitored collections involve having a monitor accompany the athlete into the toilet area, but allow the athlete to urinate in the privacy of a closed stall. An observer of the same gender as the athlete must conduct a direct observed collection. Both types of collections provide deterrence from attempted *adulteration*, substitution, or manipulation during the actual urinating process, but the direct observed collection process is the most effective means of verifying urine validity at the collection site.

Split specimen testing involves splitting a single urine void into two separate vials labeled A and B. Both are securely sealed and shipped to the laboratory. The laboratory will analyze the A sample, but will freeze and store the B sample in the event additional testing is indicated. Generally, the B sample is made available if the athlete challenges the initial drug test result and requests a second analysis. Some athletic organizations require B sample analysis on all positive results.[28,44] Single specimen collections are easier; however, providing laboratories with split samples allows for testing in rare cases when a vial may have leaked or a security seal became damaged during shipping.

In the United States, the federal government regulates drug testing through the Department of Transportation (DOT). The DOT requires agencies, transportation employers, and self-employed individuals to participate in drug and alcohol testing following very specific procedures. Non-DOT regulated companies and other organizations can adopt the DOT's collection procedures as an industry standard.[44]

Specimen Adulteration

Specimen *adulteration* is a potential problem in urine drug testing. There are a variety of substances and methods used to interfere with testing procedures that can lead to an unwarranted negative result. Any attempt to circumvent the identification of a drug in the donor's system can invalidate the process and compromise the very purpose of a drug testing program.[57] Specimen adulteration can be categorized as *in vivo* or *in vitro*. In vivo adulteration refers to the process of self-administering a substance for the purpose of altering drug test results. Athletes may attempt to mask the presence of a drug in the urine or "flush" the drug out of the body prior to the drug test collection. The most common method of in vivo adulteration is simple over hydration. These actions occur prior to arrival at the specimen collection site, making detection of the adulterating activity practically impossible.[57] Of course, by not notifying athletes prior to specimen collection, in vivo adulteration opportunities are virtually eliminated.

There are a number of substances reputed to interfere with the drug testing process when taken by the donor. Some of these adulterants can alter urinary pH, which will in turn alter the excretion profile of some drugs. As an example, amphetamine excretion rates are slowed when the urine pH is alkaline increasing the amount of time to fully excrete the drug from the system. This actually lowers the concentration levels of the drug during this time period to levels below cut-off, thus providing a negative drug test. Vitamin C, vinegar, a variety of acidic fruit juices, ibuprofen, aspirin, and golden seal root are other substances that have been ingested in an attempt to produce negative drug tests. Golden seal root is particularly popular, gaining its reputation as an adulterant because alkaloids in the plant material interfere with thin layer chromatography (TLC) tests for opiates. However, current methodologies are no longer subject to this interference.[57] Golden seal products marketed as drug testing adulterants typically involve adding large amounts of water prior to ingesting. This will create a dilute specimen. Dilution is another method of manipulating a drug test and is discussed later in this section. Diuretics do not typically interfere with a drug test, but they can dilute the concentration of a drug to an undetectable level. Including diuretic testing as part of the complete drug testing panel can circumvent this type of masking.

In vitro adulteration involves modifying samples to prevent the proper identification of a drug. This type of adulteration is accomplished directly on the sample and does not involve influencing the biological system like in vivo methods.[57] By adding a foreign substance to a urine sample, the testing process is disrupted or the actual drug present in the urine is destroyed. There are many products available that claim to guarantee a negative test result when used according to directions. These products are easily available and often sold over the Internet. Gluteraldehydes are chemical additives in products like UrinAid, Klear, Whizzies, or UrineLuck used to attempt interfering with specimen analysis, but are generally detectable during the analysis process. Other substances range from diesel fuel, which is easily detected, to Visine, which is extremely difficult to detect in urine samples with the intention of producing false-negative results. Other items include alcohol, ammonia, ascorbic acid, bleach, blood, soap, or detergent, Drano, golden seal root, lemon juice, Lime-A-Way, peroxide, salt, Vanish, and vinegar. Of course, the ideal adulterant is one that can easily be introduced into the sample, interferes with the testing process causing a negative result, and will not be detected.[57] Most contain common-

Table 14-3. Adulterants

Class	Example	Action on Specimen
Chlorine	Clorex	Oxidizer
Nitrites	Klear	Oxidizer
Peroxidase	Stealth, Stealth II	Oxidizer
Pyridinium Chlorochromate	UrineLuck, LL418, Sweet Pee's Spoiler, Randy's Klear II	Oxidizer
Acids	Amber-13, THC-Free, Urine Luck	Interference
Gluteraldehydes	UrinAid, Clear Choice	Interference
Soaps	Mary Jane SuperClean 13, Joy Lemon-Scented Dish Detergent	Interference

Substitution

Placing clean urine (from another person) in collection beaker or putting another look-alike liquid in collection beaker for processing in an attempt to produce a negative test result.

Dilution

Either adding water to a specimen in the collection beaker or ingesting copious amounts of water/fluid forcing the urine specimen to be dilute upon voiding.

ly used chemicals that laboratories can now detect by performing adulteration testing on all samples as part of standard operating procedures.

Nitrites added to urine oxidize drugs and their metabolites into undetectable by-products. Adding acid or base chemical substances to urine will greatly impact urine pH and ultimately complicate analysis. Although nitrites are normally present in urine, laboratories now screen samples for nitrite levels and determine a level >500 ng/mL to be adulterated.[44] Likewise, pH levels must be within "human" range—generally between 4.5 and 8.0. Products containing glutaraldehyde will also cause abnormal immunoassay screens; however, glutaraldehyde does not normally occur in urine and is detectable[44] (Table 14-3).

Perhaps the most common method of attempting to adulterate a urine sample is dilution. Dilution refers to the process of providing a sample for testing in which the relative concentrations of drugs or drug metabolites are below applicable cut-off levels, preventing laboratories from detecting drugs present in the specimen. Donors either externally add fluids to the sample at the collection site (in vitro) or consume copious amounts of fluids prior to providing a sample (in vivo), which results in a dilute urine specimen. To prevent dilution, individuals responsible for administering specimen collections must control athlete fluid consumption from the time of notification until an adequate sample is obtained. Fluids are provided to athletes in single serving, individually sealed containers to control fluid consumption for proper hydration purposes and to protect athletes from ingesting fluids possibly contaminated with banned drugs.

When setting up testing parameters with laboratories, organizations should request that laboratories report samples as "dilute" if creatinine is <20 mg/dL and the specific gravity is <1.003 so that drug testing administrators can obtain recollection from athletes providing dilute samples. Of course, this loophole allows athletes who are intentionally diluting samples because of

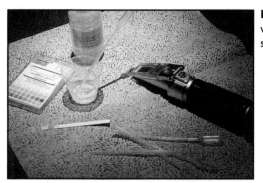

Figure 14-1. Refractometer and reagent strips, which can be used to measure specific gravity on-site.

drug use additional time to rid his/her body of the prohibited substance. By the time another sample is collected, the drug in question may not be detectable. A more effective method of preventing dilution involves measuring samples at the collection site for specific gravity. If specific gravity is too low, collectors can withhold fluids from the donor until a concentrated sample is collected, packaged, and sent to the laboratory.

Specific gravity can be measured on site using either reagent strips or a handheld refractometer (Figure 14-1). Reagent strips are not as accurate, but can provide enough information to determine urine adequacy for laboratory analysis. The hand-held refractometer is a device intended to determine the amount of solute in a solution by measuring the index of refraction (ratio of the velocity of light in a vacuum to the velocity of light in the solution). A few drops of urine are dripped on the prism with the light refracted from the boundary of sample and prism projected on a scale. The urine specific gravity between healthy men and women tends to fluctuate in range from 1.010 to 1.030.[58] Laboratories analytical methods become challenged in detecting drugs present in the specimen if specific gravity is <1.003. Collection procedures recommend rejecting any sample <1.005.

Substituting urine is another form of adulteration that can be accomplished in vitro or in more extreme cases through in vivo methods. In vitro methods of urine substitution involve concealing "clean" urine somewhere on the body and once in the restroom facility, placing the clean urine in the specimen container for drug testing. This complicated procedure is difficult, if not impossible, when performing an observed collection. However, those drug-tainted donors desperate to conceal use will go to any extreme. The process involves choosing from any number of marketed contraptions or homemade devices including the use of condoms or something as sophisticated as "The Whizzinator," a prosthetic urinating device, to carry "clean" urine into the collection site unnoticed. Not only is concealing a device problematic, but obtaining "clean" urine is yet another step to this masquerade. The donor may ask a trusting nondrug user to provide him or her with drug-free urine or may choose to purchase "clean" urine from any number of marketing suppliers. Several states are introducing laws addressing the problem of beating drug tests by making it illegal to distribute urine or sell additives for the purpose of altering drug test results. Collectors who witness attempts to adulterate a drug test are obligated to report such activities to drug testing administrators because in many programs an adulterated drug test is considered a positive drug test. However, with new anti-fraud statutes, forwarding such evidence of fraud to local authorities will initiate a criminal process. To date, these statutes do not require collectors (service providers) to notify any state authority.[59]

Specimen Analysis

Laboratory Analysis

Forensic drug testing is the process of analyzing biological specimens for illicit drugs.[59] Sports drug testing expands on this principle to include not only illicit drugs, but also many other compounds including a variety of performance-enhancing substances. Most testing for drugs of abuse is done using urine specimens and involves two procedures, screening and confirmation. Screening tests have high sensitivity (low rate of false-negative results), are fast, and less expensive, whereas confirmatory tests have high specificity (low rate of false-positive results).[4] A false-negative result refers to a negative report when a sought-after substance is actually present in a concentration greater than a predetermined cut-off level, yet not detected through the analytical method used. As an example, one might falsely conclude that cocaine was not used 24 hours ago when examining urine using thin layer chromatography as opposed to a more sensitive method.[9]

> *False negative—The laboratory reports a negative result when the specimen actually contains a substance that is being tested for, but for whatever reason is not reported as being found present in the specimen. False positive—The laboratory reports a positive result when the specimen does not actually contain the substance the laboratory reported.*

Toxicologists involved with drug testing have identified several compounds that may possibly interfere with initial absorbance readings on *immunoassay* screenings. Certain nonsteroidal anti-inflammatories (eg, tolmetin) have been known to cause significant interferences during screening, but not with GC/MS confirmation. In addition, many potential adulterants, including glutaraldehyde, have the same effect creating a false-negative result.[44] Laboratories now include screening for a number of adulterants that contribute to false-negative results and observed specimen collections virtually eliminate adulteration of samples.

A false-positive result means that a positive result is produced when the substance being sought is not present, confirmable as present, or is present at a concentration below the cut-off value.[9] A sample may screen positive, but must be considered as "presumptive positive" until confirmation specifically indicates the presence of a banned substance. Screening methods do not merely test for presence or absence of a drug, but provide a quantitative or semiquantitative result based on the specific cut-off values previously established. If a sample screens positive, it is important for a laboratory to use highly specific methods of testing for confirmation.[4]

Current standard operating procedures for federally regulated drug testing programs require laboratories to screen using *immunoassay* and confirm presumptive positives using GC/MS.[61] "Federal and state courts have supported the legal reliability of immunoassay urine drug tests either used singly or a double immunoassay test and/or confirmation by an alternate method. Immunoassays have over 20 years of successful legal history."[38]

During screening, specimens are subjected to nonspecific assays for the presence of drugs, metabolites, and related compounds.[2] Prior to testing, samples must be prepared for analytical techniques. Pretreatment of biological specimens is done to release drugs from the biological matrix; remove interfering particles; and adjust the pH, ionic strength, and concentration of the sample to allow optimum extraction.[61] Immunochemical assays are popular for screening of the more typical drugs of abuse because these assays are very sensitive, detecting nanogram quantities of drug metabolites in urine and techniques that have been extensively developed through high-volume workplace drug testing. They are rapid tests producing results in minutes. Perhaps the greatest disadvantage is the cross-reactions that occur with loosely related endogenous or exogenous substances, thus the need for specific confirmatory tests.

There are a number of different immunochemical methods available. One of the most popular immunoassay procedures is the enzyme immunoassay (EIA). The EIA is based on an enzyme bound to the drug that can also bind to a specific antibody. A newer method is fluorescent polarization immunoassay (FPIA). It is also very sensitive and rapid. Less specimen manipulation is required, but the testing procedure is more expensive. Latex agglutination testing is another screening method that is easy to use and appears to be as accurate as other immunoassay techniques.[4] If the screening process does not detect any banned substances, the test result is reported as negative. If the screening *assay* detects a compound that is consistent with a banned substance, a confirmation assay is conducted. A positive screen is confirmed or refuted by using a different assay technique. The confirmation process identifies the specific compound, minimizing a false-positive result. Although liquid and gas chromatography can be used for confirmation, GC/MS is the standard.[2]

Gas chromatography can be used for screening or for confirmation. It requires expensive equipment and personnel with specific training. A small amount of an extract from the specimen is injected into a heated chamber that immediately volatilizes the liquid and sweeps it into a column by a carrier gas. Compounds are then absorbed to a stationary phase (column). Each compound has its own retention time, the time of emergence of the compound from the column, and thus separates individual components in a mixture. A detector and recorder at the end of the column records height and area of the peak that correlates with the quantity of each compound present.[4] This procedure is generally joined by a mass spectrophotometer (MS). Mass spectrometry uses an electron beam to ionize each compound. These ions are filtered and separated electromagnetically and identified according to their mass/charge ratio. A detection system then detects the amount of each ion present as a result for the electron beam. Each substance has a unique pattern (mass spectrum) or fingerprint. Mass spectrometry is often combined with GC to produce a sensitive and specific detection system. *Gas chromatography/mass spectrometry is the "gold standard" for confirmation of positive screens.* Testing methods have become extremely sensitive, which provides organizations the opportunity to work with laboratories to determine levels of detection when testing for specific drugs.[4]

Testing for typical drugs of abuse is relatively straightforward and similar to other areas of forensic toxicology. Sports drug testing is a unique area within the field of toxicology. Both the scope of testing provided and the analytical techniques applied are among the most sophisticated in the field. A unique challenge in sports drug testing is identifying whether performance-enhancing substances occur naturally or are *exogenous* (eg, peptide hormones and testosterone).[13] When testing for these types of substances, analysis must be performed at highly specialized laboratories. Anabolic steroid testing requires a minimum of one GC/MS and one technician devoted entirely to anabolic steroid testing. In addition, interpretation of results requires a certifying scientist knowledgeable in steroid metabolism and pharmacology.

Up until 1984, samples were initially screened using radioimmunoassay (RIA) and presumptive positive samples were confirmed using GC/MS techniques. It was during the 1984 Olympic Games in Los Angeles, California that GC/MS was adopted for both screening and confirmation for anabolic steroid analysis.[12,17] RIA screening for steroid metabolite detection did not provide the sensitivity necessary to accurately detect anabolic steroids. In addition, *endogenous* testosterone was added to the IOC list of banned substances. A method has been developed for assessing whether athletes were using testosterone. The testing method involved measuring both testosterone (T) and epitestosterone (E). The normal ratio of T to E is approximately 1:1 for both males and females. Use of testosterone raises this ratio appreciably. A ratio of 6:1 or greater is considered evidence of testosterone administration and classified as a positive drug test.[13] However, limitations to the T/E ratio test, including microbial degradation, excessive alcohol consumption, and genetic and pathologic conditions complicate the interpretation of T/E results.[13] Testosterone has been the most commonly used endogenous steroid and lately its OTC precursors, such as androstenedione and DHEA, have become very popular. These substances occur naturally in the body, therefore a process that distinguishes natural from administered substances was needed. The introduction of carbon isotope ratio mass spectrometry as a complementary means of performing a single measurement on a suspect sample with a T/E >6:1 has helped resolve the issue of endogenous production.[53] Gas chromatography/combustion/isotope ratio mass spectrometry (GC/C/IRMS) is a promising approach for detecting the use of exogenous testosterone. The premise of this approach is that the relative amount of the naturally occurring carbon-13 isotope in a pharmaceutical preparation of testosterone is different than that produced from dietary precursors, thus providing the ability to distinguish between endogenous and exogenous testosterone. Although successful at identifying the carbon difference, GC/C/IRMS is extremely expensive and time consuming.

Another analytical advancement was the introduction of high resolution mass spectrometry (HRMS) at the Atlanta Olympics in 1996. Prior to the availability of HRMS, the main technique used was the benchtop GC/MS. The detection levels by GC/MS for anabolic steroids has a limit of about 10 µg/mL but with HRMS levels of detection are lowered to <1 ng/mL. These capabilities extended the detection period from last ingestion of the anabolic agent.[53] Although detection of a limited list of substances is possible using several techniques, the only technique presently available for detecting the full list of prohibited anabolic agents is the HRMS.[3]

On-Site Screening Devices

On-site urine testing, also referred to as point-of-collection urine testing, has recently been adopted in the drug testing industry. On-site testing includes both benchtop screening instruments and *immunoassay* kits at the collection site. Point-of-collection testing is an initial test conducted at the collection site for either the presence of drugs or to determine specimen validity. This type of testing can be done for both urine and oral fluid. Any on-site screening device being considered for use should be approved by the FDA and be supported by validation studies. In addition, collectors using on-site testing devices must be adequately trained and certified to administer these testing devices.[62] On-site tests produce rapid results using simple procedures and do not require sending a specimen to a laboratory. Results are available within minutes, eliminating uncertainty and substantially reducing the administrative burden posed by chain of custody. Point-of-collection testing is perceived as a strong deterrent to drug use because it decreases the time between results and consequences, providing an opportunity to promptly and positively reinforce drug-free behavior. On-site testing has other advantages including flexibility as to where testing is conducted.[38] However, on-site testing products are manufactured for workplace drug testing panels (eg, marijuana, cocaine, and amphetamines) and use SAMHSA cut-offs. These products do not include testing opportunities for most of the drugs found on sports organizations' banned drug lists. When considering on-site devices or alternative specimens for drug testing, procedures and products must have scientific acceptance and be able to withstand legal challenges. The level of services available from the supplier, including litigation support, is essential. Use of these products or procedures must be specifically described in written drug testing policies and procedures and the specimen collection and chain of custody procedures must be clearly defined.[38]

Today's technology provides many options for drug testing. It is important to remember the relationships that exist between the various methodologies. For example, the banned drug list should be considered before the type of specimen to be analyzed is selected. There are limitations to what drugs can be identified in certain specimens. In addition, the collection procedures should be carefully considered to prevent specimen adulteration challenges. Ultimately, the ability to detect drug use will only be as strong as the scientific methodologies and industry-adopted procedures being used.

Results Verification and Applying Sanctions

After receipt of drug testing results from the laboratory, it is critical to review all reports carefully for any inconsistencies and to compare these reports with chain of custody forms, ultimately matching an athlete to his/her result via specimen identification numbers. Positive results must then be reported to the athlete and discussed. Interviewing the athlete is imperative to determine whether there is an alternative medical explanation for the positive result. In many cases, a team physician or another designated medical review officer best completes this process. Ultimately, this verification process must be carried out on all positive drug tests before classifying the result as positive and applying sanctions.

An unintentional positive result may occur when an athlete is prescribed a medication or elects to take an OTC substance without knowing the medication was banned or contained a banned substance. The difficulty exists in trying to accurately determine whether the ingestion was unintentional or not. Many sports organizations support the position that any substance an athlete places into his or her body is intentional; ignorance is no excuse. This is a perfect example of how a drug testing program without education is problematic. It is critical to provide all athletes with policies, procedures, and a list of prohibited substances. In addition, all athletes should have access to resources designed to assist in determining if a medication or OTC product contains banned substances. Some organizations allow athletes to take a banned substance (eg, stimulant, β-blocker) for legitimate medical reasons if no "nonbanned" alternative exists. These exceptions to the consequences of a positive drug test result must be fully documented by the attending physician and usually reviewed by a medical review board for the sports organization.

Most positive drug tests are reviewed by adjudicating bodies such as committees of administrators, medical doctors, and athletes. When dealing with OTC drugs, athletes will often accept the result, but ask for leniency based on inadvertent use or lack of understanding of a product. Contentious cases may lead to appeals, hearings, and arbitration at the national and international level.[8] The path to final adjudication depends on the type of organization and its existing policies and procedures. The arbitration process in sports is unlike criminal or civil proceedings in a variety of ways. One area of controversy is the shift in burden of proof from the national governing body or international governing body to the athlete.[13] Once a positive result has been reported and confirmed positive through interpretation and due process, appropriate sanctions must be applied. Drug testing in sports has been criticized for alleged inefficiencies, unfairness in testing methods, and for the way sanctions have been levied. It is vital to apply appropriate sanctions consistently.

There should be a detailed description of the sanctions applied for policy violations. Penalties are generally imposed for athletes who refuse to sign a consent form, athletes who engage in criminal misconduct (eg, drug trafficking), athletes who refuse to submit to a required drug test, and athletes who test positive. Institutional penalty structures generally involve a three-tiered system of sanctions:

- First offenses involve suspension from participation until the nature and extent of the involvement with prohibited drugs can be determined. Athletes are usually referred to a substance abuse specialist for appropriate counseling and treatment, if necessary. Athletes are then allowed to return to participation, but will be required to undergo unannounced follow-up testing.

- A second offense requires immediate suspension, re-evaluation for substance abuse and/or addiction, and a predetermined period of nonparticipation. Return to participation will include evaluation by a medical doctor to determine that re-entry would not pose a health risk to the athlete.
- Third offenses result in permanently suspending the athlete from athletic participation at that institution.

Sanctions should also be included for athletes who voluntarily disclose drug use, but penalties for first offenses should be graded to encourage athletes with drug use problems to seek help.

Regardless of the drug testing entity, a process for interpreting the result of a positive drug test must be described in the written policy, completely followed, and documented. Once a drug test is deemed positive, athletes must be given the opportunity to appeal the interpretation of the positive result. The penalties or consequences must be explicitly defined in the policy and fully applied once any appeal process concludes the positive result to be final.

DEVELOPMENT OF A DRUG TESTING PROGRAM

In developing any type of program or service, the first step is to determine if a need exists. The need to drug test in sport may seem obvious because it deters athletes from using potentially dangerous substances and because it creates a level playing field; however, a needs analysis is encouraged to further support the implementation of an often-controversial program. In determining this need, athletic organizations should define the nature and the extent of any drug use problem. There are numerous national surveys and studies that have examined drug use in sport at various levels of competition, but local applicability must also be considered. Athletic organizations, such as the NCAA, survey student-athletes at member institutions periodically and provide information on drug use trends. Other methods of determining the need for drug testing include reviewing reports from staff members and campus security, engaging in focus group discussions, examining current institutional data and referral trends, and discovering evidence indicating drug use (eg, finding drug paraphernalia).

Once a needs assessment is complete, a committee or task force comprised of an attorney, physician, athletics administrator, athletic trainer, toxicologist, and possibly a coach and student-athlete should be formed. The organization's legal counsel should be involved with program development from the onset, particularly with regard to right-to-privacy statutes, which may vary from state to state.[40] The committee should submit a proposal for implementing a drug testing program to decision makers and be prepared to discuss a number of issues including constitutionality, effective methodology, confidentiality, administrative impact, and budgeting. There may be outside resources available for schools eligible for federal funding, including assistance from the United States Department of Education, Department of Health and Human Services, Partnership for Drug-Free America, and the National Institute on Drug Abuse. Private schools may be exempt from federally funded program, but may find funding opportunities through other corporations and nonprofit groups.

Once approval for drug testing is accomplished, a detailed written policy must be developed before any testing can occur. The policy should include a clear explanation of the purposes of the program, who will be tested and by what methods, which drugs will be tested for and under what conditions (eg, announced, reasonable suspicion), and what actions will be taken against those who test positive. A copy of the policy should be given to each athlete along with a written consent form that each athlete should read and sign, confirming receipt and understanding of the policy and agreement to participate in the drug testing program.[40] A list of banned substances must be developed and should be included in the policy. Athletic organizations should consider including performance-enhancing substances and illicit drugs in the banned list. The NCAA list of banned drug classes may be used if an institution wishes to adopt it for its own drug testing program.

There are numerous logistical, technical, and economic issues to consider for proper administration of a drug testing program. Administrators must determine how and when samples will be collected, secured, and transported. The appropriate personnel responsible for these duties must have a clear understanding of procedures. If the institution elects to outsource the collection of specimens to a third party, a complete description of each party's responsibilities and a description of the services being provided should be agreed upon prior to testing. If a third-party administrator is used, typically the TPA contracts with certified laboratories for specimen analysis. Often this relationship provides the institution with discounted laboratory costs because the service provider can negotiate lower pricing due to a higher testing volume. If the institution chooses to contract directly with a laboratory, there are a number of issues that need to be considered. The institution should request documentation supporting the laboratory's accreditation and certification along with staff qualifications. Depending on the credentialing agency, laboratories are required to complete proficiency programs and to maintain quality control programs. The laboratory should also provide the institution with a description of what analytical methods are available for testing samples, concentration levels of drug detection available, and how specimens are handled within the laboratory from receiving and processing to storage. The chain of custody of samples should be described along with a list of the certified scientists who will review and approve results for processing. Turnaround times for drug test results can be crucial depending on the reason for testing. Usually laboratories will provide a quote for turnaround times on negative results and another quote for turnaround times on positive results because of confirmation testing. Results reporting and maintaining confidentiality of results is critical. Laboratory pricing is usually quoted on a per sample basis and should include screening and confirmation testing and include necessary supplies and shipping of samples to the laboratory with pick-up from the collection site and delivery to the laboratory within 24 hours of collection.

Programs should be reassessed annually to maintain effectiveness. Surveying athletes who participate in drug testing programs, obtaining current national drug use trends and research, encouraging substance abuse counselor feedback, and gathering other anecdotal information will be helpful in evaluating a drug testing program. Building a consortium to fully address drug use and improve the deterrent effect strengthens the effectiveness of a program. Athletic organizations are encouraged to include the medical community, local law enforcement and municipal alliances, and other related businesses to assist in these efforts.

Drug testing cannot be the only element in an effective antidoping program. Educating athletes about the potential dangers of drug and dietary supplement use is critical and all participants must be made aware of their respective responsibilities. A drug testing program is designed to create awareness and evoke sound decision making with regard to drug use in sport. Integrity is an obvious ingredient in drug testing; it is an active process that cannot be taken for granted. Implementing a drug testing program requires the courage to draw a line between acceptable and unacceptable behavior.[8] Developing a drug testing program based on a solid, purposeful foundation and a commitment from informed and courageous individuals will produce an effective deterrent to drug use in sport and promote ethical behavior by the athletes it serves.

CURRENT AND FUTURE CHALLENGES
IN DRUG TESTING IN SPORT

Performance-enhancing substances have been used since ancient times. Athletes today use a wide range of substances from anabolic steroids and stimulants to simple medical techniques, such as blood doping to improve performance. Technical advancements have inadvertently led to new delivery of "old" drugs such as testosterone administration through nasal mists or skin patches.[23] Doping has developed into a widespread problem in competitive sport because of increased financial incentives from professional opportunities and commercialism. It is possible to earn more money as a highly paid top athlete in a short time, than over an entire conventional career.[64]

Doping in sport has grown in scientific and ethical complexity. The future limits to athletic performance will be determined more by technological advances than innate physiology of the athlete. Where do we draw the line between what is natural and what is artificially enhanced?[61] Some of the new and emerging technologies challenging the ethical fiber of sport tomorrow include gene transfer therapy, stem cell transplantation, and RBC substitutes.[65] Invariably, athletes will turn to these and other unknown doping agents in search of the competitive edge. Every time a new drug or technology is developed, an athlete determined to gain an athletic advantage finds a way to misuse or abuse that drug or technology, perverting its original intent.[6]

Controversy surrounding blood doping has been evident for >25 years. Following the 1984 Olympic Games, the IOC banned all forms of blood doping. In 1990, the organization added recombinant human erythropoietin (rhEPO) to the banned list. The IOC has now modified its definition of doping to account for the developments in biotechnology. The definition of blood doping now includes the administration of blood, RBCs, artificial oxygen carriers, and related blood products to an athlete. International testing protocol now includes both blood and urine testing to determine rhEPO use.[66]

The current use of anabolic steroids and EPO will soon be replaced by injecting genes to enhance performance and appearance. Within the next decade, genetic engineering will probably change the course of competitive sport.[23,67] The IOC Medical Commission is currently developing high-tech, anti-abuse tests that analyze blood and saliva for antibodies produced as a result of taking gene medications and is working on the creation of gene footprint detection.[23]

Despite the development of advanced drug testing systems, doping, both deliberate and inadvertent, continues to plague sport today. A particular problem is the risk of today's dietary supplement culture. An effective antidoping program must incorporate educational components in addition to testing and these educational initiatives need to be collaborative and proactive. Athletes, coaches, managers, governing bodies, and athletic trainers and other health care professionals must come together in these efforts. Technological advances cannot address what is essentially a behavioral problem.[11] Doping leads to major health problems, including death, and violates the basic principles of equal opportunity and fair play. More frequent testing and more severe punishments for doping violations by the sports associations themselves may be one way of fighting doping in sports. More thorough education of athletes on the negative effects of uncontrolled drug use may also help.[64] Educational efforts designed to encourage informed, responsible, and healthy decisions can supplement athletes' understanding and perceptions of the effectiveness of drug testing and can encourage athletes to develop decision-making skills that are internally motivated, rather than externally driven.[68] Manufacturers and suppliers of dietary supplement products containing banned substances must be must be confronted and held accountable if a victim-blaming approach is to be avoided.

ROLE OF THE ATHLETIC TRAINER

The athletic trainer plays an intricate role in sport antidoping campaigns. Whether working with youth groups or professional athletes, the athletic trainer is positioned to provide participants with direct and immediate feedback regarding the risks of using drugs regardless of their intent. It is critical for athletic trainers to become and remain knowledgeable about all types of drugs and the implications of substance use in sport. Likewise, it is extremely important for the athletic trainer to understand the application of drug education and testing programs and to be prepared to contribute in the ongoing commitment to athlete health and welfare, as well as fair play.

REFERENCES

1. Shorter F, Bowers LD. Foreword. In: Bahrke MS, Yesalis CE, eds. *Performance-Enhancing Substances in Sport and Exercise*. Champaign, Ill: Human Kinetics; 2002:v-vi.

2. Ambrose PJ. Doping control in sports—a perspective from the 1996 Olympic Games. *Am J Health Syst Pharm*. 1997;54:1053-1057.

3. Bowers LD. Athletic drug testing. *Clin Sports Med*. 1998;17:299-318.

4. Landry GL, Kokotailo PK. Drug screening in the athletic setting. *Curr Probl Pediatr*. 1994;24:344-359.

5. Green GA, Uryasz FD, Petr TA, Bray CD. NCAA study of substance use and abuse habits of college student-athletes. *Clin J Sport Med*. 2001;11:51-56.

6. Wadler G. Science and research. Presented at: First Meeting of the White House Task Force on Drug Use in Sports Proceedings; December 7, 2000; Salt Lake City, Utah.

7. Walters JP. *What You Need to Know About Drug Testing in Schools*. Washington, DC: Office of National Drug Control Policy; 2002:i-16.

8. Shults TF. The intangible elements of successful drug testing programs. *MROAlert*. 2002;131-132.

9. Wadler GI, Hainline B. *Drugs and the Athlete*. Philadelphia, Pa: FA Davis Co; 1989:197-212.

10. Yesalis CE. History of doping in sport. In: Bahrke MS, Yesalis CE, eds. *Performance-Enhancing Substances in Sport and Exercise*. Champaign, Ill: Human Kinetics; 2002:1-20.

11. Sheehan O, Quinn B. Doping in sport—a deadly game. *Irish Pharmacy Journal*. 2002;80(6):256-62. Available at: http://www.sports-drugs.com/asp/ss_features5.asp. Accessed November 29, 2002.

12. Kammerer RC. Drug testing in sport and exercise. In: Bahrke MS, Yesalis CE, eds. *Performance-Enhancing Substances in Sport and Exercise*. Champaign, Ill: Human Kinetics; 2002:323-339.

13. Bowers LD, Black R, Borts DJ. Athletic drug testing: an analyst's view of science and the law. *Ther Drug Monit*. 2000;22:98-102.

14. Uryasz FD. Historical review of NCAA involvement with drug education and drug testing. Addendum for NCAA Committee on Competitive Safeguards and Medical Aspects of Sport. March 1994.

15. National Collegiate Athletic Association Research Staff. *NCAA Study of Substance Use Habits of College Student-Athletes*. Indianapolis, Ind: National Collegiate Athletic Association; 2001:1-12.

16. International Olympic Committee. *International Olympic Committees* Web page. Available at: http://www.olympic.org/uk/organisation/commissions/medical/index_uk.asp. Accessed June 1, 2004

17. Catlin DH, Kammerer RC, Hatton CK, Sekera MH, Merdink JL. Analytical chemistry at the games of the XXIIIrd Olympiad in Los Angeles. *Clin Chem*. 1987;33:319-327.

18. International Olympic Committee. *National Olympic Committees*. Web page Available at: http://www.olympic.org/uk/organisation/noc/index_uk.asp. Accessed June 1, 2004.

19. International Olympic Committee. *International Sports Federations* Web page. Available at: http://www.olympic.org/uk/organisation/if/index_uk.asp. Accessed June 1, 2004

20. Petit GE. Form over substances: the legal context of performance-enhancing substances. In: Bahrke MS, Yesalis CE, eds. *Performance-Enhancing Substances in Sport and Exercise*. Champaign, Ill: Human Kinetics; 2002:341-350.

21. International Olympic Committee. *Protection of Athletes* Web page. Available at: http://www.olympic.org/ uk/organisation/missions/athletes_uk.asp. Accessed June 1, 2004

22. International Olympic Committee. *Court of Arbitration for Sport* Web page. Available at: http://www.olympic.org/ uk/organisation/actions/index_uk.asp. Accessed June 1, 2004.

23. Bahrke MS, Yesalis CE. Issues, concerns, and the future of performance-enhancing substances in sport and exercise. In: *Performance-Enhancing Substances in Sport and Exercise.* Champaign, Ill: Human Kinetics; 2002:351-355.

24. World Anti-Doping Agency. About WADA. http://www.wada-ama.org/en/t3.asp?p=41506. Accessed June 1, 2004.

25. National Football League Players Association. *Drug Policy* Web page. http://www.nflpa.org/members/ main.asp?subPage=Drug+Policy. Accessed June 1, 2004.

26. Johnson, Osborne, Watts, Kind, Simmons, Foley, Israel, Camp, Holden, Gekas, Culberson, Mcinnis, Houghton, Boswell, Boehlert, Castle, Pryce. House of Representatives Resolution 496. House passes resolution supporting mandatory testing of Major League Baseball players for steroids. *MROAlert.* 2002;13:10-11.

27. National Collegiate Athletic Association. *Committee on Competitive Safeguards and Medial Aspects of Sports.* Web page. Available at: http://www1.ncaa.org/eprise/main/membership/governance/assoc-wide/competitive_safeguards/index.html. Accessed June 1, 2004.

28. National Collegiate Athletic Association Research Staff. *NCAA Drug Education/Testing Survey 2001.* Indianapolis, Ind: National Collegiate Athletic Association; 2001:1-13.

29. Johnston LD, O'Malley PM, Bachman JG. *Monitoring The Future National Results on Adolescent Drug Use Overview of Key Findings, 2001.* Bethesda, Md: National Institute on Drug Abuse; 2002:3-5.

30. Goldberg L, Elliot D, MacKinnon D, et al. Drug testing athletes to prevent substance abuse: background and pilot study results of the SATURN study. *J Adolesc Health.* 2003;32:16-25.

31. Curtis R. What are the issues surrounding drug testing privacy? *Workplace Substance Abuse Advisor.* 1999; 13:3.

32. Wong GM. Drug testing in amateur athletics. In: *Essentials of Amateur Sports Law.* Westport, Conn: Praeger Publishing; 1994:711-731.

33. Niccolai FR. Legal considerations of drug testing. In: Banks R, ed. *Substance Abuse in Sport: The Realities.* Dubuque, Iowa: Kendall/Hunt Publishing Co; 1990:77-88.

34. Wong GM, Barr CA. Passing the test NCAA drug testing program gets ok from California high court. *Athletic Business.* 1994:10.13.

35. Barr CA. Busted in Boulder. *Athletic Business.* 1994;18:10,16.

36. Vernonia School District 47J v. Acton, 515 US 646 (1995). Available at: http://www/caselaw.lp. findlaw.com. Accessed March 25, 2003.

37. Board of Education of Independent School District No. 92 of Pottawatomie County et al v. Earls et al (2002). Available at: http://www/caselaw.lp.findlaw.com. Accessed June 27, 2002.

38. Evans D. *Drug Courts and On-site Drug Testing Effective Weapons in the War on Drugs.* Indianapolis, IN: Roche Diagnostics; 1995-1997.

39. Lombardo JA. Drug programs. *Clin Sports Med.* 1998;17:319-326.

40. National Collegiate Athletic Association. *NCAA drug testing Program 2002-03.* Indianapolis, Ind: National Collegiate Athletic Association; 2002:14-15.

41. Ringhofer KR, Harding ME. *Coaches Guide to Drugs In Sport.* Champaign, Ill: Human Kinetics; 1996. Available at: http://www.nfhs.org/sportsmed/drug_testing2.htm. Accessed January 2, 2003.

42. National Collegiate Athletic Association. *Drug Testing Program* Web page. Available at: http://www1. ncaa.org/membership/ed_outreach/health-safety/drug_testing/index.html. Accessed June 1, 2004.

43. Dawson RT. The war on drugs in sport. *BBC News and Views.* 2000;1:3 (published October 3, 2000). Available at: http://www.biomedcentral.com/1471-8219/1/3/abstract. Accessed November 29, 2002.

44. Shults TF. *The Medical Review Officer Handbook.* Research Triangle Park, NC: Quadrangle Research, LLC; 1999:XXI-XXIV, 3-26, 65-89, 223-237.

45. 49 CFR Part 40 [Docket OST-99-6578] RIN 2105-AC49 Department of Transportation Procedures for Transportation Workplace Drug and Alcohol Testing Programs. Washington, DC: Office of Drug and Alcohol Policy and Compliance; August 2001.

46. World Anti-Doping Agency. Science and Medicine. http://www.wada-ama.org/en/t3.asp?p=41629. Accessed November 11, 2004.

47. Federal Register: January 3, 2003;68:382-384. Available at: http://www.drugfreeworkplace.gov. Accessed January 24, 2003.

48. Kinz P, Cirimele V, Sachs H, Jeanneau T, Ludes B. Testing for anabolic steroids in hair from two body-builders. *Forensic Sci Int.* 1999;101:209-216.

49. Kintz P, Samyn N. Use of alternative specimens: drugs of abuse in saliva and doping agents in hair. *Ther Drug Monit.* 2002;24:239-246.

50. Caplan YH, Goldberger BA. Alternative specimens for workplace drug testing. *J Anal Toxicol.* 2001;25:396-399.

51. Hair test confirmation, interpretation face DTAB as major issues. *Workplace Substance Abuse Advisor.* 1999; 1:9-10.

52. Update on the War on Adulterants and Substitution. *MROAlert.* 2002;13:8.

53. Kazlauskas R, Trout G. Drugs in sports: analytical trends. *Ther Drug Monit.* 2000;22:103-109.

54. Spriet LL. Caffeine. In: Bahrke MS, Yesalis CE, eds. *Performance-Enhancing Substances in Sport and Exercise.* Champaign, Ill: Human Kinetics; 2002:267-278.

55. Rawson ES, Clarkson PM. Ephedrine as an ergogenic aid. In: Bahrke MS, Yesalis CE, eds. *Performance-Enhancing Substances in Sport and Exercise.* Champaign, Ill: Human Kinetics; 2002:289-298.

56. Mission Petroleum Carriers Inc v. Solomon. The risks of employer collecting urine specimens for its employees. *MROAlert.* 2001;12:8-11.

57. Cody JT. Adulteration of urine specimens. In: Liu RH, Goldberger BA, eds. *Handbook of Workplace Drug Testing.* Washington, DC: American Association for Clinical Chemistry; 1995:181-207.

58. Atago Company. *Clinical Refractometer Instruction Manual.* Tokyo, Japan: Atago Co. Ltd.

59. New Jersey Latest State to Pass Drug Test Anti-Fraud Statute. *MROAlert.* 2002;13:8-9.

60. Jenkins AJ. Forensic drug testing. In: Levine B, ed. *Principles of Forensic Toxicology.* Washington, DC: American Association for Clinical Chemistry; 1999:31-45.

61. Chen XH, Franke J-P, de Zeeuw RA. Principles of Solid-Phase Extraction. In: Liu RH., Goldberger BA, eds. *Handbook of Workplace Drug Testing.* Washington, DC: American Association for Clinical Chemistry; 1995:1-21.

62. Proposed Revisions to Federal Drug Testing Procedures. *MROAlert.* 2000;11:4-9.

63. Catlin DH, Murray TH. Performance-enhancing drugs, fair competition, and olympic sport. *JAMA.* 1996;276:231-237.

64. Striegel H, Vollkommer G, Dickhuth HH. Combating drug use in competitive sports: an analysis from the athletes' perspective. *J Sports Med Phys Fitness.* 2002;42:354-359.

65. Wadler GI. Future and designer drugs: emerging science and technologies. In: Bahrke MS, Yesalis CE, eds. *Performance-Enhancing Substances in Sport and Exercise.* Champaign, Ill: Human Kinetics; 2002:305-321.

66. Mendoza J. The war on drugs in sport: a perspective from the front-line. *Clin J Sport Med.* 2002;12:254-258.

67. Corrigan B. Beyond EPO. *Clin J Sport Med.* 2002;12:242-244.

68. Tricker R, Connolly D. Drugs and the college athlete: an analysis of the attitudes of student athletes at risk. *J Drug Educ.* 1997;27:105-119.

Bibliography

Karch SB. Amphetamines. In: Bahrke MS, Yesalis CE, eds. *Performance-Enhancing Substances in Sport and Exercise.* Champaign, Ill: Human Kinetics; 2002:257-265.

GLOSSARY

α-adrenergic agonists. Drugs that combine with the α-adrenergic receptor and initiate the biological response.

α-receptors. A type of adrenergic receptor. Activation by adrenergic agonists cause constriction of peripheral blood vessels, constriction of urinary sphincter, pupil dilation, and increased glycogenolysis in the liver.

α_1-receptor. A subtype of α-adrenergic receptor; when stimulated it results in peripheral vasoconstriction, pupil dilation, and contraction of urinary sphincter.

α_2-receptor. A subtype of α-adrenergic receptor located on peripheral nerve terminals; activation of these receptors inhibits the release of additional norepinephrine.

abortifacient. Producing abortion.

absorption. Refers to getting the drug into the bloodstream.

acetylsalicylic acid. Chemical name for aspirin; also abbreviated ASA.

acneiform eruptions. Resembling acne.

acid. A proton donor; a molecule capable of releasing hydrogen ions (ie, protons, H^+) in solution. Also refers to a solution with a hydrogen ion concentration high enough to give a pH <7.

acid secretion transporter. An active transport mechanism in the renal tubule cells that moves acid compounds from the blood into the renal tubule for excretion.

active drug. The structure of the drug that combines with the receptor to produce the response.

active transport. A mechanism for the transport of substances across membranes. The compound being transported attaches itself to a particular binding site of a protein transporter. The mechanism can transport against the concentration gradient but requires cellular energy.

addiction. A behavioral disorder that is characterized by obsessive drug use typically accompanied by extreme measures to obtain the drug. The driving force that causes addiction is the desire for the euphoria from the drug.

additive effects. When the response obtained from two or more drugs is equal to the sum of the responses obtained when the drugs are used individually.

adenosine receptors. Receptors to which the chemical mediator adenosine combines and may contribute to bronchoconstriction. Inhibition of adenosine receptors may be part of the mechanism of theophylline action.

adrenaline. *See* epinephrine.

adrenergic. Relating to nerve cells or fibers of the autonomic nervous system that use norepinephrine as their neurotransmitter; relating to drugs that mimic the actions of the sympathetic nervous system.

adrenergic receptor. Receptors to which epinephrine and norepinephrine combine to initiate a sympathetic response. Drugs that combine with the same receptors either mimic (agonist) or inhibit (antagonist) the sympathetic response.

adulteration. The alteration of any substance by the deliberate addition of a component not ordinarily part of the substance.

adverse drug reaction (ADR). Any undesirable response from a drug. These reactions can range from dry mouth to life-threatening organ damage. Some ADRs are not dose-related. A broader term than side effect.

affinity component. The first phase of the drug-receptor interaction; refers to the strength of the chemical binding interaction between the drug and the receptor. The second phase of this interaction causes the biological response (see efficacy component).

agonist. A drug capable of combining with a receptor and activating the transduction mechanism to initiate the biological response.

albumin. The plasma protein with the largest concentration in the blood. Many drugs bind to albumin, which increases the drug's volume of distribution.

aldosterone. A mineral corticosteroid hormone that causes reabsorption of sodium and water by the renal tubule and increased potassium excretion.

aldosterone antagonist. A drug that blocks the effects of aldosterone to cause a response that is opposite of the effects of aldosterone, such as increased sodium excretion and potassium retention.

aldosterone antagonism. The physiological effect of an aldosterone antagonist.

alkylated. *See* alkylation.

alkylation. Substitution of an alkyl radical for a hydrogen atom.

allergic reaction. An exaggerated immune response initiated by the exposure to certain drugs or other chemicals and causing effects ranging from skin rash to life-threatening anaphylaxis. Typically not dose-related effects.

allergic rhinitis. Hypersensitivity reaction in response to inhaled allergens.

allyl isothiocyanate. A compound used as a counterirritant.

amino acid. Organic compounds containing nitrogen, carbon, hydrogen, and oxygen; building blocks of protein.

anabolic. *See* anabolism.

anabolism. Energy requiring reactions whereby small molecules are built up into larger ones.

analgesic. A drug that is used to alleviate pain without causing the loss of consciousness.

androgen. A general term for male sex hormones that produce male sex characteristics; testosterone is a specific example and is the major androgen produced in the body.

androgenic. *See* androgen; having a masculinizing effect.

androgenic-anabolic steroids (AASs). Derivatives of the male hormone testosterone, which produce both masculinizing (androgenic) and tissue-building (anabolic) effects.

angina. A type of coronary heart disease in which the coronary arteries are not able to supply sufficient oxygen to the heart muscle.

angioneurotic edema. A rare condition in which rapid swelling in the nose, throat, and larynx may lead to death if not treated; it occurs more frequently in African Americans than in Caucasians.

angiotensin. Either of two forms of a peptide (angiotensin I or angiotensin II) associated with regulation of blood pressure

angiotensin I. A peptide produced by the action of renin on angiotensinogen and is converted to angiotensin II.

angiotensin II. A peptide hormone produced from the action of angiotensin-converting enzyme (ACE) on angiotensin I; produces vasoconstriction and triggers the release of aldosterone to increase blood pressure.

angiotensin II receptor blockers. Drugs that combine with the angiotensin II receptor to prevent the response of angiotensin II.

angiotensin-converting enzyme (ACE). An enzyme that catalyzes the conversion of angiotensin I to angiotensin II and also the inactivation of bradykinin. Angiotensin-converting enzyme is present in cells of blood vessels and is therefore readily available to catalyze the formation of angiotensin II.

angiotensinogen. A glycoprotein that is continuously produced by the liver; converted by renin to angiotensin I.

antacid. A pharmacologic agent used to neutralize the acidity of hydrochloride acid released by the stomach. Common agents include sodium bicarbonate, magnesium hydroxide, aluminum hydroxide, and calcium carbonate.

antagonist. A drug that reduces the effect of another drug.

antagonistic effect. When the use of a second drug reduces the effect of another drug.

antibiotic. A drug used to treat bacterial infections although the origin of the term is broader and sometimes refers to any antimicrobial agent.

antibody. A protein produced by certain cells in the body in response to a specific antigen; the antibody combines with the antigen to neutralize, inhibit, or destroy it. Also called an immunoglobulin (Ig).

anticholinergic. Generally refers to antagonistic to the action of parasympathetic nerve fibers although broadly may also refer to antagonism of other cholinergic nerve fibers.

anticholinergic effects. Refers to a group of adverse effects that are similar to the effects from drugs in the pharmacological category called anticholinergic drugs, which inhibit the parasympathetic nervous system. Anticholinergic effects include blurred vision, constipation, dry mouth, decreased sweating, urinary retention, and increased heart rate.

antihistamine. A pharmacologic agent used to treat allergic reactions by inhibiting the effects of histamine.

antiemetics. A pharmacological agent used to treat nausea or vomiting.

antigen. A substance that is recognized as foreign by the immune system, activates the immune system by inducing the production of antibodies, and reacts with immune cells or their products.

antihyperuricemic. A pharmacological agent that reduces enhanced blood concentration of uric acid.

antimicrobial. Any drug used to treat any microorganism, bacteria, fungi, or virus.

antipyretic. A pharmacological agent used to reduce fever.

antiseptics. Products applied to tissue such as hands or a site of injection or incision to kill or inhibit the growth of microorganisms.

antitussive. Drugs that suppress a cough.

anxiolytic. Drug that relieves anxiety.

arachidonic acid. Unsaturated fatty acid that is the starting point (substrate) for the biosynthesis of several groups of compounds (eicosanoids). These compounds are metabolites of arachidonic acid, which contribute to the inflammatory response.

assay. To examine; to subject to analysis to determine purity.

asthma. A chronic inflammatory disease of the airways. The inflammation results in obstruction of the airways from bronchoconstriction, edema, and excessive mucus production.

β-adrenergic agonists. Drugs that combine with the β-adrenergic receptor and initiate a biological response.

β-adrenergic antagonists. Another name for β-blocker drugs; *see* β-blocker.

β-adrenergic receptors. Receptors through which the sympathetic nervous system is activated along with β-receptors. Principal subtypes are β_1 and β_2.

β-agonist. Drug or hormone that combines with the β-adrenergic receptors to activate a transduction mechanism to initiate a response.

β-blocker. Drugs that combine with the β-adrenergic receptor but do not initiate a transduction mechanism and therefore prevent the corresponding agonist response; primary effects include decreased heart rate and force of contraction.

β-lactam. A class of broad-spectrum antibiotics that are structurally and pharmacologically related to the penicillins and cephalosporins.

β-lactamases. A group of enzymes that inactivate some penicillins and cephalosporins by breaking apart a key chemical structure of these antibiotics.

β_1-adrenergic receptors. The subtype of β-adrenergic receptor found principally in the heart.

β_1-blockers. Drugs that combine with β_1-receptors but do not initiate a transduction mechanism and therefore prevent the corresponding agonist response; primary effects include decreased heart rate and force of contraction.

β_1-receptors. Another name for β_1-adrenergic receptor.

β_2-agonists. Drugs that combine with the β_2-receptor and mimic certain sympathetic responses such as bronchodilation. The most effective drugs for treatment of an acute asthma attack are the short-acting β_2-agonists administered by inhalation. Short-acting refers to the duration of action, but these drugs also have a short onset of action. Long-acting β_2-agonists are used for long-term control but not for quick relief.

β_2-receptors. A type of adrenergic receptor that is predominant in the skeletal muscle, liver, and bronchial smooth muscle.

bacteremia. Presence of viable bacteria in the circulating blood.

bactericidal. A drug that kills bacteria.

bacteriostatic. Drugs that slow the normal growth rate of the bacteria so that the patient's immune system has a better opportunity to eliminate the infecting organisms.

banned substance. Any substance foreign to the body or any physiological substance prohibited from use by an athletic or sport governing body during competition and/or training, and if present in a urine and/or blood sample, would result in some form of penalty.

Barrett's esophagus. A premalignant change in epithelial cells of the esophagus, which significantly increases the risk of esophageal cancer.

baroreceptors. Receptors that are stimulated by changes in blood pressure and initiate the baroreceptor reflex as a compensation mechanism; specifically found in the wall of the auricles of the heart, vena cava, aortic arch, and carotid sinus.

baroreceptor reflex. An automatic response stimulated by baroreceptors in an attempt to maintain blood pressure. Causes constriction of arterioles and veins and increases heart rate in response to a drop in blood pressure; the opposite responses occur when blood pressure rises sharply.

base. A proton acceptor; a molecule capable of binding with hydrogen ions. Also refers to a solution with a hydrogen ion concentration low enough to give a pH >7.

basophil. Type of white blood cell.

benzodiazepine. Compounds, that as a group, have many uses, such as to treat insomnia, anxiety, alcohol withdrawal syndrome, various seizures, as well as muscle spasm; some drugs in this group are significantly more effective for one or more of these therapeutic uses than others; all benzodiazepines have an abuse potential and thus are controlled substances (schedule IV) and all cause central nervous system depression and thus produce drowsiness.

beta-blocker. *See* β-blocker.

bioavailability. The portion of a drug dose that reaches the systemic circulation and thus has an opportunity to produce a biological effect.

bioequivalent. When the amount and rate of a drug entering the blood stream is approximately the same for two or more formulations of the drug.

biotransformation. *See* drug metabolism.

bismuth. A trivalent metallic element in which several of its salts are used in medicine, such as bismuth subsalicylate (Pepto-Bismol) used to treat diarrhea and as a component in the drug regimen for *Helicobacter pylori*-induced peptic ulcers.

bisphosphonate drugs. Drugs with a particular phosphate structure; used to treat and prevent osteoporosis.

blood-brain barrier. A term used to describe the inability of most ions and large molecules to pass from the blood to the central nervous system. This selectivity occurs in part because of the tight junction between the endothelial cells of the capillaries that supply the brain.

bradykinin. A peptide hormone that is formed during inflammation. It contributes to the pain response but also has vasodilation properties, which contribute to reducing blood pressure.

breath-actuated metered dose inhaler (MDI). Used in asthma treatment. The technique to operate this inhaler is somewhat of a cross between MDI and dry powder inhaler (DPI); a propellant is used to expel the drug but it is not activated until the patient inhales.

calcium channel blockers. Drugs that inhibit the influx of calcium into the cells of arterial smooth muscle and cardiac muscle, resulting in peripheral vasodilation, decreased heart rate and force of contraction, and dilation of arterioles of the heart.

camphor. A compound used as a stimulant, carminative, expectorant, and diaphoretic.

capsicum. A compound used as a gastric stimulant and counterirritant.

capsules. Two-piece gelatin containers that are oblong or bullet-shaped. The drug and inactive ingredients are placed in one piece of the container and the second piece acts as the cap.

cardiac remodeling. Process that changes the shape, size, and effectiveness of the heart as a result of cardiac injury.

catabolic. The breaking down in the body of complex chemical compounds into simpler ones.

catecholamine. Any of several compounds occurring naturally in the body, including dopamine, epinephrine, and norepinephrine, that function as hormones or as neurotransmitters in the sympathetic nervous system. They are derived from the amino acid tyrosine and resemble one another chemically in having an aromatic portion (catechol) to which an amine or nitrogen-containing group is attached. They have a marked effect on the nervous and cardiovascular systems, metabolic rate, temperature, and smooth muscle.

chain of custody. Used to describe the process of documenting the handling of a specimen from the time an athlete provides a specimen and the collector processes the specimen, through shipping to the laboratory, during the testing at the laboratory, and until the results are reported by the lab.

chemical mediators. Compounds that are released by one cell type, attach to the receptor of a second cell type, and affect the response of that second cell.

chemotactic mediator. Chemical compound that causes movement of selected cells to the site of inflammation.

chemotaxis. Attraction of phagocytes by a chemical stimuli as a result of an inflammatory or immune response.

cholinesterase. An enzyme that inactivates acetylcholine.

cholesterol. Steroid found in animal fats as well as in most body tissues, made by the liver. Located in cell membranes and used in the synthesis of steroid hormones and bile salts.

cholestyramine. A drug used to decrease blood cholesterol. It is taken prior to meals, is not absorbed from the gastrointestinal tract, and increases the excretion of bile acids, which are made from cholesterol.

cholinergic. Relating to nerve cells or fibers that use acetylcholine as their neurotransmitter; denoting an agent that mimics the action of acetylcholine.

cholinergic receptor. Receptor to which acetylcholine binds.

chromatography. A process in which a chemical mixture carried by a liquid or gas is separated into components as a result of differential distribution of the solutes as they flow around or over a stationary liquid or solid phase.

chronotropic. Affecting the rate of rhythmic movements such as the heart beat.

Churg-Strauss syndrome. Rare but has also been noted with the use of leukotriene-receptor antagonist. This syndrome involves vasculitis, which primarily affects the respiratory tract during its early stages and can progress to become life threatening.

clearance rate. A measure of the efficiency of the metabolism and excretion of a drug.

competitive antagonist. A drug that combines with the same receptor as the agonist but does not activate the transduction mechanism. When the competitive antagonist is binding to the receptor, it prevents the agonist from binding to that receptor, thus reducing the effect of the agonist.

complement system. A group of blood-borne proteins, which, when activated, enhance the inflammatory and immune responses and can lead to the lysis of invading microorganisms.

conjugation. The addition of another molecule (eg, glucuronic or sulfuric acid) to a drug (primarily in the liver) to terminate the biological activity of the drug and prepare it for excretion.

controlled substance. Any drug or other substance, or immediate precursor, included in schedule I, II, III, IV, or V as defined by the Controlled Substance Act. These include narcotics, stimulants, depressants, hallucinogens, anabolic steroids, and chemicals used in the illicit production of these drugs. The term does not include distilled spirits, wine, malt beverages, or tobacco.

coronaviruses. A category of RNA viruses that can cause the symptoms of the common cold.

corticosteroids. Steroid hormones released by the adrenal cortex; synthetic corticosteroids are used for their anti-inflammatory effect.

COX-1. A form of the cyclooxygenase enzyme that is produced in most tissues. It catalyzes the synthesis of several arachidonic acid metabolites (ie, eicosanoids), which are important to the normal physiology in those tissues.

COX-2. A form of the cyclooxygenase enzyme that is primarily activated at the site of inflammation and tissue injury. It catalyzes the synthesis of several arachidonic acid metabolites (ie, eicosanoids), which contribute to the pain and inflammation.

Crohn's disease. An inflammatory disease usually affecting the small and large intestines but can affect any part of the digestive tract. Ulcerative lesions affect all layers of the intestinal wall. Treatment includes antibiotics, immunosuppressive drugs, and in some cases, removal of the affected part of the intestine.

cross-reactivity. When patients who experience a hypersensitivity reaction from drugs in one category are also likely to experience a similar adverse response from drugs in another category because the drug categories share a common chemical characteristic.

cross-tolerance. The development of diminished therapeutic and/or adverse effects (tolerance) to additional drugs as a result of tolerance from another drug.

Cushing's syndrome. Condition caused by a hypersecretion of glucocorticoids characterized by spindly legs, "moon face," "buffalo hump," pendulous abdomen, flushed facial skin, poor wound healing, hyperglycemia, osteoporosis, weakness, hypertension, and increased susceptibility to disease.

cyclooxygenase (COX). An enzyme found in virtually all cells and uses arachidonic acid as substrate to initiate the production of several chemical mediators. Isoforms are COX-1 and COX-2.

cysteine. An amino acid that is a component of many proteins but also is a component of some leukotrienes referred to as cysteinyl leukotrienes.

cytokine. Generic term for nonantibody proteins, such as interleukins and tumor necrosis factor, released by a certain cell population on contact with a specific antigen; they act as intercellular chemical mediators, as in the generation of immune response.

decongestant. Having the property of reducing nasal congestion by constriction of blood vessels and decreasing mucosal edema in the nasal passage through β-adrenergic agonist activity.

dependence. Occurs as a result of cellular changes within the body in response to continual exposure to the drug.

digoxin. A drug used to treat congestive heart failure; it increases the force of contraction without increasing heart rate.

disease-modifying antirheumatic drugs (DMARDs). Drugs that are able to delay or stop the progression of rheumatoid arthritis, but it takes weeks to months for the effects of DMARDs to develop.

disinfectants. Products applied to inanimate objects, such as surgical areas or instruments, to kill or inhibit the growth of microorganisms.

dissolution. The process of dissolving.

distribution. Refers to the movement of the drug throughout the body to the various compartments. Besides blood, these compartments include the central nervous system, cells (eg, muscle, adipose, liver, kidney), excretory fluids (eg, urine, bile, sweat), and plasma proteins (primarily albumin).

diuresis. Excretion of urine; commonly denotes production of large quantities of urine.

diuretic. A pharmacologic agent designed to increase the amount of water in the urine thereby removing excess water from the body; commonly used to treat fluid retention and hypertension.

DNA (deoxyribonucleic acid). A nucleic acid in the shape of a double helix found in all living cells; carries the organism's hereditary information.

dose-response curve. *See* dose-response principle.

dose-response effect. When the magnitude of the effect being measured increases as the dose increases.

dose-response principle. As the concentration of drug increases, more receptors are occupied by the drug, producing a greater effect until the dose is high enough that all of the receptors are occupied and therefore additional drug does not produce additional effect; maximal response is achieved.

dosage form. Physical form in which the drug exists for administration, such as tablet, capsule, solution for injection.

dosing interval. The time period between doses.

drug. A chemical that has demonstrated to be effective for the prevention or treatment of a disease.

drug interaction. Occurs when one drug increases or decreases the effect of another drug.

drug metabolism. The chemical alteration of the drug by one or more enzymes in the body with an associated change in pharmacological activity. *See* biotransformation.

drug resistance. A change in the susceptibility of the organism to a particular drug or group of drugs so that drugs that were once effective against the microorganism are no longer effective.

dry powder inhaler (DPI). A device used to administer drugs by inhalation. The drug exists as a dry powder and a controlled amount is released when the patient inhales deeply from the device. Used for delivery of asthma medications to the lungs. DPIs provide an alternative to the use of pressurized gases. As the patient inhales deeply, the process of inhalation through the inhaler draws the powdered drug into the lungs. The drug is contained in a capsule or other package form which the inhaler breaks open during use to allow the powder to be inhaled.

duration of action. The time between onset and termination of action, and represents the length of time the drug produces its effect.

dynorphins. A family of peptides found in the central nervous system that act as a painkiller. Also see endorphins.

dyslipidemia. Elevated blood lipid beyond normal range; most commonly as elevated cholesterol or triglycerides.

dysphoria. A feeling of unpleasantness or discomfort.

ED50 (effective dose). The dose of drug that is effective in producing 50% of a specified response.

efficacy component. The second phase of the drug-receptor interaction and the phase that produces the biological response. The first phase of this interaction is the ability of the drug to chemically bind to the receptor (see affinity component).

eicosanoids. Physiologically active substances derived from arachidonic acid (ie, the prostaglandins, leukotrienes, prostacyclin, and thromboxanes).

elixirs. Sweetened and flavored solutions of ethanol and water containing one or more drugs.

emulsions. Liquids usually consisting of small droplets of oil dispersed in water. The oil may be the drug or may be used to dissolve a lipid-soluble drug.

endogenous. Arising from inside of the body.

endorphins. As β-endorphins, a family of peptides in the central nervous system that act as a pain killer. Also used as a broader term to collectively refer to β-endorphins, enkephalins, and dynorphins.

enkephalins. A family of peptides found in the central nervous system that act as a painkiller. Also see endorphins.

enteric coating. Coating on the outside of a solid dosage form that does not allow it to dissolve in the acidity of the stomach and is intended to delay the release of the drug until it reaches the small intestine.

enterohepatic. Blood circulation from small intestine directly to the liver.

eosinophils. Type of white blood cell.

epinephrine. Also known as adrenaline. A hormone secreted by the adrenal glands in response to stress or fear. Stimulates alpha and beta adrenergic receptors, resulting in increased heart rate, increased metabolism, and improved breathing.

equipotent dose. The dose of one drug adjusted so that it gives the same response as the dose of a similar drug. If 20 mg of one drug gives the same response as 10 mg of a similar drug, these two doses are equipotent.

erythema. Redness of the skin.

esters. Usually formed by the reaction between an acid and an alcohol with elimination of water.

excretion. Process whereby the drug and metabolites of metabolism are eliminated from the body.

exogenous. Arising or produced outside of the body.

expectorants. A drug that decreases the viscosity of lower respiratory tract secretions so that they can be moved out of the respiratory tract more efficiently by coughing.

facilitated diffusion. A membrane transport mechanism that combines the characteristics of passive diffusion and active transport. It requires a carrier protein but it does not use energy.

first pass effect. The inactivation of drugs by enzymes in the intestinal cells or liver before the drug enters the general circulation, thus decreasing the bioavailability of the drug.

flora. Various bacteria and other microorganisms that normally inhabit an individual without causing disease.

formulation. The total composition of a drug product and nature of the dosage form, including the inactive ingredients and the means by which the ingredients are put together.

free drug. Drug that is not bound to albumin and is free to bind at its site of action.

gamma amino butyric acid (GABA). A neurotransmitter that is widely distributed in the central nervous system and involved in inhibiting responses that would otherwise cause pain, depression, and convulsions.

ganglion. Collection of nerve cell bodies outside the central nervous system.

gas chromatography. Chromatography in which a sample mixture is vaporized and injected into a stream of carrier gas moving through a column containing a stationary phase composed of a liquid or particulate solid and is separated into its component compounds according to their affinity for the stationary phase.

gastrin. A hormone produced in the pyloric regions of the stomach that stimulates the production of gastric acid.

gastroesophageal reflux disease (GERD). A chronic condition that exists when heartburn occurs regularly (ie, more than twice a week).

glomerulus. A tuft of capillaries surrounded by the Bowman's capsule forming part of the nephron and aids in filtration of the blood.

gluconeogenesis. The process by which glucose is made from amino acids or lactic acid.

glycogenolysis. The process of converting glycogen to glucose.

glycoside. A term referring to a drug that contains a sugar and a nonsugar component bonded together (eg, digoxin).

gout. Inflammation and joint pain as a result of elevated uric acid blood concentration.

gram-negative. Bacteria that do not retain dye from a gram stain laboratory test.

gram-positive. Bacteria that retain dye from a gram stain laboratory test.

H_1-receptors. One of the three types of histamine receptors; found in the respiratory tract and near peripheral blood vessels. Antihistamines that block the H_1-receptor were on the market for decades prior to H_2-blockers and thus, historically, any reference to antihistamines without specifying the receptor type is generally understood to be referring to antihistamines that block the H_1-receptor.

H_2-receptors. One of the three types of histamine receptors; located primarily on stomach cells; activation causes an increased production of stomach acid.

H_3-receptors. One of the three types of histamine receptors; located in the central nervous system. Their function is not clearly understood and there are no drugs clinically available that are known to specifically block these receptors.

half-life ($t\frac{1}{2}$). The time required for the amount of drug in the body (as measured in the blood, serum, or plasma) to be reduced by one-half.

HDL (high-density lipoprotein) cholesterol. Considered to be the "good cholesterol"; a specific lipoprotein in the blood that removes cholesterol from the blood, thereby protecting against heart disease. The HDL cholesterol is considered "good" because cholesterol in the blood is captured by the HDL particles and thus the cholesterol is no longer able to deposit in unwanted places such as the interior of blood vessels.

heart block. A condition in which the impulse from the atria to the ventricles is partially or totally prevented. If untreated, the ventricles fail to contract.

heartburn. Also called acid indigestion, results from the contact of gastric acid, and to some extent bile and pepsin, with the esophageal mucosa.

heart failure. Also know as congestive heart failure. With this condition the heart cannot pump with enough force to adequately supply blood to the tissues.

Helicobacter pylori (*H. pylori*). A gram-negative bacteria that promotes peptic ulcer disease and is the most common cause of gastric and duodenal ulcers.

hiatal hernia. This condition exists when the stomach partially sits in the chest cavity because of a weakness in the diaphragm. Can also be the cause of GERD.

hirsutism. Excessive growth of body and facial hair, especially in women.

histamine. Substance found in many cells, especially mast cell, basophils, and platelets released during inflammatory and immune responses or tissue injury and causes vasodilation and increased vascular permeability.

histamine (H_2)-receptor antagonists (H_2RAs). Also known as H_2-blockers, are competitive antagonists to histamine receptors on the stomach parietal cells. These drugs suppress gastric acid secretion and are effective in treating mild heartburn, GERD, and peptic ulcer disease.

hydrolyzed. Process by which water is used to split a substance into smaller molecules.

hydrophilic. Means "love water." Drugs that are more water soluble in an aqueous environment, such as blood or urine, because the polar and ionized chemical groups form bonds with water molecules. They do not dissolve readily in lipid environments such as membranes.

hydrophobic. Means "fear water." Drugs that have more nonpolar than polar chemical characteristics. They have low water solubility, but dissolve readily in the lipid environments of membranes. *See also* lipophilic.

hyperkalemia. Too much potassium in the blood.

hypokalemia. Deficiency of potassium in the blood.

hypothalamic-pituitary-adrenal (HPA) axis. A physiological control mechanism in which the amount of cortisol produced by the adrenal gland is regulated based on the amount of cortisol the hypothalamus detects in the blood. If there is a sufficient amount in the blood, the hypothalamus sends a hormone signal to the pituitary, which sends a hormone signal to the adrenal gland to decrease cortisol production. Excessive inhibition of cortisol production occurs (adrenal suppression) when corticosteroid therapy lasts for more than several days. If adrenal suppression occurs, the corticosteroid dosage must be gradually decreased to give the adrenal gland time to begin making cortisol, otherwise fatal deficiency of corticosteroid may result.

idiopathic. Unknown cause.
IgE (immunoglobulin E). Antibodies located on the surface of mast cells in the airways.
IgE antibodies. A type of immunoglobulin located on mast cells and basophils. When IgE antibodies combine with specific antigens, they initiate an allergic response by causing the release of chemical mediators from these cells.
immune cells. Any type of cell that contributes to the immune response by synthesizing antibodies, releasing chemical mediators, or removing foreign substances.
immunoassay. An analytical method used for the detection and analysis of the presence of hormones or other substances.
induce. To initiate, cause, or bring about.
induction. *See* induce.
inflammatory bowel disease (IBD). A term that refers to two similar diseases: Crohn's disease and ulcerative colitis.
inotropic. Influencing the contractility of muscular tissue.
intrinsic efficacy. The ability of the drug to cause a response as a result of interacting with the receptor.
ion. Any positively or negatively charged particle; usually formed when a substance, such as a salt, dissolves and dissociates.
ionization. Dissociation into ions with a positive and negative charge.
irritable bowel syndrome (IBS). A common disorder in which the colon, for no apparent reason, is more sensitive to stimuli than normal.
isoenzymes. *See* isozymes.
isoform. Different forms of an enzyme that vary slightly in chemical structure but catalyze the same reaction. Also called isoenzymes or isozymes.
isozymes. Two or more enzymes that catalyze the same reaction, but may be differentiated by variations in physical properties.

kinin system. A group of blood proteins that when activated, enhance the inflammatory and immune responses, increase vascular permeability, and contribute to the pain response.

lactose. A disaccharide found in dairy milk.
LD50 (lethal dose). The dose that will cause death in 50% of the population as extrapolated from animal data.
LDL (low-density lipoprotein) cholesterol. Considered the "bad" cholesterol; a specific lipoprotein that carries cholesterol in the blood and deposits it at tissues. The LDL cholesterol is considered "bad" because high levels of LDL cause the deposit of cholesterol in unwanted places, such as the interior of blood vessels, and is associated with heart disease and atherosclerosis.

leukotriene modifiers (also called antileukotrienes). A group of long-term control medications used to treat asthma. They can be subdivided into drugs that block the leukotriene receptor (leukotriene-receptor antagonists) and drugs that decrease the synthesis of leukotrienes (leukotriene-synthesis inhibitors).

leukotrienes (LTs). Products of arachidonic acid metabolism by the lipoxygenase pathway. They serve as chemical mediators of inflammation, allergic reactions, and asthma.

lipase. A fat-splitting enzyme; it releases fatty acids from triglyceride molecules.

lipolysis. The breakdown of fat.

lypolytic. *See* lypolysis.

lipophilic. Means "love lipid." Drugs that have more nonpolar than polar chemical characteristics. They have low water solubility, but dissolve readily in the lipid environments of membranes. *See also* hydrophobic.

loading dose. One or more doses that are higher than the maintenance dose and administered at the beginning of therapy for the purpose of achieving the desirable therapeutic concentration quicker.

maintenance dose. Repetitive use of the same dose of a drug at the same dosing interval.

mast cells. Cells found in connective tissue along blood vessels that produce a variety of chemical mediators during inflammation. Chemical mediators include arachidonic acid metabolites that cause vessel dilation and increased permeability, and chemotactic factors that attract phagocytic cells to the site of inflammation.

mast cell stabilizers. Pharmacological agents used to treat asthma by inhibiting the release of inflammatory mediators for mast cells.

macrophages. Phagocytic cells that phagocytize tissue cells, bacteria, and other foreign debris.

mechanism of action. The biochemical changes that occur to cause the observed effects from a drug.

menthol. An alcohol obtained from peppermint oil or other mint oils; used as an antipruritic and topical anesthetic.

metabolic alkalosis. An increase in blood pH, resulting in a pH more basic compared to normal, due to an imbalance in one or more biochemical processes.

metabolites. Product of the reaction of a parent drug or substrate interacting with a metabolizing enzyme.

metered dose inhaler (MDI). Used for delivery of asthma medications to the lungs. The drug is contained in a pressurized container with a metering valve to control the amount of drug released as a mist during each use. A propellant is used to force the metered amount of drug from the inhaler each time the device is actuated.

molecular weight. The weight of a molecule determined by adding the atomic weight of each atom that comprises the molecule; the larger the molecular weight the larger the size of the molecule. Most drugs have a molecular weight 100 to 1000; drugs that are proteins being the primary exception.

monoamine oxidase (MAO). An enzyme that inactivates norepinephrine and epinephrine.

monoamine oxidase inhibitors (MAOIs). A group of drugs that are categorized therapeutically as antidepressant drugs, although they also have some other uses. Monoamine oxidase inhibitors have a significant drug interaction with sympathomimetics; MAOIs inhibit the inactivation of sympathomimetics, enhancing their activity and causing a potentially dangerous exaggerated hypertensive response. They also exhibit anticholinergic adverse effects.

mononuclear cells. Phagocytic cells having only one nucleus and include macrophages and monocytes. They engulf and remove debris from site of inflammation, injury, and immune response.

muscarinic receptor. Another name for cholinergic receptor at the site where the parasympathetic nerve innervates the tissue.

myocardial infarction. An ischemic heart disease. Occlusion of a coronary artery prevents sufficient blood from reaching a portion of the heart muscle, thus causing death of some heart cells.

narcotic. Used in a legal context to refer to any controlled substance.

narcotic analgesic. Another term used to refer to opioids. They can produce a state of narcosis (drowsiness or sleep) and relieve pain.

nebulizer. A device used to deliver liquid medication as an extremely fine cloud; useful in delivering medication to the deep part of the respiratory tract. These devices are larger than MDIs or DPIs and are used primarily in hospitals and clinics, or in homes if the patient is unable to use inhalers.

nephron. The active filtering unit of the kidney that consists of the glomerulus and renal tubule.

neutrophils. Most common type of white blood cell and ingests bacteria.

nifedipine. A calcium channel blocking agent that causes coronary vasodilator but minimal effect on the heart (ie, it is selective).

nociceptors. Afferent nerves responsible for sensing pain.

nonsteroidal anti-inflammatory drugs (NSAIDs). A group of anti-inflammatory drugs that is not from the steroid family; used to reduce inflammation and pain.

noradrenaline. *See* norepinephrine.

norepinephrine. A hormone secreted by the adrenal medulla that produces actions similar to those that result from sympathetic stimulation.

nucleic acid. Class of organic molecules that include DNA and RNA.

onset of action. The time it takes for the concentration of drug molecules at the site of action to become large enough to cause a noticeable biological response.

opiates. Drugs that are obtained from the opium poppy, opium being the extract from the plant. Morphine and codeine are two of the components of opium and thus are opiates.

opioids. A broader term than "opiates" and refers to drugs that have effects similar to the opiates. Oxycodone (OxyContin) and meperidine (Demerol) are two examples.

organelle. Small cellular structures that perform specific metabolic functions for the cellular functions (eg, ribosomes, mitochondria).

orthostatic hypotension. Also called postural hypotension. A decrease in blood pressure upon standing from a sitting or supine position due to an insufficient automatic baroreceptor reflex.

oxidation. Addition of oxygen to or removal of hydrogen from a molecule.

parasympathetic. Division of the autonomic nervous system that oversees digestion, elimination, and glandular function.

parasympathomimetics. Drugs that mimic the parasympathetic nervous system.

parent drug. The drug reacting with a metabolizing enzyme and converted to metabolites. *See* substrate.

parenteral route. The use of an intravenous, intramuscular, or subcutaneous injection to administer a drug.

parietal cells. Cells of the stomach that produce hydrochloric acid.

passive diffusion. Refers to the drug penetrating through the membrane due to the solubility of the drug in the membrane and is the transport mechanism of greatest impact for most drugs; does not require cellular energy.

peak expiratory flow (PEF). A pulmonary function test that determines the maximum flow rate of forced expiration that the patient can achieve at that time.

peak flow meter (PFM). Hand-held device used to determine peak expiratory flow.

pepsin. The principle digestive enzyme of the gastric juice.

pepsinogen. The inactive form of pepsin; it is produced by stomach cells and released in the stomach in response to autonomic regulation. The acid pH of the stomach catalyzes the conversion of pepsinogen to pepsin.

peptide. Any sequence of amino acids joined by peptide bonds. Proteins are larger peptides.

perforation. An abnormal opening in an organ or body tissue from disease or injury.

perioral dermatitis. A rash that occurs around the mouth.

peristalsis. Progressive, wavelike contractions that move foodstuffs through the gastrointestinal tract.

phagocytosis. Engulfing of foreign debris by phagocytic cells.

pharmacodynamics. The study of the impact of drugs on the body. The primary focus of pharmacodynamics is on the molecular mechanism by which drugs exert their therapeutic and adverse effects.

pharmacokinetics. The study of the impact of the body on drugs. The primary focus of pharmacokinetics is on the rate and extent to which drugs are absorbed into the bloodstream, distributed throughout the body, metabolized, and finally excreted.

pharmacology. The effect of drugs on the body and the effect of the body on drugs.

phosphodiesterases. An enzyme that inactivates second messengers such as cyclic AMP.

phospholipase A_2. An enzyme that catalyzes the intracellular release of arachidonic acid from the membrane-bound phospholipid.

phospholipids. Modified lipid containing phosphorous.

pills. Small, spherical, solid dosage forms that are rarely used any more. The drug and inactive ingredients are rolled together rather than being compressed.

placebo. A dosage form that contains no active ingredient (eg, capsules filled with lactose).

placebo effect. Either a therapeutic or adverse response that can not be attributed to the pharmacological effect of the drug.

plasma protein systems. Biochemical sequences that produce several proteins with specific important functions in the inflammatory response; blood clotting, kinin, and complement systems.

platelet-activating factor. A phospholipid chemical mediator produced by a variety of cells including platelets, neutrophils, mast cells, and vascular endothelial cells. Platelet-activating factor causes vasodilation, increases vascular permeability, and platelet aggregation.

polar compounds. Drugs or other chemical compounds that have predominately polar characteristics, which increase their solubility in water.

polar conjugated metabolites. Drugs that have been made more polar by a conjugation reaction as part of the drug metabolism process.

polarity. A chemical characteristic of a molecule that increases the water solubility of the molecule.

polypeptide. A peptide formed by the union of an indefinite number of amino acids.

potency. Compares the dose of a drug required to produce a particular effect relative to the dose of another drug that acts by a similar mechanism to produce that same effect.

prodrug. The inactive form of a drug that is administered with the intent of a metabolic reaction converting the drug (biotransformation) to a form that has pharmacologic action (ie, active form).

progestin. A general term for female hormones that produce some or all of the biological changes produced by progesterone.

prostacyclin (PGI$_2$). A derivative of prostaglandin that is a natural inhibitor of platelet aggregation and is also a vasodilator.

prostaglandins (PGs). A group of lipid-based chemical messenger synthesized from arachidonic acid (ie, eicosanoids) by most tissue cells, which acts locally as a hormone-like substance.

proton pump. Actively transports hydrogen ions (protons = H$^+$) into the stomach to combine with chloride ions to form hydrochloric acid (HCl).

proton pump inhibitor (PPI). Drugs that inhibit the production of gastric acid by inhibiting the H$^+$, K$^+$ ATPase mechanism that releases the acid into the gastric lumen.

protozoa. A eukaryotic microorganism, characteristically unicellular and motile. Many are parasites of animals.

pruritus. Itching.

radioimmunoassay. Immunoassay of a substance that has been radioactively labeled.

rate of solubility. Rate that a drug becomes dissolved; it impacts the rate of absorption as drugs must be dissolved to be absorbed.

receptor. Any macromolecule that has specific chemical characteristics allowing it to selectively bind to drugs or hormones. Typically receptors, when activated by an agonist, have the ability to initiate a signaling mechanism (*see* transduction mechanisms), which ultimately produces a biological response.

receptor antagonist. *See* competitive antagonist.

recombinant. A microbe, or strain, that has received chromosomal parts from different parental strains.

renal tubule. Part of the nephron into which filtered fluid passes.

renin. An enzyme released by the kidney into the plasma where it produces angiotensin from angiotensinogen (angiotensinogen ——> angiotensin I); also referred to as angiotensinogenase.

renin-angiotensin system. A series of enzyme reactions initiated by renin and resulting in the production of angiotensin II, which causes the release of aldosterone. Plays an important role in regulating blood pressure.

renin-angiotensin-aldosterone system. *See* renin-angiotensin system.

Reye's syndrome. A rare, but potentially fatal disorder mainly affecting children and teens, characterized by vomiting, disorientation, lethargy, and liver damage following a viral infection. May be linked to the use of aspirin in the treatment of viral infection.

rheumatoid arthritis. A common systemic inflammatory disease caused by an autoimmune response, possibly initiated as a result of a bacterial or viral infection.

rhinoviruses. Category of viruses for which >100 specific viruses have been identified and are associated with the common cold in human beings.

ribosomes. Cytoplasmic organelles at which proteins are synthesized.

RNA (ribonucleic acid). Nucleic acid that contains ribose rather than deoxyribose; acts in protein synthesis.

rubefacient. Causing redness of the skin due to cutaneous vasodilation; a counterirritant that produces erythema when applied to the skin surface.

sarcolemma. Membrane of a muscle fiber.

second messenger system. An example of a transduction mechanism; a series of reactions initiated inside a cell in response to a receptor being activated on the cell surface by a drug or hormone (the first messenger). The series of reactions is the messenger system that allows the drug or hormone to cause a biological response inside the cell without entering the cell.

serotonin. Also called 5-hydroxytryptamine (5-HT). A neurotransmitter important for regulating many functions including sleep, mood, pain, appetite, gastrointestinal motility, and as a chemical mediator affecting inflammation.

side effects. Expected undesirable responses based on the pharmacologic action of the drug. Dose-related effects (ie, larger doses will increase the frequency of the undesirable effects).

site of action. The molecular site where the drug has a significant chemical interaction to produce a biological effect.

sitz bath. A shallow bath of warm water, usually for therapy, which allows for immersion of buttocks and hips. The tub is usually shaped to allow the legs to be out of water.

spirometer. A gasometer that measures respiratory gases; device to measure lung capacity by measuring the volume of air exhaled.

steady-state concentration. The concentration of drug in the blood that is reached when a dose of drug is given at regular dosing intervals and the clearance rate is equal to the rate of absorption. Steady-state is reached after the drug has been given for a time equivalent to 4 to 5 half-lives of the drug.

streptococcal. Gram-positive bacteria that cause a variety of diseases, including scarlet, fever, pneumonia, and strep throat.

substance P. A neurotransmitter that is thought to be involved in pain sensation at peripheral sites.

substrate. The compound that reacts with and is chemically changed by an enzyme. A broader term than parent drug. Encompasses all substances that are converted to product by an enzyme.

superinfection. A second infection that develops during the treatment of an initial infection as a result of the antibiotic used to treat the initial infection but also kills a sufficient number of normal flora in the gastrointestinal, respiratory, or urinary tract, allowing for the increased growth of resistant microorganisms that cause the second infection.

suspension. Liquid dosage form in which a solid (the drug) is dispersed (not dissolved) throughout the liquid.

sympathetic. Division of the autonomic nervous system that activates the body to cope with some stressor (eg, danger, excitement, etc); the fight, fright, and flight responses.

sympathomimetics. Drugs that mimic the sympathetic nervous system.

synergistic effects. When the response obtained from two or more drugs is greater than what would be expected by adding the responses obtained when the drugs are used individually.

syrups. Sweetened and flavored aqueous solutions containing one or more drugs. They contain little or no alcohol and thus are particularly suitable for children, as well as for adults who have difficulty swallowing tablets or capsules.

T lymphocytes. Also called T cells. A lymphocyte that becomes immunocompetent in the thymus gland and differentiates into one of several kinds of effector cells that function in cell-mediated immunity.

tablets. Solid dosage forms, most of which are prepared by compressing the powders into the desired shape.

TD50 (toxic dose). The dose that will produce a specific toxic effect in 50% of the population.

theophylline. A long-term control medication for treatment of asthma. Not used as much as newer drugs because of the greater risk of toxicity and lower effectiveness.

therapeutic drug monitoring. Measuring the blood (or serum or plasma) concentration of a drug; usually done with drugs that have a low therapeutic index.

therapeutic index (TI). The ratio of the dose that causes a specified toxic effect compared to the dose that causes a specified therapeutic effect. The larger the TI, the greater the margin of safety.

therapeutic range. The range between the lowest and the highest desired concentration of a drug in the blood (or serum or plasma). The range of a drug concentration that will produce the desired effects without the unwanted side effects.

therapeutic window. *See* therapeutic range.

therapeutics. The study of the parameters that determines the most appropriate therapy for a patient. It considers the parameters necessary to individualize treatment for the specific patient, including all of the patient's diseases, all of the drugs the patient may be using, the dosage regimen of each drug, and the impact of potential adverse effects.

thermogenic. Producing heat in the body as a result of increased metabolic reactions.

thromboxanes (TX). Formed from arachidonic acid (ie, eicosanoids) and cause platelet aggregation and vasoconstriction.

tolerance. The diminished response to a drug as a result of continued use.

transdermal. A type of dosage form in which the drug is placed on the surface of the skin and the drug passes into the bloodstream to produce a systemic effect.

transduction mechanism. Any of several mechanisms that allows a drug or hormone on the outside of the cell to have an effect on the inside of the cell, ultimately causing the biological response (see Figure 3-2). Usually a series of reactions inside the cell is initiated when a receptor is activated.

tricyclic antidepressants. A group of drugs characterized chemically by a specific three-ring structure and pharmacologically by their ability to relieve depression. Besides their therapeutic use as antidepressants, they are noted for anticholinergic and sedative adverse effects.

triturate. To accomplish trituration, which is reducing a substance to a fine power.

tumor necrosis factor (TNF). Protein cytokine chemical mediators produced by macrophages, T lymphocytes, and other cells. There are two TNFs; TNF-α and TNF-β. Tumor necrosis factor contributes to the inflammatory and immune response, especially against bacteria, by promoting neutrophil infiltration, activating several cell types, including the production of other cytokines, and activating the complement and blood coagulation systems.

ulcerative colitis. An inflammatory bowel disease of the colon and rectum.

ulcerogenic effect. Anything that contributes to ulcer formation.

vasculitis. Inflammation of a blood vessel of a lymphatic vessel.

volume of distribution. The apparent space in the body that is available to the drug; the more extensive distribution, the larger the volume of distribution.

Pharmacological Abbreviations

a, a	before		C	Celsius
aa, aa, aa	of each		c	with
a.c.	before meals		CAD	coronary artery disease
ACE	angiotensin-converting enzyme		cal	calorie
ad	to, up to		cap, caps	capsule
a.d.	right ear		CBC	complete blood cell count
ad lib	as desired, freely		cc	cubic centimeter
ADH	antidiuretic hormone		CHF	congestive heart failure
a.l.	left ear		cm	centimeter
ALT	alanine aminotransferase		CNS	central nervous system
alt. h.	alternate hours		CO_2	carbone dioxide
AM	in the morning, before noon		comp	compound
amp	ampul		cont	continue
amt	amount		COPD	chronic obstructive pulmonary disease
aq.	water			
aq. dest.	distilled water		CPK	creatine phosphokinase
ASA	acetylsalicylic acid (aspirin)		CPR	cardiopulmonary resuscitation
ASAP	as soon as possible		CrCl	creatinine clearance
AST	aspartate aminotransferase (SGOT)		CSF	cerebrospinal fluid
			CV	cardiovascular
a.u.	each ear			
AV	artrioventricular		d	day
			d/c	discontinue
bid	twice a day		D5W	5% glucose in distilled water
bin	twice a night		dil	dilute
BM	bowel movement		disp	dispense
B/P	blood pressure		dist	distilled
BS	beats per minute		DC	discontinue
BSA	body surface area		DX	diagnosis
BUN	blood urea nitrogen		DW	dextrose water; distilled water

ECG	electrocardiogram (EKG)		LT	leukotriene
EEG	electroencephalogram		LUQ	left upper quadrant
EENT	ear, eye, nose, and throat			
elix	elixir		M	meter
			m^2	square meter
F	Fahrenheit		MAOI	monoamine oxidase inhibitor
FBS	fasting blood sugar		MI	myocardial infarction
FDA	United States Food and Drug Administration		min	minute
			µg	microgram
fl, fld	fluid		mEq.	milliequivalent
			mg	milligram
g	gram		mL	milliliter
gal	gallon			
GI	gastrointestinal		Na	sodium
gr	grain		neg	negative
gtt	drop		ng	nanogram
			non rep	do not repeat, no refills
h	hour		NPO	nothing by mouth
H_2	histamine-2		NS	normal saline
Hgb	hemoglobin			
HR	heart rate		O_2	oxygen
hs	at bedtime		OD	right eye
			o.n.	every night
ID	intradermal		OR	operating room
IgG	immunoglobulin G		os	left eye
IM	intramuscular		OU	both eyes
INF	infusion		oz	ounce
INH	inhalation			
inj	injection		p	per
IV	intravenous		p	after
			pc	after meals
K	potassium		per	by
kcal	kilocalorie		pH	hydrogen ion concentration
kg	kilogram		PM	afternoon; evening
			PO	by mouth
L	liter		p.r.	by rectum
LA	long acting		p.r.n.	as needed, when necessary
lb	pound		pt	pint
LDH	lactic dehydrogenase		pulv	a powder
LE	lupus erythematosus		PVC	premature ventricular contraction
LFT	liver function test		pwd	powder
liq	liquid			
LLQ	left lower quadrant		q.	each, very
LOC	level of consciousness		qAM	every morning

q.d.	every day	supp	suppository
q.h.	every hour	syr.	syrup
q.2h	every 2 hours		
q.3h	every 3 hours	tab.	tablet
q.4h	every 4 hours	tbs, tbsp, T	tablespoon
q.6h	every 6 hours	t.i.d.	three times a day
q.12h	every 12 hours	tinct., tr.	Tincture
q.i.d.	four times a day	tsp	teaspoon
q.o.d.	every other day		
q.o.h.	every other hour	U	unit supplied
qPM	every night	u	unit ordered
q.s.	quantity sufficient; as much as needed	u.d.	as directed
		µg	microgram; one-millionth of a gram.
qt	quart		
		ung	ointment
RBC	red blood cell count or red blood cell	USP	United States Pharmacopeia
		ut dict	as directed
rep.	repeat	UTI	urinary tract infection
Rx	a medical prescription	UV	ultraviolent
s	without	vol	volume
sc	subcutaneous		
sig	label, or let it be printed	WBC	white blood cell count
sl	sublingual	wk	week
sol., soln.	solution	wt	weight
solv	dissolve		
SQ, sq.	subcutaneous(ly)	y	year
SR	slow release		
ss	one half	>	greater than
STAT, stat	immediately	<	less than
subq.	subcutaneous		

BIBLIOGRAPHY/SUGGESTED READING

AHFS Drug Handbook. 2nd ed. Philadelphia, Pa: Lippincott Williams & Wilkins. Bethesda, Md: American Society of Health-System Pharmacists; 2003.

Covington TR, eds. *Nonprescription Drug Therapy: Guiding Patient Self-Care.* St. Louis, Mo: Facts and Comparisons; 2002.

DiPiro JT, Talbert RL, Yee GC, et al. *Pharmacotherapy: A Pathophysiologic Approach.* 5th ed. New York, NY: McGraw-Hill; 2002.

Drug Facts and Comparisons. St Louis, Mo: Facts and Comparisons.

Berardi RR, DeSimone EM, Newton GD, et al. *Handbook of Nonprescription Drugs.* 13th ed. Washington, DC: American Pharmaceutical Association; 2002.

Hardman JG, Limbird LE, eds. *Goodman & Gilman's The Pharmacological Basis of Therapeutics.* 10th ed. New York, NY: McGraw-Hill; 2001.

Herfindal ET, Gourley DR, eds. *Textbook of Therapeutics: Drug and Disease Management.* 7th ed. Baltimore, Md: Lippincott Williams & Wilkins; 2000.

Lacy CF, Armstrong LL, Goldman MP, Lance LL, eds. *Drug Information Handbook.* Hudson, Ohio: Lexi-Comp Inc; 2003.

Lance LL, Lacy CF, Armstrong LL, Goldman MP, eds. *Drug Information Handbook for the Allied Health Professional.* 10th ed. Hudson, Ohio: Lexi-Comp Inc; 2003.

Lehne RA. *Pharmacology for Nursing Care.* 4th ed. Philadelphia, Pa: WB Saunders; 2001.

McCance KL, Huether SE, eds. *Pathophysiology: The Biologic Basis for Disease in Adults and Children.* 3rd ed. St. Louis, Mo: Mosby-Year Book Inc; 1998.

PDR for Nonprescription Drugs and Dietary Supplements. 24th ed. Montvale, NJ: Medical Economics Co Inc; 2003.

Physicians' Desk Reference. 56th ed. Montvale, NJ: Medical Economics Co Inc; 2002.

Index